Pancreatic Cancer

Editors

DOUGLAS A. RUBINSON
MATTHEW B. YURGELUN

HEMATOLOGY/ONCOLOGY
CLINICS OF NORTH AMERICA

www.hemonc.theclinics.com

Consulting Editors
GEORGE P. CANELLOS
EDWARD J. BENZ JR

October 2022 • Volume 36 • Number 5

ELSEVIER

1600 John F. Kennedy Boulevard • Suite 1800 • Philadelphia, Pennsylvania, 19103-2899

http://www.theclinics.com

HEMATOLOGY/ONCOLOGY CLINICS OF NORTH AMERICA Volume 36, Number 5
October 2022 ISSN 0889-8588, ISBN 13: 978-0-323-98655-7

Editor: Stacy Eastman
Developmental Editor: Ann Gielou M. Posedio

Hematology/Oncology Clinics (ISSN 0889-8588) is published bimonthly by Elsevier Inc., 360 Park Avenue South, New York, NY 10010-1710. Months of issue are February, April, June, August, October, and December. Business and Editorial Offices: 1600 John F. Kennedy Blvd., Ste. 1800, Philadelphia, PA 19103–2899. Customer Service Office: 3251 Riverport Lane, Maryland Heights, MO 63043. Periodicals postage paid at New York, NY and at additional mailing offices. Subscription prices are $470.00 per year (domestic individuals), $1190.00 per year (domestic institutions), $100.00 per year (domestic students/residents), $495.00 per year (Canadian individuals), $100.00 per year (Canadian students/residents), $1232.00 per year (Canadian institutions) $563.00 per year (international individuals), $1232.00 per year (international institutions), and $255.00 per year (international students/residents). International air speed delivery is included in all *Clinics* subscription prices. All prices are subject to change without notice. **POSTMASTER:** Send address changes to *Hematology/Oncology Clinics of North America*, Elsevier Health Sciences Division, Subscription Customer Service, 3251 Riverport Lane, Maryland Heights, MO 63043. Customer Service (orders, claims, online, change of address): Elsevier Health Sciences Division, Subscription **Customer Service, 3251 Riverport Lane, Maryland Heights, MO 63043. Tel: 1-800-654-2452 (U.S. and Canada); 314-447-8871 (outside U.S. and Canada). Fax: 314-447-8029. E-mail: journalscustomerservice-usa@elsevier.com (for print support); journalsonlinesupport-usa@elsevier.com (for online support).**

Reprints. For copies of 100 or more, of articles in this publication, please contact the Commercial Reprints Department, Elsevier Inc., 360 Park Avenue South, New York, New York 10010-1710; Tel.: 212-633-3874, Fax: 212-633-3820, E-mail: reprints@elsevier.com.

Hematology/Oncology Clinics of North America is covered in *MEDLINE/PubMed (Index Medicus), EMBASE/ Excerpta Medica, and BIOSIS.*

Contributors

CONSULTING EDITORS

GEORGE P. CANELLOS, MD
William Rosenberg Professor of Medicine, Department of Medical Oncology, Dana-Farber Cancer Institute, Boston, Massachusetts, USA

EDWARD J. BENZ Jr, MD
Professor, Pediatrics, Richard and Susan Smith Professor, Medicine, Professor, Genetics, Harvard Medical School, President and CEO Emeritus, Office of the President, Dana-Farber Cancer Institute, Boston, Massachusetts, USA

EDITORS

DOUGLAS A. RUBINSON, MD, PhD
Assistant Professor of Medicine, Harvard Medical School, Gastrointestinal Cancer Center, Dana-Farber Cancer Institute, Boston, Massachusetts, USA

MATTHEW B. YURGELUN, MD
Assistant Professor of Medicine, Harvard Medical School, Gastrointestinal Cancer Center, Dana-Farber Cancer Institute, Boston, Massachusetts, USA

AUTHORS

ELHAM AFGHANI, MD, MPH
Assistant Professor of Medicine, Johns Hopkins School of Medicine, Baltimore, Maryland, USA

ANNE ARONSON, MPH
Henry D. Janowitz Division of Gastroenterology, Icahn School of Medicine at Mount Sinai, New York, New York, USA

CHAD A. BARNES, MD
LaBahn Pancreatic Cancer Program, Medical College of Wisconsin, Milwaukee, Wisconsin, USA

WILLIAM J. CHAPIN, MD
Department of Medicine, Division of Hematology-Oncology, Perelman School of Medicine, Abramson Cancer Center, University of Pennsylvania, Philadelphia, Pennsylvania, USA

ETHAN CHEN
Brigham and Women's Hospital, Boston, Massachusetts, USA

ANU CHITTENDEN, MS
Licensed Genetics Counselor, Dana-Farber Cancer Institute, Center for Cancer Genetics and Prevention, Boston, Massachusetts, USA

ANA DE JESUS-ACOSTA, MD
Department of Oncology, The Sidney Kimmel Comprehensive Cancer Center, Johns Hopkins School of Medicine, Baltimore, Maryland, USA

RICHARD F. DUNNE, MD, MS
Department of Medicine, Wilmot Cancer Institute, Assistant Professor of Medicine, University of Rochester Medical Center, Rochester, New York, USA

SUJANA GOTTUMUKKALA, MD
Department of Radiation Oncology, University of Texas Southwestern, Dallas, Texas, USA

SIGURDIS HARALDSDOTTIR, MD, PhD
Landspitali University Hospital, University of Iceland, Iceland

KUNAL JAJOO, MD
Brigham and Women's Hospital, Harvard Medical School, Boston, Massachusetts, USA

AAKIB KHALED
Medical Student, Georgetown University School of Medicine, Washington, DC, USA

ALISON P. KLEIN, PhD, MHS
Professor of Oncology, Medicine and Pathology, Sidney Kimmel Comprehensive Cancer Center, Johns Hopkins School of Medicine, Professor of Epidemiology, Johns Hopkins Bloomberg School of Public Health, Baltimore, Maryland, USA

ARIELLE J. LABINER, MHS
Henry D. Janowitz Division of Gastroenterology, Icahn School of Medicine at Mount Sinai, New York, New York, USA

MU-HAN LIN, PhD
Department of Radiation Oncology, University of Texas Southwestern, Dallas, Texas, USA

AIMEE L. LUCAS, MD, MS
Henry D. Janowitz Division of Gastroenterology, Icahn School of Medicine at Mount Sinai, New York, New York, USA

FLORENCIA MCALLISTER, MD
Department of Clinical Cancer Prevention, Department of Gastrointestinal Medical Oncology, Department of Immunology, Clinical Cancer Genetics Program, The University of Texas MD Anderson Cancer Center, Houston, Texas, USA

CHIRAYU MOHINDROO, MD
Department of Clinical Cancer Prevention, The University of Texas MD Anderson Cancer Center, Houston, Texas, USA; Department of Internal Medicine, Sinai Hospital of Baltimore, Baltimore, Maryland, USA

MAYSSAN MUFTAH, MD
Brigham and Women's Hospital, Harvard Medical School, Boston, Massachusetts, USA

RYAN D. NIPP, MD, MPH
University of Oklahoma Health Sciences Center, Stephenson Cancer Center, Oklahoma City, Oklahoma, USA

SAHAR NISSIM, MD, PhD
Dana-Farber Cancer Institute, Brigham and Women's Hospital, Harvard Medical School, Boston, Massachusetts, USA

MARCUS NOEL, MD
Associate Professor of Medical Oncology, MedStar Georgetown University Hospital, Washington, DC, USA

CHUNJOO PARK, PhD
Department of Radiation Oncology, University of Texas Southwestern, Dallas, Texas, USA

MUNEEB REHMAN, MD
Hematology and Medical Oncology Fellow, MedStar Georgetown University Hospital, Washington, DC, USA

KIM A. REISS, MD
Department of Medicine, Division of Hematology-Oncology, Perelman School of Medicine, Abramson Cancer Center, University of Pennsylvania, Philadelphia, Pennsylvania, USA

ERIC J. ROELAND, MD
Division of Hematology/Oncology, Oregon Health & Science University, Assistant Professor of Medicine, Knight Cancer Institute, Portland, Oregon, USA

MICHAEL ROSENTHAL, MD, PhD
Department of Imaging, Dana-Farber Cancer Institute, Brigham and Women's Hospital, Harvard Medical School, Boston, Massachusetts, USA

SAMER SALAMEKH, MD
Department of Radiation Oncology, University of Texas Southwestern, Dallas, Texas, USA

NINA N. SANFORD, MD
Department of Radiation Oncology, University of Texas Southwestern, Dallas, Texas, USA

MALVI SAVANI, MD
Division of Hematology/Oncology, Department of Medicine, University of Arizona Cancer Center, Tucson, Arizona, USA

KHOSCHY SCHAWKAT, MD, PhD
Department of Imaging, Dana-Farber Cancer Institute, Brigham and Women's Hospital, Harvard Medical School, Boston, Massachusetts, USA

RACHNA T. SHROFF, MD, MS
Division of Hematology/Oncology, Department of Medicine, Chief, Section of GI Medical Oncology, University of Arizona Cancer Center, Associate Professor of Medicine, University of Arizona College of Medicine-Tucson, Tucson, Arizona, USA

SUSAN TSAI, MD, MHS
LaBahn Pancreatic Cancer Program, Medical College of Wisconsin, Professor, Department of Surgery, Milwaukee, Wisconsin, USA

Contents

Pancreatic cancer is one of the most lethal cancers in the world; it is a silent disease in which symptoms do not present until advanced stages, thereby reducing the 5-year survival rate to 10%. The global burden of pancreatic cancer has doubled over the past 25 years despite advancements in medicine. This review aims to discuss the global trends and disparities in pancreatic cancer, as well as the up-to-date literature on the known risk factors. A better understanding of these risk factors will reduce mortality by providing opportunities to screen these patients as well as counseling on lifestyle modifications.

Pancreatic ductal adenocarcinoma (PDAC) is associated with complex changes in body composition. Visceral obesity and type 2 diabetes mellitus are established risk factors for developing PDAC; however, clinical and metabolic features of PDAC commonly lead to cancer cachexia, a hypermetabolic syndrome characterized by weight loss secondary to muscle and adipose tissue wasting. Reduction in muscle mass in patients with PDAC is associated with poorer survival in patients undergoing surgical resection and increased chemotherapy toxicity. Although no standardized treatment exists, a multidisciplinary, tailored, symptom-based approach is recommended to improve outcomes and quality of life for patients with PDAC and cachexia.

Imaging and endoscopy play several important roles in the diagnosis and management of pancreatic ductal adenocarcinoma (PDAC). Computed tomography (CT) and endoscopic ultrasound play complimentary roles in the initial diagnosis and pathologic confirmation of PDAC. Endoscopy can also be used to manage biliary obstruction and gastrointestinal complications. MRI and fluorodeoxyglucose-PET-CT are typically used as problem-solving tools for complex cases. Neoadjuvant chemotherapy and surgery are often selected based on imaging findings related to vascular involvement by tumors and invasion of adjacent structures. Posttreatment surveillance imaging is used to monitor for complications, local recurrence, and systemic metastasis.

Pancreatic ductal adenocarcinoma (PDAC) is an aggressive disease with high mortality, largely due to late stage at diagnosis. Approximately 10% to 15% are hereditary, and detection of early stage PDAC or precursor lesions through pancreatic surveillance programs may improve outcomes. Current surveillance is annual, typically with endoscopic ultrasound and/ or magnetic resonance imaging.

Germline genetic variants implicated in increasing lifetime risk of pancreatic cancer (PDAC) have been identified in ~4% to 10% of cases. Clinical features such as family history have poor sensitivity in identifying carriers of these risk variants. Genetic testing for these germline variants has potential to guide risk assessment and surveillance recommendations in high-risk individuals to promote prevention and early detection measures. Furthermore, identification of novel germline variants can offer important insights into pathogenesis that may inform precision medicine approaches. This article reviews current understanding of germline mutations associated with PDAC risk and implications of genetic testing.

Pancreatic cancer is a fatal malignancy that is projected to emerge as the second leading cause of cancer-related death in the United States. Despite the critical advances in surgical strategies, radiographic techniques, and systemic therapy, the treatment modality has remained largely unchanged over the past two decades eliciting a dire need for clinical trials in improving quality of life and prolonging survival in this patient population. Emergence of innovative strategies including novel combination chemotherapy, immunotherapy, vaccines, small compound drugs, among others is avenues under investigation to improve perioperative outcomes in localized pancreatic cancer.

The management of localized pancreatic cancer (PC) has evolved significantly in the last decade, moving away from prioritizing surgery as the primary treatment modality to embracing the need for preoperative (neoadjuvant) multimodality therapy to achieve durable disease-free control. Neoadjuvant therapy is currently recommended for all patients with borderline and locally advanced PC, and is being increasingly utilized in patients with resectable disease as well. When assessing operability the following 3 factors should be considered: clinical stage of disease, response to neoadjuvant therapy, and patient performance status. Patients who demonstrate a response to neoadjuvant therapy may benefit significant from surgical resection.

Current indications for radiotherapy in pancreatic cancer vary by surgical resectability status of the tumor. Radiation is generally not used pre-operatively for resectable tumors, but may be given adjuvantly particularly in settings of a close or positive surgical margin. For borderline resectable tumors, pre-operative radiation has been shown to improve surgical parameters including lowering nodal positivity and positive margin rates. For locally advanced unresectable tumors, radiation can improve local control, give patients an interval off of chemotherapy and provide symptomatic relief. Multidisciplinary discussion is critical for choosing the best modality and sequencing of care for patients with pancreatic cancer. Prospective trials with appropriately chosen endpoints and meticulous radiotherapy quality assurance are needed to best define populations with pancreatic cancer most likely to benefit from radiotherapy.

Advanced pancreatic cancer remains one of the deadliest malignancies in 2022. Although there has been significant progress in treatment options with improved outcomes in many cancers, this growth has been slow in pancreatic cancer. This article examines specific components of approved first- and second-line therapies for advanced pancreatic cancer treatment and their effectiveness and concludes with a brief exploration of future directions for targeted therapies.

Pancreatic ductal adenocarcinoma (PDAC) has a poor prognosis, with a mere ~10% of patients in the United States surviving 5 years from the time of diagnosis. Until recently, the treatment for advanced PDAC differed little based on patient or tumor characteristics. However, recent breakthroughs have identified subgroups of patients who benefit from novel, biomarker-driven therapies. We review the data and role for PARP inhibitors and for other biomarker-directed therapies, including for patients with NTRK fusions, NRG1 fusions, mismatch repair deficiency, and KRAS p.G12C mutations.

Pancreatic neuroendocrine tumors (pNETs) represent a relatively rare disease; however, the incidence has been increasing during the last 2 decades. Next generation sequencing has greatly increased our understanding of driver mutations in pNETs. Sporadic pNETs have consistently presented with mutations in MEN1, DAXX/ATRX, and genes related to the mammalian target of rapamycin pathway. Inherited pNETs have traditionally been associated with multiple endocrine neoplasia type 1, von Hippel-Lindau

Individuals with pancreatic adenocarcinoma experience a complex constellation of palliative and supportive care needs. Notably, when caring for patients with pancreatic adenocarcinoma, clinicians must carefully assess and address these individuals' palliative and supportive care needs, as these can have important implications related to their treatment experience and care outcomes. Importantly, prior research has consistently demonstrated the benefits of palliative and supportive care interventions for patients with cancer to help address symptom burden, illness understanding, coping mechanisms, and informed decision making. However, much of this research did not specifically tailor the interventions to the unique concerns of a pancreatic cancer population. Thus, an urgent need exists to design and conduct rigorous research with the goal of enhancing care delivery and outcomes for the highly symptomatic population of individuals with pancreatic adenocarcinoma.

HEMATOLOGY/ONCOLOGY CLINICS OF NORTH AMERICA

THE CLINICS ARE AVAILABLE ONLINE!
Access your subscription at:
www.theclinics.com

Preface

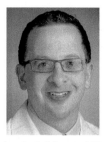 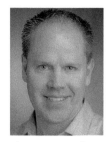

Douglas A. Rubinson, MD, PhD   Matthew B. Yurgelun, MD
Editors

Pancreatic cancer is a disease whose name has too long been equated with a death sentence. Unfortunately, decades of disappointing progress in attempting to improve therapeutic and early diagnostic approaches for pancreatic cancer throughout the twentieth century have led to this well-earned notoriety. The barriers that have historically hindered major clinical advances in pancreatic cancer are well known, and a full enumeration of such factors could, sadly, extend over pages.

The reviews assembled for this issue of *Hematology/Oncology Clinics of North America* will seek to articulate many of these barriers while describing the ongoing, frequently cross-institutional and cross-discipline collaborative efforts to overcome them. Overall, in reading this collection of articles, we are heartened to see a field that is truly changing the narrative about this malignancy, which has too long been defined by patient suffering and stasis in clinical progress. The data and expertise compiled within these pages demonstrate how decades of painstaking research are now being translated into real-world advances, which are already dramatically altering patients' outcomes for the better. At the same time, it is also now becoming clearer how to build on both the successes and the scientific frustrations of the past in ways that will continue to change the landscape of how pancreatic cancer is treated, detected, resected, cured, and ultimately prevented.

The progress described herein would not have been possible without an incredible worldwide network of researchers across academia and industry, spanning both the clinic and the laboratory. Furthermore, the tireless efforts and passion of patient advocates, family members, and the individuals themselves directly affected by pancreatic cancer are at the core of such advancement. In reading this collection of reviews, it is hard not to believe that pancreatic cancer research stands at the brink of great success. While it may be tempting to damn such optimism as blind hope or naïveté, the

Hematol Oncol Clin N Am 36 (2022) xiii–xiv
https://doi.org/10.1016/j.hoc.2022.08.007
0889-8588/22/© 2022 Published by Elsevier Inc.

real-world advances made against pancreatic cancer in recent years validate this confidence as being well justified.

Douglas A. Rubinson, MD, PhD
Harvard Medical School
Gastrointestinal Cancer Center
Dana-Farber Cancer Institute
450 Brookline Avenue
Boston, MA 02215, USA

Matthew B. Yurgelun, MD
Harvard Medical School
Gastrointestinal Cancer Center
Dana-Farber Cancer Institute
450 Brookline Avenue
Boston, MA 02215, USA

E-mail addresses:
douglas_rubinson@dfci.harvard.edu (D.A. Rubinson)
matthew_yurgelun@dfci.harvard.edu (M.B. Yurgelun)

Pancreatic Adenocarcinoma
Trends in Epidemiology, Risk Factors, and Outcomes

Elham Afghani, MD, MPH[a], Alison P. Klein, PhD, MHS[a,b,]*

KEYWORDS

- Pancreatic cancer • Pancreatic Adenocarcinoma • Risk Factors • Epidemiology
- Trend

KEY POINTS

- The prevalence of Pancreatic cancer is expected to increase due to longer lifespans, urbanization of countries worldwide, and increased exposure to modifiable risk factors.
- Cigarette Smoking, diabetes, obesity and heavy alcohol are modifiable risk factors that increase risk of pancreatic cancer while hereditary predisposition is a nonmodifiable risk factor.
- Knowledge of modifiable and nonmodifiable risk factors may lead to screening for early detection.

INTRODUCTION

There are several types of pancreatic cancer, but the most common type is pancreatic adenocarcinoma, which comprises 90% of all pancreatic cancer diagnoses. This review focuses on the epidemiology of adenocarcinoma of the pancreas and includes studies limited to pancreatic adenocarcinomas or studies of all pancreatic cancer combined, where the vast majority of patients have adenocarcinoma of the pancreas.

Globally, pancreatic cancer is the 12th most common cancer and the 7th most common cause of cancer-related death.[1] By 2025, it is projected to be the third leading cause of cancer-related deaths in Europe.[2] Pancreatic cancer accounts for 2.6% of all new cancer diagnoses, 4.7% of all new cancer deaths,[1] and 12.7% of all deaths due to gastrointestinal-related cancers in the world.[3] In the United States, it accounts

This work was supported by Meitar Global IPMN Foundation, NCI RO1CA154823, U01CA247283, NCI P50 CA62924 and P30CA006973, and the Sol Goldman Pancreatic Cancer Research Center.
^a Johns Hopkins School of Medicine, 1830 E Monument Street, Room 436, Baltimore, MD 21205, USA; ^b Sidney Kimmel Comprehensive Cancer Center, Johns Hopkins School of Medicine, Johns Hopkins Bloomberg School of Public Health, 1550 Orleans Street, Baltimore, MD 21231, USA
* Corresponding author.
E-mail address: aklein1@jhmi.edu

Hematol Oncol Clin N Am 36 (2022) 879–895
https://doi.org/10.1016/j.hoc.2022.07.002
0889-8588/22/© 2022 Elsevier Inc. All rights reserved.

hemonc.theclinics.com

for 3.2% of all new cancer cases and 8% of all cancer deaths, and a lifetime risk of 1.7.[4] The incidence is highest in Western Europe with rates of 8.6 per 100,000, followed by Northern America at 8.0 per 100,000, Central and Eastern Europe at 7.5 per 100,000, and Northern Europe at 7.4 per 100,000. The incidence is lowest in Southeast Asia, with rates of 1.3 per 100,000.[5] In the United States, the incidence of pancreatic cancer has been increasing at a rate of 1% per year. Pancreatic cancer is the fourth leading cause of death in men and women.[6] The increasing trend is largely due to longer life spans, urbanization of countries worldwide, and exposure to increased modifiable risk factors. Countries with a very high and high human developmental index (HDI) and gross domestic product per capita have a higher number of pancreatic cancers.[5,7] Regions with very high and high HDI had age-standardized rates of 7.9 and 4.6 per 100,000, respectively, compared with 1.8 and 1.2 per 100,000 in regions with low and medium HDI, respectively.[5] Increased prevalence of lifestyle risk factors, increased availability of imaging, heightened health awareness, and longer life expectance have led to the higher incidence and mortality of pancreatic cancer.[8]

The incidence of pancreatic cancer increases with age (**Fig. 1**). Despite the median age of pancreatic cancer being 71 years in the United States, there has been an increase in incidence in younger patients. The average annual percent change in pancreatic cancer incidence increased with decreasing age, from 0.77% (95% confidence interval [CI], 0.57–0.98) for ages 45 to 49 years to 2.47% (1.77–3.18) for ages 30 to 34 years, and 4.34% (3.19–5.50) for ages 25 to 29 years.[9] Although this is partly due to the increase in younger patients, there is also an increase in the prevalence of modifiable risk factors in this population.

Mortality from pancreatic cancer also varies depending on the part of the world and is highest in Western Europe, North America, and Central and Eastern Europe and lowest in Middle Africa and South Central Asia.[5] Mortality is highest in regions with

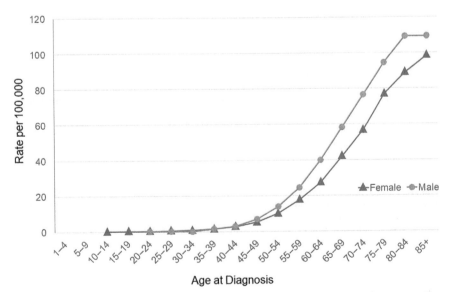

Fig. 1. Surveillance, Epidemiology and End Results (SEER) incidence rates by age at diagnosis, 2014 to 2018. (*Adapted from* SEER Database, National Cancer Institute. https://seer.cancer.gov/statfacts/html/pancreas.html Web site. Accessed December 18, 2021.)

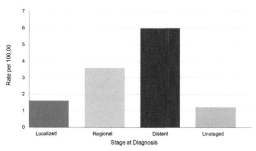

Fig. 2. Surveillance, Epidemiology and End Results (SEER) 5-year age-adjusted incidence rates, 2014 to 2018 by stage of diagnosis. (*Adapted from* SEER Database, National Cancer Institute. https://seer.cancer.gov/statfacts/html/pancreas.html Web site. Accessed December 18, 2021.)

very high and high HDI.[5] Survival rates for pancreatic cancer remain low despite recent improvements in overall 5-year survival from 2% from 1975 to 1979 to 10% in the United States and Europe in 2019.[7] The low survival rates are due to 52% of cases being diagnosed as metastatic disease (stage IV) with a 5-year survival rate of 3% in the United States, whereas only 11% of cases being diagnosed as stage I or localized cancer, with a 5-year survival rate of 41.6%[4] (**Figs. 2** and **3**). Among patients who undergo surgical resection, the 5-year survival rate is approximately 15% to 25%.[10,11] A large study involving multiple national databases, including the Surveillance, Epidemiology and End Results (SEER) and national cancer registries of Netherlands, Belgium, Norway, and Slovenia, provided age-stratified survival rates based on the stage of disease. It was found that the 3-year survival rate of those with stage I to II disease was 20% to 34% if age was less than 60 years, 14% to 25% if age was between 60 and 69 years, and 9% to 13% if age was greater than or equal to 70 years, whereas the survival rates for those with stage III to IV disease were 2% to 5%, 1% to 2%, and less than 1%, respectively. Alternatively, 3-year survival after resection for stage I to II disease was 23% to 39% if age was less than 60 years, 16% to 31% if age was between 60 and 69 years, and 17% to 30% if age was greater than or equal to 70 years, whereas the survival rates for those with stage III to IV disease were 23% to 39%, 16% to 31%, and 17% to 30%, respectively.[11]

There exists gender and racial differences in pancreatic cancer rates. The age-standardized incidence of pancreatic cancer is 5.7 per 100,000 in men and 4.1 per

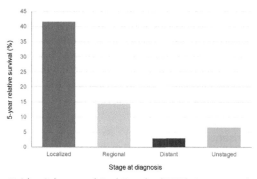

Fig. 3. Surveillance, Epidemiology and End Results (SEER) 5-year survival by stage of diagnosis, 2011 to 2017. (*Adapted from* SEER Database, National Cancer Institute. https://seer.cancer.gov/statfacts/html/pancreas.html Web site. Accessed December 18, 2021.)

100,000 in women.[7] There has been a recent increase in incidence rates of pancreatic cancer in women and men, which is likely due to an increase in life expectancy and increase prevalence of obesity.[12] In the United States, since 2000, incidence rates from pancreatic cancer have been increasing at a rate of 0.9% annually in men and 0.8% in women.[4] Since 2000, the death rate from pancreatic cancer has been increasing at a rate of 0.3% annually in men and 0.2% in women.[4]

Cancer occurrence, diagnosis, and outcome vary substantially between racial and ethnic groups. This variation is likely attributable to socioeconomic barriers, access to care, exposures to risk factors, barriers to cancer prevention and early detection, and treatment. In the United States, age-adjusted incidence rates were higher in blacks at 15.8 per 100,000 compared with that in whites at 13.7 per 100,000, in Hispanics at 12.4 per 100,000, and in Asians at 10.5 per 100,000 in 2018.[4] Although understudied, the increased risk in blacks has been suggested to be primarily due to differences in the prevalence of established risk factors such as smoking, high body mass index (BMI), and diabetes,[13] as well as the decreased likeliness of being evaluated by a health professional and be enrolled in clinical trials in pancreatic cancer.[14,15] Nevertheless, although survival rates of most cancers are usually lower for blacks compared with whites, that of pancreatic cancer is the same for the 2 groups.[6] Data on pancreatic cancer among Hispanics are limited. However, based on the SEER database, there has been an increase in pancreatic cancer among Hispanics since 1974.[16] The few published data have conflicting results, with 1 showing worse outcomes[17] and others showing better outcomes among Hispanics compared with non-Hispanics.[18] Studies on pancreatic cancer in Asians have shown heterogeneity within this group. In a study evaluating the incidence of pancreatic cancer in the California Cancer Registry, the investigators found that Japanese and Koreans have pancreatic cancer risk as high as non-Hispanic whites, whereas Chinese, Filipinos, and South Asians have a similar low risk as non-Hispanic American Indians/Alaska Natives.[19] In addition, a recent study found higher morbidity after resection in Asians and individuals reporting Hispanic ethnicity.[20]

Risk Factors

Cigarette smoking

Cigarette smoking is a well-established risk factor for pancreatic cancer.[21–25] A meta-analysis assessing the impact of smoking on the risk of pancreatic cancer reported a 48% relative increase in ever-smokers compared with never-smokers and an excess risk of 82% in current smokers compared with 17% in former smokers. Risk decreased for increasing time from cessation, reaching the level of nonsmokers after 20 years.[26] The elevated risk of mortality in smokers diagnosed with pancreatic cancer is independent of alcohol use, BMI, and history of diabetes.[27] Smoking has also been associated with a younger onset of pancreatic cancer.[28] Although there has been a decrease in the prevalence of cigarette smoking in much of Europe and North America,[29] the prevalence rates in Asia[30] and other parts of the world remain high.

Diabetes

The association between diabetes and pancreatic cancer is intricate. Diabetes is both a risk factor and a consequence of pancreatic cancer. In a large cohort study of young and middle-aged subjects who attended routine health screening programs in Korea, individuals with diabetes had a 2-fold risk increase for pancreatic cancer mortality.[31] Studies evaluating the Mayo Clinic population initially indicated that up to 1% of newly diagnosed diabetic patients develop pancreatic cancer within 3 years of their diabetes diagnosis.[32] However, studies conducted within the VA system have shown a lower risk of less than 0.3% within 3 years of diagnosis.[33] A recent study found that those with new-onset diabetes, defined as less than or equal to 4 years, had an age-adjusted risk of 2.97 (95% CI, 2.31–3.82), whereas the risk of those with long-standing diabetes, defined as greater than 4 years, was 2.16 (95% CI, 1.78–2.60) compared with those without diabetes.[34] However, the time interval from diagnosis of new-onset diabetes to pancreatic cancer has been a topic of debate, with earlier studies showing stronger associations between diabetes and pancreatic cancer when the diabetes was less than or equal to 4 years[35] and a more recent study suggesting within the first year of diagnosis.[36]

Obesity

Obesity, defined by BMI greater than or equal to 30, has increased substantially world-wide between 1975 and 2016.[37] Obesity is associated with a cascade of other conditions, such as hyperglycemia, insulin resistance, and hypercholesterolemia. Elevated cholesterol has been shown to have a linear dose-response relation to the risk of pancreatic cancer, with 1 meta-analysis indicating that the risk of pancreatic cancer increased by 8% with 100 mg/d of cholesterol intake.[38,39] Several other studies have also shown an increased risk of pancreatic cancer with increased BMI.[40–42]

Temporal onset of changes in BMI has also been studied in the risk of pancreatic cancer. Some studies have suggested that weight gain after age 50 years is associated with an increased risk of pancreatic cancer,[43] whereas others suggest in early life.[44] Obesity among children has grown substantially. A population-based study of 51,505 children found that the most rapid weight gain was between 2 and 6 years of age, and 90% of children who were obese at the age of 3 years were overweight or obese in adolescence.[45] A recent study of data from 20 pooled prospective cohorts suggests that excess body weight during early adulthood (ages 18–21 years) could be a more important influence on pancreatic cancer risk than weight gain later in life.[46]

Alternatively, weight loss has also been implicated but likely as a result of an underlying pancreatic cancer rather than as a risk factor. In a large cohort study, Yuan and colleagues[34] found that compared with those with no weight loss, participants who reported a 0.45- to 1.8-kg weight loss had an age-adjusted hazard ratio (HR) for pancreatic cancer of 1.25 (95% CI, 1.03–1.52), those with a 2.25- to 3.6-kg weight loss had an age-adjusted HR of 1.33 (95% CI, 1.06–1.66), and those with more than an 3.6-kg weight loss had an age-adjusted HR of 1.92 (95% CI, 1.58–2.32). In addition, those with new-onset diabetes accompanied by weight loss of 0.45 to 3.6 kg had an HR 3.61 (95% CI, 2.15–6.10) and those with weight loss of more than 3.6 kg had an HR of 6.75 (95% CI 4.55–10.00). The risk was further increased in older individuals, those with healthy weight before weight loss, and those with unintentional weight loss. Co-occurrence of these symptoms should be recognized by clinicians because this group may benefit from early detection strategies.

Alcohol

Alcohol has a variety of effects on the pancreas, and the effects are dose dependent. A pooled analysis of data from the PanC4 found a statistically significant increased risk of pancreatic cancer among heavy alcohol drinkers defined by 9 or more drinks/d compared with drinkers taking less than 1 drink/d (odds ratio [OR], 1.6; 95% CI, 1.2–2.2).[47] A meta-analysis of 19 prospective studies found that light (0–12 g/d) to moderate ($\geq$12–24 g/d) alcohol intake had little or no effect on the risk of pancreatic cancer, whereas high intake ($\geq$24 g/d) was associated with an increased risk (Relative Risk (RR), 1.15; 95% CI, 1.06–1.25).[48] Other studies have corroborated these findings.[49,50] Analysis of the NIH-AARP Diet and Health study and American Cancer

Society Prevention Study II reported a relative risk of 1.32 to 1.45 in pancreatic cancer among those who drink more than 3 drinks/d.[51,52] Other studies have indicated that binge drinking increases the risk of pancreatic cancer by 2.5 times.[53] The underlying mechanism for the risk of pancreatic cancer with alcohol is likely its association with pancreatitis and the generation of toxic metabolites that lead to pancreatic carcinogenesis.[54]

Pancreatitis

Pancreatitis is both a modifiable and nonmodifiable risk factor, depending on the cause. Smoking, alcohol, hypertriglyceridemia, and genetic mutations are common causes of pancreatitis. There are 2 types of pancreatitis. Acute pancreatitis is an acute inflammation of the pancreas triggered by one or more factors. Acute pancreatitis is a risk factor for pancreatic cancer and can also be a symptom of underlying pancreatic cancer. A meta-analysis of retrospective and prospective studies evaluating the association between acute pancreatitis and pancreatic cancer risk found an effect estimate of 2.07 (95% CI, 1.36–2.78) during a 10-year follow-up. Further subgroup analysis showed a relative risk of 7.81 (95% CI, 5.00–12.19) for pancreatic cancer in patients with acute pancreatitis compared with healthy controls. The strongest association was found within the first year after acute pancreatitis (effect estimate, 23.47 [95% CI, 3.26–43.68]) and diminished over time, such that after greater than 10 years following acute pancreatitis there was only a slightly increased OR of 1.17 (95% CI, 0.78–1.57).[55] Similar findings were observed in data from the Danish National Patient Registry, Civil Registration System, and Danish Cancer Registry.[56] The relative hazard of pancreatic cancer in individuals with acute pancreatitis was 19.3 (95% CI, 14.6–25.4) within the 2 years following the pancreatitis diagnosis but continued to be elevated (adjusted relative hazard, 2.02; 95% CI, 1.57–2.61) for patients followed beyond 5 years. The investigators also adjusted for alcohol- and smoking-related conditions and Charlson Comorbidity Index and excluded patients with chronic pancreatitis (CP). This study found that those with idiopathic cause of acute pancreatitis were associated with the highest risk of pancreatic cancer with an adjusted HR of 2.52 (95% CI, 1.83–3.47).[56]

CP is defined as progressive inflammatory and fibrotic changes leading to irreversible structural damage, causing impairments in endocrine and exocrine functions. Patients with CP have a cumulative risk for pancreatic cancer of 1.8% (95% CI, 1–2.6) and 4% (95% CI, 2–5.9) 10 and 20 years after diagnosis, respectively.[57] A more recent meta-analysis found that although CP increases the risk of pancreatic cancer by 16-fold, the risk decreases over time. The risk after 5 years of diagnosis was 7.9-fold (95% CI, 4.26–14.66) and decreased to 3.5-fold (95%C 1.69–7.38) at 9 years suggesting closer follow-up in the first few years following CP diagnosis.[58]

There are several suggested mechanisms of pancreatitis increasing the risk of pancreatic cancer. Obstruction of the pancreatic duct, such as by a tumor, is a risk factor for the development of acute pancreatitis. Alcohol consumption and smoking are risk factors for acute pancreatitis and CP as well as pancreatic cancer. Chronic inflammation increases the possibility of development of mutations within cells, most commonly KRAS mutations, which are found in pancreatic intraepithelial neoplasia, one of the most common precursor lesions to pancreatic cancer.[59]

Allergy

The immune system's role in the development of pancreatic cancer is of increasing interest. Individuals with a personal history of allergies have been shown to be protective against pancreatic cancer.[59] Studies have found that those with asthma, nasal allergies, hay fevers, and other related symptoms have a lower risk of pancreatic cancer.[60-63] A recent exhaustive analysis found an inverse relationship between pancreatic cancer risk, severity, and duration. Furthermore, an increased asthma severity was associated with a reduced risk of pancreatic cancer.[60] The mechanism is unknown, but the underlying hypothesis is that individuals with active immune systems may have increased tumor immunity as a result of sustained elevated levels of IgE,[60] and the ability to survey the pancreas with the innate and adaptive antigen-specific immune system such as NK, NK-T, $\gamma\delta$, and $\alpha\beta$ T cells.[64,65] Genetic factors and gene-environmental interactions have also been shown to play a role. Atopy-related genetic variants have been associated with reduced pancreatic cancer risk.[65] However, further studies are needed for us to understand the underlying mechanism.

Microbiome

The microbiome has been extensively studied in its role in inflammation and carcinogenesis, with the speculation that the microbiota plays an essential role in activating, training, and modulating the host immune response.[66] Periodontal disease and oral microbiome have been shown to have increased the risk of pancreatic cancer.[67,68] Studies evaluating *Helicobacter pylori* in the risk of pancreatic cancer have been inconsistent.[69-71] Studies evaluating fecal microbiota have been limited.[69] Distinct intratumor microbiome has also been shown to promote pancreatic cancer through mutations of protumorigenic genes, inflammation, immune suppression, and treatment resistance.[72] Proteobacteria, *Fusobacterium nucleatum*, Bacteroidetes, and Firmicutes have shown to dominate the microbiome of pancreatic cancer.[72-76]

Table 1		
Germline genetic mutations and familial pancreatic cancer associated with pancreatic cancer		
	Risk of Developing Pancreatic Cancer	**Lifetime Risk of Developing Pancreatic Cancer**
Germline mutations		
STK-11	76–140	11%–32%
PRSS1	50–80	7.2%–40%
CFTR	1.82	—
CPA1	3.7	Not defined
CPB1	9.5	Not defined
CDKN2A	9–47	17%
MLH1 MSH2 MSH6 PMS2	9–11	3.7%
BRCA1	2.7–4.1	3.6%
BRCA2	3.5–10	10%
PALB2	6	Not defined
ATM	2.7	Not defined
Familial pancreatic cancer		
3 or more FDRs	32	38.5%
2 FDRs	6.4	8%–12%
1 FDR	4.6	4.7%

Abbreviation: FDR, first-degree relative.

Family History of Cancer

Up to 10% of patients with pancreatic cancer report having a close relative with pancreatic cancer,[77,78] and heritability estimates for pancreatic cancer range from 21% for array-based heritability[79] to 36% in twin studies.[80] Both rare high-risk genetic variants and common variants have been associated with pancreatic cancer. Many of the high-risk genetic variants are associated with established hereditary cancer syndromes. These and the associated risk of pancreatic cancer are detailed in the following sections and **Table 1**.

Individuals with a family history of pancreatic cancer have an increased risk. Still, the risk is variable and depends on the number of family members affected and their relationship with affected family members. Individuals with a single close relative have approximately a 1.8 to 2.5 fold increases risk for pancreatic cancer.[81-83] Familial pancreatic cancer (FPC) is defined as kindred where there has been a diagnosis of pancreatic cancer in at least 2 close relatives (parent and child or sibling pair). At-risk relatives in FPC families who have at least 1 close relative (sibling, parent, or child with pancreatic cancer) have a 6.8-fold (95% CI, 4.5–9.8) increased risk of pancreatic cancer,[84,85] whereas those with 3 or more close relatives with pancreatic cancer have a 17-fold increased risk (95% CI, 7.3–33.5).[81] Approximately 15% to 20% of patients with a family history of pancreatic cancer will have a pathogenic genetic variant identified as the likely basis for their increased risk of pancreatic cancer when undergoing multigene clinical genetic testing; this is in contrast to 5% to 10% of all patients with pancreatic cancer (unselected for family history).

High-risk genes/syndromes associated with pancreatic cancer

Hereditary breast-ovarian cancer has been associated with an increased risk of pancreatic cancer. Several gene mutations associated with DNA repair have been implicated, including BRCA1, BRCA2, PALB2, and ATM.

Individuals with pathogenic variants in the BRCA1 gene have up to a 3-fold increased risk of pancreatic cancer with a lifetime risk of up to of 3.6%.[86] Pathogenic variants in BRCA1 have been reported in 0.35% to 1% of patients with pancreatic cancer.[87-89] Pathogenic variants in the BRCA2 gene are more common in patients with pancreatic cancer, occurring in 2% to 7% of patients with pancreatic cancer unselected for family history and up to 16% of patients from families with 3 or more pancreatic cancers. The risk of pancreatic cancer in BRCA2 pathogenic variant carriers has been estimated to be 4- to 6-fold higher than in noncarriers.[90-93] The PALB2 protein, like its binding partner BRCA2, acts to repair double-stranded DNA breaks, and pathogenic variants in the PALB2 gene are associated with an increased risk of pancreatic cancer. Pathogenic variants in PALB2 are uncommon, with prevalence estimates less than 1% in patients with pancreatic cancer, but large population studies are showing risk estimates ranging from 2.5 to 3.5.[94,95]

Pathogenic variants in the ATM gene, named due to the syndrome that occurs among individuals with homozygous germline pathogenic variants in the gene, are present in 1% to 3% of patients with pancreatic cancer.[87,96-98] The risk of pancreatic cancer in ATM pathogenic variant carriers has been estimated to be 9.5% (95% CI, 5.0%–14.0%) by age 80 years, with an overall relative risk of 6.5 (95% CI, 4.5–9.5) compared with noncarriers.[99]

Inherited pathogenic variants in the CDKN2A gene, commonly associated with familial atypical multiple mole melanoma syndrome, are often associated with a high risk of melanoma, respiratory tract tumors, soft tissue tumors, basal and squamous cell carcinomas, and pancreatic cancer.[100] Pancreatic cancer is the second most common cancer after melanoma in these patients, with a 12- to 38-fold increased risk and a lifetime risk of 17%.[87,101]

Lynch syndrome is an autosomal dominant syndrome most commonly associated with early-onset colorectal cancer and endometrial cancer due to mutations in DNA mismatch repair genes (MSH2, MLH1, MSH6, PMS2, EPCAM). Individuals with Lynch syndrome have a 9- to 11-fold increased risk of pancreatic cancer[102,103] with a cumulative risk of 3.7% by the age of 70 years.[103]

Peutz-Jeghers syndrome (PJS) is an autosomal dominant hamartomatous polyposis syndrome involving the *STK11/LKB1* gene. Pathogenic variants in the STK11 gene are very rare and observed in greater than 0.5% of patients with pancreatic cancer. However, individuals with PJS have an extremely high risk of pancreatic cancer of 36% by age 64 years.[104]

As discussed earlier, genetic variants may also contribute to the development of acute pancreatitis and CP, thereby increasing the risk of pancreatic cancer. The risk depends on the genes involved.

Hereditary pancreatitis is associated with recurrent acute pancreatitis and CP at a young age, in addition to endocrine and exocrine pancreatic insufficiency. The risk of pancreatic cancer has been estimated to be as high as 30% to 40% by age 70 years in some forms of hereditary pancreatitis, such as in individuals with pathogenic variants in the *PRSS1* gene, which result in premature trypsin activation and autosomal dominant pancreatitis.[105–107]

In addition to pathogenic variants in PRSS1, variation in other genes has also been suggested to be involved in pancreatic cancer risk in the setting of pancreatitis. However, the risk of pancreatitis and pancreatitis cancer is less strong in these families; this includes variation in the pancreatic secretory enzymes *CPA1* and *CPB1,* particularly variants associated with endoplasmic reticulum stress phenotype, which are more common in patients with pancreatic cancer compared with control populations.[108,109] Common genetic variation in the *CTRB2* locus has been associated with both pancreatitis and pancreatic cancer.[110,111] In addition, genetic variation in the CFTR gene, which encodes the cystic fibrosis transmembrane conductance regulator protein, can cause acute pancreatitis and CP without causing pulmonary issues and has been associated with early-onset CP. However, some studies have also shown an increased risk of pancreatic cancer, but this finding is not consistent.[112]

Common variants. In addition to the high-risk variants associated with pancreatic cancer, as detailed earlier, all of which more than double the risk of pancreatic cancer yet rarely occur in healthy individuals, common genetic variants (that occur in >1%– 5% of healthy individuals of all ages) have also been associated and occur more frequently among individuals with pancreatic cancer. The first large-scale genome-wide association study (GWAS) for pancreatic cancer identified that individuals with genetic variants causing non-O versus O blood group were associated with an increased risk of pancreatic cancer. Subsequent studies examining the blood antigens themselves[113] found that those with blood groups A, AB, or B were more likely to develop pancreatic cancer with an adjusted hazards ratio for incident pancreatic cancer being 1.32 (95% CI, 1.02–1.72) for blood group A, 1.51 (95% CI, 1.02–2.23) for blood group AB, and 1.72 (95% CI, 1.25–2.38) for blood group B and that smoking may further increase these risks.[114,115] A GWAS identified a variant at the ABO locus 9q34 to pancreatic carcinogenesis. This initial GWAS study was followed by larger, better-powered studies both in European ancestry and in East Asian populations, including a recent, large-scale meta-analysis of 421 patients with European ancestry with pancreatic cancer and 426 controls.[113] To date, GWAS studies have identified primary associations at 1q32.1, 1p36.33, 2p13.3, 3q29, 5p15.33, 7p14.1, 8q21.11 8q24.21, 9q34.2, 13q12.2, 13q22.1, 16q23.1, 17q12, 17q25.1,18q21.32, and 22q12.1 in European ancestry individuals; 6p25.3, 12p11.21, 7q36.2, 13q12.2, 13q221, and 16p12.3 in Japanese populations; and 21q21.3, 5p13.1, 21q22.3, 22q13.32, and 10q26.11 in Chinese populations.[110,116,117] Subsequent studies of these GWAS data including transcriptome-wide association studies,[118] pathway-based approaches,[119] as well as mendelian randomization studies have provided further insight into the genetic basis of pancreatic cancer and the relationship between the genes underlying the connection between pancreatic cancer and some of the risk factors discussed previously.

SUMMARY

There has been a significant increase in pancreatic cancer globally despite advancements in diagnostic and therapeutic interventions when compared with other cancers, which have been declining. Mortality continues to be high among those with pancreatic cancer. The increase in pancreatic cancer cases is attributed to the modifiable and nonmodifiable risk factors described in this review. Further studies are needed to solidify the association between other risk factors and pancreatic cancer. Health initiatives aimed at smoking cessation and obesity may reduce the incidence of pancreatic cancer. Screening for early detection in those with genetic predisposition have already been implemented. Further studies are needed on the role of risk-modifying agents in reducing the risk of pancreatic cancer.

CLINICS CARE POINTS

- Pancreatic cancer is the 12th most common cause of cancer in the world and currently the 7th most common cause of cancer-related death.
- Survival rates remain low due to late diagnosis of pancreatic cancer despite advancement in medicine.
- Modifiable risk factors including ciagerette smoking, obesity and heavy alcohol use have been associated with increased risk of pancreatic cancer. However there are nonmodifable risk factors as well, including hereditary predisposition and common genetic variants.
- There is evidence that microbiome and immune system may also play a role as a risk factor for pancreatic cancer.

REFERENCES

1. Sung H, Ferlay J, Siegel RL, et al. Global cancer statistics 2020: GLOBOCAN estimates of incidence and mortality worldwide for 36 cancers in 185 countries. CA Cancer J Clin 2021;71(3):209–49.
2. Ferlay J, Partensky C, Bray F. More deaths from pancreatic cancer than breast cancer in the EU by 2017. Acta Oncol 2016;55(9–10):1158–60.
3. Arnold M, Abnet CC, Neale RE, et al. Global Burden of 5 Major Types of Gastrointestinal Cancer. Gastroenterology 2020;159(1):335–49.e15.
4. SEER Database. Available at: https://seer.cancer.gov/statfacts/html/pancreas.html Web site. Accessed December 18, 2021.
5. World Health Organization. Global cancer observatory. Available at: https://gco.iarc.fr/. Accessed January/9/21.

6. Siegel RL, Miller KD, Fuchs HE, et al. Cancer statistics, 2021. CA Cancer J Clin 2021;71(1):7–33.

7. Khalaf N, El-Serag HB, Abrams HR, et al. Burden of pancreatic cancer: from epidemiology to practice. Clin Gastroenterol Hepatol 2021;19(5):876–84.

8. Klein AP. Pancreatic cancer: a growing burden. Lancet Gastroenterol Hepatol 2019;4(12):895–6.

9. Sung H, Siegel RL, Rosenberg PS, et al. Emerging cancer trends among young adults in the USA: analysis of a population-based cancer registry. Lancet Public Health 2019;4(3):e137–47.

10. He J, Ahuja N, Makary MA, et al. 2564 resected periampullary adenocarcinomas at a single institution: trends over three decades. HPB (Oxford) 2014; 16(1):83–90.

11. Huang L, Jansen L, Balavarca Y, et al. Stratified survival of resected and overall pancreatic cancer patients in Europe and the USA in the early twenty-first century: a large, international population-based study. BMC Med 2018;16(1): 125–9.

12. Huang J, Lok V, Ngai CH, et al. Worldwide burden of, risk factors for, and trends in pancreatic cancer. Gastroenterology 2021;160(3):744–54.

13. Silverman DT, Hoover RN, Brown LM, et al. Why do Black Americans have a higher risk of pancreatic cancer than White Americans? Epidemiology 2003; 14(1):45–54.

14. Hue JJ, Katayama ES, Markt SC, et al. A nationwide analysis of pancreatic cancer trial enrollment reveals disparities and participation problems. Surgery 2021. S0039-6060(21)00983-1 [pii].

15. Eskander MF, Gil L, Beal EW, et al. Access denied: inequities in clinical trial enrollment for pancreatic cancer. Ann Surg Oncol 2021. https://doi.org/10. 1245/s10434-021-10868-4.

16. Gordon-Dseagu VL, Devesa SS, Goggins M, et al. Pancreatic cancer incidence trends: evidence from the Surveillance, Epidemiology and End Results (SEER) population-based data. Int J Epidemiol 2018;47(2):427–39.

17. Nipp R, Tramontano AC, Kong CY, et al. Disparities in cancer outcomes across age, sex, and race/ethnicity among patients with pancreatic cancer. Cancer Med 2018;7(2):525–35.

18. Fagenson AM, Grossi SM, Musgrove K, et al. Ethnic and racial disparities of pancreatic adenocarcinoma in Florida. HPB (Oxford) 2020;22(5):735–43.

19. Liu L, Zhang J, Deapen D, et al. Differences in pancreatic cancer incidence rates and temporal trends across asian subpopulations in california (1988-2015). Pancreas 2019;48(7):931–3.

20. Pastrana Del Valle J, Mahvi DA, Fairweather M, et al. Associations of gender, race, and ethnicity with disparities in short-term adverse outcomes after pancreatic resection for cancer. J Surg Oncol 2021. https://doi.org/10.1002/jso.26748.

21. Iodice S, Gandini S, Maisonneuve P, et al. Tobacco and the risk of pancreatic cancer: a review and meta-analysis. Langenbecks Arch Surg 2008;393(4): 535–45.

22. Bosetti C, Lucenteforte E, Silverman DT, et al. Cigarette smoking and pancreatic cancer: an analysis from the International Pancreatic Cancer Case-Control Consortium (Panc4). Ann Oncol 2012;23(7):1880–8.

23. Lynch SM, Vrieling A, Lubin JH, et al. Cigarette smoking and pancreatic cancer: a pooled analysis from the pancreatic cancer cohort consortium. Am J Epidemiol 2009;170(4):403–13.

24. Maisonneuve P, Marshall BC, Lowenfels AB. Risk of pancreatic cancer in patients with cystic fibrosis. Gut 2007;56(9):1327–8.

25. Momi N, Kaur S, Ponnusamy MP, et al. Interplay between smoking-induced genotoxicity and altered signaling in pancreatic carcinogenesis. Carcinogenesis 2012;33(9):1617–28.

26. Lugo A, Peveri G, Bosetti C, et al. Strong excess risk of pancreatic cancer for low frequency and duration of cigarette smoking: a comprehensive review and meta-analysis. Eur J Cancer 2018;104:117–26.

27. Ben QW, Liu J, Sun YW, et al. Cigarette smoking and mortality in patients with pancreatic cancer: a systematic review and meta-analysis. Pancreas 2019; 48(8):985–95.

28. Weissman S, Takakura K, Eibl G, et al. The diverse involvement of cigarette smoking in pancreatic cancer development and prognosis. Pancreas 2020; 49(5):612–20.

29. Marcon A, Pesce G, Calciano L, et al. Trends in smoking initiation in Europe over 40 years: a retrospective cohort study. PLoS One 2018;13(8):e0201881.

30. Yang JJ, Yu D, Wen W, et al. Tobacco smoking and mortality in asia: a pooled meta-analysis. JAMA Netw Open 2019;2(3):e191474.

31. Kim NH, Chang Y, Lee SR, et al. Glycemic status, insulin resistance, and risk of pancreatic cancer mortality in individuals with and without diabetes. Am J Gastroenterol 2020;115(11):1840–8.

32. Chari ST, Leibson CL, Rabe KG, et al. Probability of pancreatic cancer following diabetes: a population-based study. Gastroenterology 2005;129(2):504–11.

33. Gupta S, Vittinghoff E, Bertenthal D, et al. New-onset diabetes and pancreatic cancer. Clin Gastroenterol Hepatol 2006;4(11):1366–72 [quiz: 1301.

34. Yuan C, Babic A, Khalaf N, et al. Diabetes, weight change, and pancreatic cancer risk. JAMA Oncol 2020;6(10):e202948.

35. Huxley R, Ansary-Moghaddam A, Berrington de Gonzalez A, et al. Type-II diabetes and pancreatic cancer: a meta-analysis of 36 studies. Br J Cancer 2005; 92(11):2076–83.

36. Huang BZ, Pandol SJ, Jeon CY, et al. New-onset diabetes, longitudinal trends in metabolic markers, and risk of pancreatic cancer in a heterogeneous population. Clin Gastroenterol Hepatol 2019. S1542-3565(19)31383-31387.

37. NCD Risk Factor Collaboration (NCD-RisC). Worldwide trends in body-mass index, underweight, overweight, and obesity from 1975 to 2016: a pooled analysis of 2416 population-based measurement studies in 128.9 million children, adolescents, and adults. Lancet 2017;390(10113):2627–42.

38. Chen H, Qin S, Wang M, et al. Association between cholesterol intake and pancreatic cancer risk: evidence from a meta-analysis. Sci Rep 2015;5:8243.

39. Bluher M. Obesity: global epidemiology and pathogenesis. Nat Rev Endocrinol 2019;15(5):288–98.

40. Carreras-Torres R, Johansson M, Gaborieau V, et al. The role of obesity, type 2 diabetes, and metabolic factors in pancreatic cancer: a mendelian randomization study. J Natl Cancer Inst 2017;109(9). https://doi.org/10.1093/jnci/djx012.

41. Arslan AA, Helzlsouer KJ, Kooperberg C, et al. Anthropometric measures, body mass index, and pancreatic cancer: a pooled analysis from the Pancreatic Cancer Cohort Consortium (PanScan). Arch Intern Med 2010;170(9):791–802.

42. Larsson SC, Orsini N, Wolk A. Body mass index and pancreatic cancer risk: a meta-analysis of prospective studies. Int J Cancer 2007;120(9):1993–8.

43. Stolzenberg-Solomon RZ, Graubard BI, Chari S, et al. Insulin, glucose, insulin resistance, and pancreatic cancer in male smokers. JAMA 2005;294(22): 2872–8.

44. Nogueira L, Stolzenberg-Solomon R, Gamborg M, et al. Childhood body mass index and risk of adult pancreatic cancer. Curr Dev Nutr 2017;1(10). https://doi.org/10.3945/cdn.117.001362.

45. Geserick M, Vogel M, Gausche R, et al. Acceleration of BMI in early childhood and risk of sustained obesity. N Engl J Med 2018;379(14):1303–12.

46. Genkinger JM, Kitahara CM, Bernstein L, et al. Central adiposity, obesity during early adulthood, and pancreatic cancer mortality in a pooled analysis of cohort studies. Ann Oncol 2015;26(11):2257–66.

47. Lucenteforte E, La Vecchia C, Silverman D, et al. Alcohol consumption and pancreatic cancer: a pooled analysis in the International Pancreatic Cancer Case-Control Consortium (PanC4). Ann Oncol 2012;23(2):374–82.

48. Wang YT, Gou YW, Jin WW, et al. Association between alcohol intake and the risk of pancreatic cancer: a dose-response meta-analysis of cohort studies. BMC Cancer 2016;16:212.

49. Korc M, Jeon CY, Edderkaoui M, et al. Consortium for the study of chronic pancreatitis, diabetes. Tobacco and alcohol as risk factors for pancreatic cancer. Best Pract Res Clin Gastroenterol 2017;31(5):529–36.

50. Genkinger JM, Spiegelman D, Anderson KE, et al. Alcohol intake and pancreatic cancer risk: a pooled analysis of fourteen cohort studies. Cancer Epidemiol Biomarkers Prev 2009;18(3):765–76.

51. Jiao L, Silverman DT, Schairer C, et al. Alcohol use and risk of pancreatic cancer: the NIH-AARP Diet and Health Study. Am J Epidemiol 2009;169(9): 1043–51.

52. Gapstur SM, Jacobs EJ, Deka A, et al. Association of alcohol intake with pancreatic cancer mortality in never smokers. Arch Intern Med 2011;171(5):444–51.

53. Gupta S, Wang F, Holly EA, et al. Risk of pancreatic cancer by alcohol dose, duration, and pattern of consumption, including binge drinking: a population-based study. Cancer Causes Control 2010;21(7):1047–59.

54. Yadav D, Lowenfels AB. The epidemiology of pancreatitis and pancreatic cancer. Gastroenterology 2013;144(6):1252–61.

55. Liu J, Wang Y, Yu Y. Meta-analysis reveals an association between acute pancreatitis and the risk of pancreatic cancer. World J Clin Cases 2020;8(19): 4416–30.

56. Kirkegard J, Cronin-Fenton D, Heide-Jorgensen U, et al. Acute pancreatitis and pancreatic cancer risk: a nationwide matched-cohort study in denmark. Gastroenterology 2018;154(6):1729–36.

57. Lowenfels AB, Maisonneuve P, Cavallini G, et al. Pancreatitis and the risk of pancreatic cancer. International Pancreatitis Study Group. N Engl J Med 1993;328(20):1433–7.

58. Kirkegard J, Mortensen FV, Cronin-Fenton D. Chronic pancreatitis and pancreatic cancer risk: a systematic review and meta-analysis. Am J Gastroenterol 2017;112(9):1366–72.

59. Lohr M, Kloppel G, Maisonneuve P, et al. Frequency of K-ras mutations in pancreatic intraductal neoplasias associated with pancreatic ductal adenocarcinoma and chronic pancreatitis: a meta-analysis. Neoplasia 2005;7(1):17–23.

60. Gomez-Rubio P, Zock JP, Rava M, et al. Reduced risk of pancreatic cancer associated with asthma and nasal allergies. Gut 2017;66(2):314–22.

61. Maisonneuve P, Lowenfels AB, Bueno-de-Mesquita HB, et al. Past medical history and pancreatic cancer risk: results from a multicenter case-control study. Ann Epidemiol 2010;20(2):92–8.

62. Turner MC, Chen Y, Krewski D, et al. Cancer mortality among US men and women with asthma and hay fever. Am J Epidemiol 2005;162(3):212–21.

63. Olson SH, Hsu M, Satagopan JM, et al. Allergies and risk of pancreatic cancer: a pooled analysis from the Pancreatic Cancer Case-Control Consortium. Am J Epidemiol 2013;178(5):691–700.

64. Gandini S, Lowenfels AB, Jaffee EM, et al. Allergies and the risk of pancreatic cancer: a meta-analysis with review of epidemiology and biological mechanisms. Cancer Epidemiol Biomarkers Prev 2005;14(8):1908–16.

65. Cotterchio M, Lowcock E, Bider-Canfield Z, et al. Association between Variants in Atopy-Related Immunologic Candidate Genes and Pancreatic Cancer Risk. PLoS One 2015;10(5):e0125273.

66. Rajagopala SV, Vashee S, Oldfield LM, et al. The human microbiome and cancer. Cancer Prev Res (Phila) 2017;10(4):226–34.

67. Fan X, Alekseyenko AV, Wu J, et al. Human oral microbiome and prospective risk for pancreatic cancer: a population-based nested case-control study. Gut 2018; 67(1):120–7.

68. Michaud DS, Izard J, Wilhelm-Benartzi CS, et al. Plasma antibodies to oral bacteria and risk of pancreatic cancer in a large European prospective cohort study. Gut 2013;62(12):1764–70.

69. Guo Y, Liu W, Wu J. Helicobacter pylori infection and pancreatic cancer risk: a meta-analysis. J Cancer Res Ther 2016;12(Supplement):C229–32.

70. Schulte A, Pandeya N, Fawcett J, et al. Association between Helicobacter pylori and pancreatic cancer risk: a meta-analysis. Cancer Causes Control 2015; 26(7):1027–35.

71. Ding SZ, Goldberg JB, Hatakeyama M. Helicobacter pylori infection, oncogenic pathways and epigenetic mechanisms in gastric carcinogenesis. Future Oncol 2010;6(5):851–62.

72. Tijeras-Raballand A, Hilmi M, Astorgues-Xerri L, et al. Microbiome and pancreatic ductal adenocarcinoma. Clin Res Hepatol Gastroenterol 2021;45(2): 101589.

73. Ren Z, Jiang J, Xie H, et al. Gut microbial profile analysis by MiSeq sequencing of pancreatic carcinoma patients in China. Oncotarget 2017;8(56):95176–91.

74. Pushalkar S, Hundeyin M, Daley D, et al. The Pancreatic Cancer Microbiome Promotes Oncogenesis by Induction of Innate and Adaptive Immune Suppression. Cancer Discov 2018;8(4):403–16.

75. Thomas RM, Gharaibeh RZ, Gauthier J, et al. Intestinal microbiota enhances pancreatic carcinogenesis in preclinical models. Carcinogenesis 2018;39(8): 1068–78.

76. Nejman D, Livyatan I, Fuks G, et al. The human tumor microbiome is composed of tumor type-specific intracellular bacteria. Science 2020;368(6494):973–80.

77. Brand R, Borazanci E, Speare V, et al. Prospective study of germline genetic testing in incident cases of pancreatic adenocarcinoma. Cancer 2018; 124(17):3520–7.

78. Permuth-Wey J, Egan KM. Family history is a significant risk factor for pancreatic cancer: results from a systematic review and meta-analysis. Fam Cancer 2009;8(2):109–17.

79. Chen F, Childs EJ, Mocci E, et al. Analysis of heritability and genetic architecture of pancreatic cancer: a PanC4 study. Cancer Epidemiol Biomarkers Prev 2019; 28(7):1238–45.

80. Lichtenstein P, Holm NV, Verkasalo PK, et al. Environmental and heritable factors in the causation of cancer–analyses of cohorts of twins from Sweden, Denmark, and Finland. N Engl J Med 2000;343(2):78–85.

81. Brune KA, Lau B, Palmisano E, et al. Importance of age of onset in pancreatic cancer kindreds. J Natl Cancer Inst 2010;102(2):119–26.

82. Amundadottir LT, Thorvaldsson S, Gudbjartsson DF, et al. Cancer as a complex phenotype: pattern of cancer distribution within and beyond the nuclear family. PLoS Med 2004;1(3):e65.

83. Schenk M, Schwartz AG, O'Neal E, et al. Familial risk of pancreatic cancer. J Natl Cancer Inst 2001;93(8):640–4.

84. Klein AP, Brune KA, Petersen GM, et al. Prospective risk of pancreatic cancer in familial pancreatic cancer kindreds. Cancer Res 2004;64(7):2634–8.

85. Ghadirian P, Liu G, Gallinger S, et al. Risk of pancreatic cancer among individuals with a family history of cancer of the pancreas. Int J Cancer 2002;97(6): 807–10.

86. Thompson D, Easton DF, Breast Cancer Linkage Consortium. Cancer incidence in BRCA1 mutation carriers. J Natl Cancer Inst 2002;94(18):1358–65.

87. Hu C, Hart SN, Polley EC, et al. Association between inherited germline mutations in cancer predisposition genes and risk of pancreatic cancer. JAMA 2018;319(23):2401–9.

88. Yurgelun MB, Chittenden AB, Morales-Oyarvide V, et al. Germline cancer susceptibility gene variants, somatic second hits, and survival outcomes in patients with resected pancreatic cancer. Genet Med 2019;21(1):213–23.

89. Shindo K, Yu J, Suenaga M, et al. Deleterious germline mutations in patients with apparently sporadic pancreatic adenocarcinoma. J Clin Oncol 2017;35(30): 3382–90.

90. Hahn SA, Greenhalf B, Ellis I, et al. BRCA2 germline mutations in familial pancreatic carcinoma. J Natl Cancer Inst 2003;95(3):214–21.

91. van Asperen CJ, Brohet RM, Meijers-Heijboer EJ, et al. Cancer risks in BRCA2 families: estimates for sites other than breast and ovary. J Med Genet 2005; 42(9):711–9.

92. Risch HA, McLaughlin JR, Cole DE, et al. Population BRCA1 and BRCA2 mutation frequencies and cancer penetrances: a kin-cohort study in Ontario, Canada. J Natl Cancer Inst 2006;98(23):1694–706.

93. Brose MS, Rebbeck TR, Calzone KA, et al. Cancer risk estimates for BRCA1 mutation carriers identified in a risk evaluation program. J Natl Cancer Inst 2002; 94(18):1365–72.

94. Casadei S, Norquist BM, Walsh T, et al. Contribution of inherited mutations in the BRCA2-interacting protein PALB2 to familial breast cancer. Cancer Res 2011; 71(6):2222–9.

95. Yang X, Leslie G, Doroszuk A, et al. Cancer risks associated with germline PALB2 pathogenic variants: an international study of 524 families. J Clin Oncol 2020;38(7):674–85.

96. Swift M, Chase CL, Morrell D. Cancer predisposition of ataxia-telangiectasia heterozygotes. Cancer Genet Cytogenet 1990;46(1):21–7.

97. Swift M, Sholman L, Perry M, et al. Malignant neoplasms in the families of patients with ataxia-telangiectasia. Cancer Res 1976;36(1):209–15.

98. Geoffroy-Perez B, Janin N, Ossian K, et al. Cancer risk in heterozygotes for ataxia-telangiectasia. Int J Cancer 2001;93(2):288–93.

99. Hsu FC, Roberts NJ, Childs E, et al. Risk of pancreatic cancer among individuals with pathogenic variants in the ATM gene. JAMA Oncol 2021;7(11):1664–8.

100. Oldenburg RA, de Vos tot Nederveen Cappel WH, van Puijenbroek M, et al. Extending the p16-Leiden tumour spectrum by respiratory tract tumours. J Med Genet 2004;41(3):e31.

101. Goldstein AM, Struewing JP, Fraser MC, et al. Prospective risk of cancer in CDKN2A germline mutation carriers. J Med Genet 2004;41(6):421–4.

102. Win AK, Lindor NM, Winship I, et al. Risks of colorectal and other cancers after endometrial cancer for women with Lynch syndrome. J Natl Cancer Inst 2013; 105(4):274–9.

103. Kastrinos F, Mukherjee B, Tayob N, et al. Risk of pancreatic cancer in families with Lynch syndrome. JAMA 2009;302(16):1790–5.

104. Giardiello FM, Brensinger JD, Tersmette AC, et al. Very high risk of cancer in familial Peutz-Jeghers syndrome. Gastroenterology 2000;119(6):1447–53.

105. Lowenfels AB, Maisonneuve P, DiMagno EP, et al. Hereditary pancreatitis and the risk of pancreatic cancer. International Hereditary Pancreatitis Study Group. J Natl Cancer Inst 1997;89(6):442–6.

106. Howes N, Lerch MM, Greenhalf W, et al. Clinical and genetic characteristics of hereditary pancreatitis in Europe. Clin Gastroenterol Hepatol 2004;2(3):252–61.

107. Whitcomb DC, Gorry MC, Preston RA, et al. Hereditary pancreatitis is caused by a mutation in the cationic trypsinogen gene. Nat Genet 1996;14(2):141–5.

108. Roberts NJ, Norris AL, Petersen GM, et al. Whole genome sequencing defines the genetic heterogeneity of familial pancreatic cancer. Cancer Discov 2016; 6(2):166–75.

109. Tamura K, Yu J, Hata T, et al. Mutations in the pancreatic secretory enzymes CPA1 and CPB1 are associated with pancreatic cancer. Proc Natl Acad Sci U S A 2018;115(18):4767–72.

110. Klein AP, Wolpin BM, Risch HA, et al. Genome-wide meta-analysis identifies five new susceptibility loci for pancreatic cancer. Nat Commun 2018;9(1):556.

111. Gao J, Zhu F, Lv S, et al. Identification of pancreatic juice proteins as biomarkers of pancreatic cancer. Oncol Rep 2010;23(6):1683–92.

112. McWilliams RR, Petersen GM, Rabe KG, et al. Cystic fibrosis transmembrane conductance regulator (CFTR) gene mutations and risk for pancreatic adenocarcinoma. Cancer 2010;116(1):203–9.

113. Amundadottir L, Kraft P, Stolzenberg-Solomon RZ, et al. Genome-wide association study identifies variants in the ABO locus associated with susceptibility to pancreatic cancer. Nat Genet 2009;41(9):986–90.

114. Wolpin BM, Chan AT, Hartge P, et al. ABO blood group and the risk of pancreatic cancer. J Natl Cancer Inst 2009;101(6):424–31.

115. Wolpin BM, Kraft P, Gross M, et al. Pancreatic cancer risk and ABO blood group alleles: results from the pancreatic cancer cohort consortium. Cancer Res 2010; 70(3):1015–23.

116. Wu C, Miao X, Huang L, et al. Genome-wide association study identifies five loci associated with susceptibility to pancreatic cancer in Chinese populations. Nat Genet 2011;44(1):62–6.

117. Lin Y, Nakatochi M, Hosono Y, et al. Genome-wide association meta-analysis identifies GP2 gene risk variants for pancreatic cancer. Nat Commun 2020; 11(1):3175-w.

118. Zhong J, Jermusyk A, Wu L, et al. A transcriptome-wide association study identifies novel candidate susceptibility genes for pancreatic cancer. J Natl Cancer Inst 2020;112(10):1003–12.
119. Walsh N, Zhang H, Hyland PL, et al. Agnostic pathway/gene set analysis of genome-wide association data identifies associations for pancreatic cancer. J Natl Cancer Inst 2019;111(6):557–67.

The Interplay Among Pancreatic Cancer, Cachexia, Body Composition, and Diabetes

Richard F. Dunne, MD, MS[a],*, Eric J. Roeland, MD[b]

KEYWORDS

- Cachexia • Diabetes • Pancreatic cancer • Adiposity • Weight loss • Muscle

KEY POINTS

- Cachexia, a syndrome of weight loss and reduced muscle mass, is common in pancreatic cancer and is associated with poorer survival and chemotherapy toxicity.
- Metabolic changes associated with pancreatic cancer cachexia and pancreatic cancer-associated diabetes occur early in the disease process, sometimes years before cancer diagnosis.
- Early dietician referral, prompt replacement of pancreatic enzymes, and involving palliative care specialists for symptom management are likely to improve outcomes in pancreatic cancer cachexia.

INTRODUCTION

The incidence of pancreatic ductal adenocarcinoma (PDAC) is increasing, and PDAC is expected to become the second leading cause of cancer death in the United States by 2030.[1] Poor survival rates are driven by PDAC's advanced stage at diagnosis when palliative chemotherapy is the only viable treatment option.[2] Furthermore, patients with PDAC often suffer from cachexia, which contributes to poor outcomes in this disease.[3] Cancer cachexia is a hypermetabolic syndrome of progressive weight and muscle loss (with or without fat loss) resulting in impaired physical function, poor quality of life, and adverse clinical outcomes that cannot be reversed by nutritional support alone.[4] Consensus diagnostic criteria for cancer cachexia include greater than 5% weight loss over the prior 6 months and greater than 2% weight loss with a body mass index (BMI) less than 20 kg/m^2 or skeletal muscle mass below the fifth percentile.[4] Thought to be most prevalent in this cancer type, cachexia affects over 80% of

[a] Department of Medicine, Wilmot Cancer Institute, University of Rochester Medical Center, 601 Elmwood Avenue, Box 704, Rochester, NY 14642, USA; [b] Division of Hematology/Oncology, Oregon Health and Science University, Knight Cancer Institute, 3181 SW Sam Jackson Park Road, Portland, OR 97239, USA
* Corresponding author.
E-mail address: richard_dunne@urmc.edu

Hematol Oncol Clin N Am 36 (2022) 897–910
https://doi.org/10.1016/j.hoc.2022.07.001
0889-8588/22/© 2022 Elsevier Inc. All rights reserved.

patients with PDAC,[5] including many with localized disease.[3,6] Recognizing and treating cachexia promptly may improve outcomes, as stabilizing weight in patients with advanced PDAC is associated with improved survival.[7] Nonetheless, up to a third of patients with PDAC die from complications of cachexia.[8] With no currently available standardized therapeutic strategies,[9] improving understanding and, consequently, the treatment of cachexia remains an urgent unmet need. This article reviews metabolic factors, including diabetes mellitus, pertinent to the care of patients with PDAC, with a particular focus on cachexia and its pathophysiology, symptomatology, clinical outcomes, and treatment.

PATHOPHYSIOLOGY AND PRECLINICAL PANCREATIC DUCTAL ADENOCARCINOMA CACHEXIA MODELS

Cachexia's pathophysiology is caused by a negative energy balance characterized by decreased energy intake combined with an elevated resting energy expenditure and hypermetabolism that cause the breakdown of muscle and adipose tissue.[10] A proinflammatory state, resulting from tumor-secreted cytokines and the host response, drives the development of cachexia. However, specific mechanisms and their interplay remain uncertain. A more in-depth discussion of cachexia pathophysiology has been published previously.[10] In the past decade, several key findings in preclinical and human studies have provided insight into why cachexia is so pervasive in PDAC compared with other tumor types. Although thought of by many as a late stage event, PDAC cachexia likely occurs early in the disease process. Patients diagnosed with PDAC were found to have elevated plasma levels of branched-chain amino acids several years prior to their clinical diagnosis.[11] Preclinical models suggest that these early changes are caused by muscle breakdown driven by mutant KRAS specific to pancreatic tumors.[11] Additionally, pancreatic exocrine insufficiency caused by pancreatic tumor infiltration is an early cachexia driver in preclinical models.[12] Recently, inflammatory changes in the brain have been detected in PDAC cachexia mouse models, particularly in specific regions of the hypothalamus that regulate anorexia, tissue catabolism, and sickness behavior.[13,14] With these recent advances and others, one can expect the underlying mechanisms of PDAC cachexia to be further elucidated, ultimately leading to the development of more effective and precise therapies.

CACHEXIA, MUSCLE WASTING AND ADIPOSITY-RELATED CLINICAL OUTCOMES IN PANCREATIC DUCTAL ADENOCARCINOMA
Cachexia Symptoms and the Patient Experience

Patients with PDAC-associated cachexia experience a wide range of symptoms, including functional, physical, social, and emotional impairments (**Fig. 1**).[15] Reduction in physical function and physical activity are hallmark characteristics of cachexia and have been demonstrated in multiple clinical trials involving patients with PDAC specifically.[8,16,17] Symptoms of pain, dyspnea, fatigue, and loss of appetite, all of which those with PDAC and cachexia experience more frequently than those without cachexia,[18] are common contributors to reduced functional status. In fact, fatigue and poor appetite are cited as the most distressing cachexia symptoms for patients with PDAC.[15,18]

Upwards of 60% of patients with PDAC cachexia do not meet expected daily energy intake requirements, which ultimately leads to malnutrition.[18] There are multiple contributors to malnutrition in patients with cachexia, but several are more prominent in patients with PDAC. Mechanical obstruction leading to vomiting and dysphagia

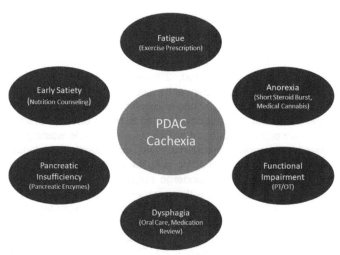

Fig. 1. PDAC cachexia. The patient experience and management strategies. OT, occupational therapy; PDAC, pancreatic ductal adenocarcinoma; PT, physical therapy.

from the primary tumor or metastatic omental disease is a relatively unique challenge of PDAC. Secondly, chemotherapy and supportive management strategies for PDAC can exacerbate dysphagia and cause food avoidance. Xerostomia, secondary to frequent use of opioids and antiemetics, and stomatitis, secondary to 5-fluorouracil based-therapies and complications of gastrointestinal surgery, are common in PDAC cachexia.[18,19] Thirdly, pancreatic insufficiency, which is widespread after pancreaticoduodenectomy (Whipple procedure) and occurs in half of patients with advanced PDAC, results in abdominal pain, diarrhea, malabsorption, and malnutrition.[20] Lastly, patients who undergo resection of PDAC can experience delayed gastric emptying for weeks or months following surgery and often develop long-standing early satiety.[21,22] Symptom management approaches will be discussed in detail.

Cachexia can also negatively impact patients socially and emotionally. Anorexia can particularly alter dynamics within the family, creating tension regarding food preparation and meals.[23] Mood disturbance is also prevalent in patients with PDAC and cachexia. More than 40% of patients experience a reduced sense of well-being, depression, and anxiety.[18] Although not always the focus in the oncology clinic, evaluating for emotional distress and routine inclusion of psychosocial experts are vital practices when caring for patients with PDAC cachexia.

Surgical Outcomes

Standardized ubiquitous assessments for weight loss in the oncology clinic are uncommon, resulting in sparse retrospective data utilizing cachexia-specific outcomes in PDAC. Consequently, surrogate endpoints, particularly skeletal muscle and fat mass, are often used. Improved technology that accurately quantifies skeletal muscle and fat mass through analysis of archived computed tomography (CT) scans, further bolstered by artificial intelligence algorithms,[24] has resulted in an increased interest in body composition-related oncology research over the past decade.

Preoperative sarcopenia, usually measured by the cross-sectional muscle area at the third lumbar vertebral body by CT slice and controlled for height,[25] is one of the most common variables evaluated in PDAC body composition studies. Sarcopenia, a skeletal muscle disorder characterized by progressive skeletal muscle wasting and weakness,[26] is prevalent in patients with PDAC at any stage, ranging from 20% to 65% in patients undergoing surgical resection.[6] Although conflicting single-institution studies have been reported, 2 recently published meta-analyses with more than 4000 patients who underwent resection for PDAC found that patients with preoperative sarcopenia experienced significantly worse survival.[6,27] Another clinical scenario related to poor outcomes is sarcopenic obesity, which describes a patient who is overweight (because of adiposity) with muscle wasting. Patients with sarcopenic obesity undergoing resection of PDAC consistently experience poorer survival outcomes.[6,28] Higher visceral adipose tissue content is also negatively associated with survival in patients who undergo surgery for PDAC.[28] Interestingly, in a single-institution study of patients with operable and advanced PDAC, those who experienced visceral adipose tissue wasting at the most accelerated rates also experienced shorter survival times.[29]

Body composition and its association with PDAC postoperative complications and surgical morbidity have also been examined. There is inconsistent evidence linking preoperative sarcopenia and postoperative complications, including pancreatic fistula formation.[6,28] In contrast, sarcopenic obesity and high visceral adipose tissue volumes are more closely associated with surgical complications, including higher rates of major complications, pancreatic fistula formation, and surgical site infections.[28,30,31] It has been suggested that visceral adiposity is a significant contributor to cancer surgery morbidity and mortality because of the excess production of proinflammatory adipokines and cytokines that can alter immune response, recovery, and wound healing.[30,32] Higher complication rates and poorer survival in patients with sarcopenia and adiposity in PDAC have led to multiple studies evaluating the role of prehabilitation to minimize these negative effects. A systematic review revealed that these programs may improve PDAC surgical outcomes, although standard approaches are not well-established.[33]

Chemotherapy Outcomes

Sarcopenia is observed at the initiation of chemotherapy in upwards of 65% of patients with advanced PDAC,[12,34] although evidence of sarcopenia as an independent prognostic biomarker in this setting has been conflicting. In several retrospective studies of patients receiving palliative gemcitabine-based chemotherapy, baseline sarcopenia was significantly associated with poorer overall survival when controlling for other prognostic factors.[35,36] In contrast, several other retrospective studies in which patients received various chemotherapy regimens showed no significant association between baseline sarcopenia and survival.[12,34] Ongoing, progressive sarcopenia during chemotherapy is common, and cytotoxic chemotherapy may further cause direct injury to skeletal muscle.[37] A longitudinal analysis of patients receiving palliative-intent chemotherapy for PDAC showed that muscle loss, particularly that seen 2 to 4 months after baseline, was associated with poorer survival.[38] Conversely, a separate study showed no significant association between muscle loss and survival in patients receiving palliative chemotherapy, but did find that those with sarcopenic obesity had the poorest survival.[39]

Similar to observations among other tumor types,[40] sarcopenia in patients with PDAC is associated with increased chemotherapy toxicity. In 2 studies of patients receiving gemcitabine-based chemotherapy, prechemotherapy sarcopenia was associated with more grade 3 or greater chemotherapy toxicities. One of these studies, a propensity-matched cohort study of patients with PDAC on first-line gemcitabine and nab-paclitaxel, found that those with pretreatment sarcopenia received significantly fewer cycles of chemotherapy compared to those with preserved muscle mass (5 vs 9 cycles).[36] In a separate study evaluating patients with advanced PDAC receiving FOLFIRINOX (folinic acid, fluorouracil, irinotecan hydrochloride, and oxaliplatin), both high visceral adipose tissue volume and sarcopenic obesity were significantly associated with a higher incidence of hematologic toxicity; no association was seen with hematologic toxicity and sarcopenia alone.[41] Body surface area dosing is thought to be, at least in part, responsible for increases in chemotherapy toxicity in those with sarcopenic obesity. Fat-free mass, a body compartment with a significant volume of distribution for cytotoxic drugs, correlates poorly with body surface area in patients with sarcopenic obesity, posing a risk of unpredictable tolerability.[42]

In summary, PDAC body composition research demonstrates that sarcopenia and sarcopenic obesity at diagnosis portend a poorer prognosis and increased treatment toxicity. Sarcopenia, however, is common in PDAC, and cross-sectional evaluation of skeletal muscle mass alone may be inadequate to risk-stratify patients. Longitudinal changes in weight and muscle over time, incorporating visceral adiposity measurements, patient-reported symptoms, and collecting functional outcomes would further enhance understanding of the complex interplay between body composition and PDAC. A practical approach to implement an assessment within the clinic may include evaluating body mass index (BMI), tracking changes in weight, and a brief functional assessment that evaluates muscle strength like the 5-chair-stand test.[43] This approach could guide the practicing oncologist and help predict who may be at greater risk for chemotherapy toxicity and/or early death.

Obesity, Diabetes, and Pancreatic Cancer

Long-standing obesity and adiposity are risk factors for developing PDAC. A prospective cohort study found that increasing BMI (starting as early as age 18) and longer periods of obesity (>25 years) were associated with a greater risk of PDAC.[44] Commonly associated with obesity, diabetes, specifically type 2 diabetes mellitus, is also a well-established independent risk factor for PDAC.[45] Increases in insulin levels[46] to overcome insulin resistance and concomitant increases in insulin-like growth factor-1 (IGF-1) levels[47] that occur in patients with obesity and/or diabetes are likely carcinogenic metabolic changes occurring in these patients. Additionally, metabolic changes related to PDAC can lead to new-onset diabetes, which has been described as a dual causality phenomenon.[48] A registry study found that after PDAC resection, 57% of patients with new-onset diabetes (<2 years before PDAC diagnosis) experienced resolution of their diabetes, while no patients with long-standing diabetes experienced resolution.[49] This effect of tumor removal on diabetes suggests that PDAC tumors have a paraneoplastic impact on glucose metabolism (reviewed more in-depth previously).[48]

A hallmark of PDAC-associated diabetes is its relatively rapid onset and its detection, on average, approximately 6.5 months before PDAC diagnosis.[50] Furthermore, three-quarters of patients with PDAC and diabetes were diagnosed with diabetes within the 2 years before their cancer diagnosis.[51] A population-based cohort study found that 0.85% of those diagnosed with diabetes after the age of 50 had PDAC within the next 3 years, an incidence approximately 8 times higher than the general population.[50] Another case-control study found elevated fasting blood glucose levels in patients with PDAC about 2.5 to 3 years before the clinical detection of PDAC.[52] Fasting blood glucose levels then become progressively higher at each 6-month interval leading up to diagnosis. Building on these findings, researchers developed a risk model indicating that patients with diabetes and advanced age with escalating blood glucose levels and weight loss are at significant risk of PDAC in the next 3 years.[53]

Researchers have attempted to link PDAC cachexia with new-onset PDAC-associated diabetes, given that both clinical scenarios commonly result in significant weight loss. A large observational study of patients with PDAC found no statistically significant difference in rates of cachexia between patients with diabetes and those without diabetes.[54] Skeletal muscle mass was also similar in patients with and without diabetes. Furthermore, in the nearly 60% of patients in the cachexia cohort, those with diabetes did not exhibit significantly more weight or muscle loss than those without diabetes. Examining metabolic changes before PDAC diagnosis remains an evolving field, and researchers hope to integrate these data to develop more specific guidelines for screening high-risk populations.

ASSESSMENT AND MANAGEMENT CONSIDERATIONS FOR PANCREATIC DUCTAL ADENOCARCINOMA CACHEXIA
Early Recognition

The international consensus definition of cachexia described a spectrum of precachexia, cachexia, and refractory cachexia.[4] Unfortunately, many clinicians still consider cachexia only in end-stage patients with severe emaciation and malnutrition when cachexia-focused interventions have little impact.[4] This late identification complicates the education of patients and caregivers, because it lacks a modern view of the early signs and symptoms of cachexia, including anorexia, poorly controlled symptoms, fatigue, and weight loss of any degree. Consequently, clinicians, patients, and caregivers must be educated about these early signs of cachexia to allow for early intervention.[55]

The authors recommend routine collection of patient-reported outcomes (PROs) to capture these early changes, starting at diagnosis. Systematic PRO collection ensures that these symptoms are reviewed in real time and trigger a clinical response.[56] Clinicians can use validated PROs, including a general and disease-specific validated questionnaire (eg, Functional Assessment of Cancer Therapy-General [FACT-G][57] and FACT-Hepatobiliary [FACT-Hep]) and align these PROs with other clinical and research priorities.[58] Clinicians can also ask registered dietitians what screening tools they use (eg, Patient-Generated Subjective Global Assessment Short-Form,[59] Mini Nutrition Assessment Short-Form [MNA][60]) and use these tools to capture nutrition-related data at predefined intervals. Optimal treatment of cancer cachexia requires team members from various specialties, several of which are understaffed in many cancer centers. Routine PRO collection may identify those patients in the greatest need of these limited resources.

Symptom Management

Before improving a patient's appetite and food intake, clinicians must treat any reversible symptoms (eg, pancreatic insufficiency, nausea, pain, diarrhea, or constipation). When symptoms are chronic, complex, or deteriorating, seek consultation from symptom experts such as palliative care specialists. Moreover, in the authors' clinical experience, patients may underreport their symptom burden directly to their treating oncologist, fearing that cancer treatment may be reduced, delayed, or stopped. Routinely integrating palliative care in managing patients with advanced cancer is evidence based and may provide a space where patients feel more comfortable reporting the severity of their symptoms.[61]

Anorexia and Weight Loss

Patients and caregivers frequently request drugs targeting cancer cachexia-related symptoms, including poor appetite and weight loss. Overall, evidence is insufficient to endorse any pharmacologic intervention to improve cancer cachexia outcomes.[62] In fact, there is no US Food and Drug Administration-approved medication to treat cancer cachexia. Off-label agents clinicians prescribe most frequently to target appetite and weight loss include dexamethasone, megestrol acetate, and cannabinoids (dronabinol and medicinal cannabis). Although these agents can improve appetite and weight,[63–65] they also have associated adverse effects that clinicians should carefully consider. For example, corticosteroids have many well-established adverse effects, including insomnia, impaired wound healing, immunosuppression, hyperglycemia, and insulin resistance, which is especially problematic in patients with PDAC and diabetes. If clinicians consider using corticosteroids, the authors recommend using them for short 3- to 5-day intervals to maximize benefits and minimize risks. Alternatively, megestrol acetate may increase weight and appetite, but it also increases the risk of thromboembolic events, edema, adrenal suppression, and death.[66] Cannabinoids may worsen fatigue, confusion, dizziness, and falls,[67] especially in the many patients with PDAC who are chronically ill, frail, or elderly.

The ROMANA studies evaluated anamorelin (a selective oral ghrelin analog) to treat cancer cachexia in patients with non-small cell lung cancer (NSCLC) and weight loss.[68] In more than 900 patients, anamorelin increased lean body mass (LBM) compared with placebo, but it did not improve handgrip strength, the coprimary endpoint with LBM. Therefore, anamorelin did not receive approval in the United States or Europe. In contrast, anamorelin received regulatory approval in Japan after investigators found that anamorelin improved LBM compared with placebo in advanced NSCLC and in a single-arm trial in patients with gastrointestinal (colorectal, gastric, or pancreatic) cancers.[69,70]

Fatigue and Exercise

As described previously, fatigue is a highly prevalent symptom in patients with cancer cachexia that does not respond to increased rest. Cancer-related fatigue results in decreased physical activity or mental capacity and has been reported in up to 80% of patients receiving chemotherapy and radiotherapy.[71] The causes of cancer-related fatigue are multifactorial, and an in-depth assessment should first focus on identifying possible reversible underlying causes (eg, hypothyroidism or anemia). Patients and caregivers frequently request medications to alleviate fatigue; however, aside from short courses of corticosteroids,[72] no drug has shown improved outcomes over placebo, exercise, and/or psychological interventions.[73] Exercise is safe and feasible in patients with PDAC and cachexia.[74] Current exercise prescription guidelines focus broadly on initiating and maintaining an exercise program consisting of cardiovascular endurance and resistance training.[49] Therefore, the authors recommend referring patients to physical therapy and cancer-specific exercise programs to tailor programs to their needs if available.

Nutritional Counseling and Malabsorption

Evidence indicates that early referrals to registered dietitians who prescribe individualized nutrition plans for patients with advanced cancer reduce weight loss and mortality while improving function and quality of life.[75,76] However, clinicians often refer patients with cachexia late, after they have experienced severe anorexia, greater than 10% weight loss, and multiple poorly controlled symptoms.[77] Late referrals and underuse of dietitian expertise may be due to limited access. Most settings currently have 1 dietitian for every 2300 patients or more, despite evidence suggesting a ratio of 1:120 or less improves nutritional outcomes.[78] Therefore, oncologists must advocate for self-sustaining business models to ensure consistent access to dietitians, including telemedicine-based models of care delivery.[79]

Pancreatic exocrine insufficiency, noted previously as frequent in PDAC, is characterized by vague abdominal pain, increased gas, and steatorrhea. In the proximal small intestine, exogenous pancreatic enzymes can replace the physiologic digestive secreted by the pancreas, catalyzing the hydrolysis of fats to monoglycerol and fatty acids, protein into peptides and amino acids, and starch into dextrans and short-chain sugars. Pancreatic enzymes should be taken with the first bite of food and are typically initiated at doses of 500 lipase units per kilogram of body weight per meal and gradually increased based on clinical symptoms, degree of steatorrhea, and fat content of the diet.[80]

Ongoing Interventional Trial Research

Cancer cachexia remains a critical area of ongoing research, including pharmacologic and multimodal interventions. Most recently, growth differentiation factor-15 has been widely explored as a biomarker of cancer growth and cachexia and a therapeutic target at the glial cell-derived neurotrophic factor family receptor alpha-like in the brainstem, including in pancreatic cancer.[81] Additional pharmacologic interventions under early-phase investigation include Janus kinase inhibitors,[82] selective beta-blockers,[83] and melanocortin-4 receptor antagonists.[84] Furthermore, given the multifactorial nature of cancer cachexia, multimodal interventions combining nutrition and exercise are also underway.[85,86] The authors eagerly look forward to their results and anticipate ongoing investigations in the pathophysiology of cancer cachexia, and, with optimism, expect these efforts to lead to more successful interventions.

SUMMARY

Patients with PDAC often suffer from cancer cachexia, a loss of weight and muscle mass with or without fat loss, which results in reduced physical function, chemotherapy toxicity, impaired quality of life, and poorer survival. Patients with PDAC are particularly at risk for cachexia because of reduced oral intake caused by mechanical obstruction by a tumor or surgical intervention, pancreatic insufficiency, and a heightened proinflammatory state. Prompt recognition and intervention are critical; mitigating weight and muscle mass changes may improve cancer-related outcomes. Incipient PDAC-induced metabolic changes that trigger cachexia and PDAC-associated DM likely occur years before clinical detection of PDAC; research in these 2 areas could lead to improved screening and early detection strategies. As further development of pharmacologic therapies targeting its underlying biology is awaited, cachexia treatment should include comprehensive symptom-based multidisciplinary care.

CLINICS CARE POINTS

- Early dietician referral for those with cachexia reduces weight loss, and weight stabilization is associated with improved mortality in advanced PDAC.

- Pancreatic insufficiency is a driver of cachexia and is common in PDAC; clinical assessment for pancreatic insufficiency in PDAC should be universal and, if diagnosed, should be promptly addressed with pancreatic enzymes.
- Evidence supports exercise as a better treatment for cancer-related fatigue compared with pharmacologic agents. Exercise is safe and feasible in PDAC.

DISCLOSURE

R.F. Dunne has served on recent advisory boards for Helsinn Healthcare S.A. and Exelixis, Inc. E.J. Roeland has served as a consultant for Asahi Kasei Pharmaceuticals, DRG Consulting, Napo Pharmaceuticals, and American Imaging Management. Additionally, he has served on recent advisory boards for Heron Pharmaceuticals, Pfizer, Vector Oncology, and Helsinn Pharmaceuticals. He has also served as a member on data safety monitoring boards for Oragenics, Inc., Galera Pharmaceuticals, and Enzychem Lifesciences Pharmaceutical Company.

REFERENCES

1. Rahib L, Smith BD, Aizenberg R, et al. Projecting cancer incidence and deaths to 2030: the unexpected burden of thyroid, liver, and pancreas cancers in the United States. Cancer Res 2014;74(11):2913–21.
2. Park W, Chawla A, O'Reilly EM. Pancreatic cancer: a review. JAMA 2021;326(9): 851–62.
3. Bachmann J, Heiligensetzer M, Krakowski-Roosen H, et al. Cachexia worsens prognosis in patients with resectable pancreatic cancer. J Gastrointest Surg 2008;12(7):1193–201.
4. Fearon K, Strasser F, Anker SD, et al. Definition and classification of cancer cachexia: an international consensus. Lancet Oncol 2011;12(5):489–95.
5. Stewart GD, Skipworth RJ, Fearon KC. Cancer cachexia and fatigue. Clin Med (Lond) 2006;6(2):140–3.
6. Mintziras I, Miligkos M, Wachter S, et al. Sarcopenia and sarcopenic obesity are significantly associated with poorer overall survival in patients with pancreatic cancer: systematic review and meta-analysis. Int J Surg 2018;59:19–26.
7. Davidson W, Ash S, Capra S, et al. Weight stabilisation is associated with improved survival duration and quality of life in unresectable pancreatic cancer. Clin Nutr 2004;23(2):239–47.
8. Bachmann J, Ketterer K, Marsch C, et al. Pancreatic cancer related cachexia: influence on metabolism and correlation to weight loss and pulmonary function. BMC Cancer 2009;9:255.
9. Dunne RF, Loh KP, Williams GR, et al. Cachexia and sarcopenia in older adults with cancer: a comprehensive review. Cancers (Basel) 2019;11(12):1861.
10. Baracos VE, Martin L, Korc M, et al. Cancer-associated cachexia. Nat Rev Dis Primers 2018;4:17105.
11. Mayers JR, Wu C, Clish CB, et al. Elevation of circulating branched-chain amino acids is an early event in human pancreatic adenocarcinoma development. Nat Med 2014;20(10):1193–8.
12. Danai LV, Babic A, Rosenthal MH, et al. Altered exocrine function can drive adipose wasting in early pancreatic cancer. Nature 2018;558(7711):600–4.

13. Burfeind KG, Michaelis KA, Marks DL. The central role of hypothalamic inflammation in the acute illness response and cachexia. Semin Cell Dev Biol 2016;54: 42–52.

14. Burfeind KG, Zhu X, Norgard MA, et al. Microglia in the hypothalamus respond to tumor-derived factors and are protective against cachexia during pancreatic cancer. Glia 2020;68(7):1479–94.

15. Labori KJ, Hjermstad MJ, Wester T, et al. Symptom profiles and palliative care in advanced pancreatic cancer: a prospective study. Support Care Cancer 2006; 14(11):1126–33.

16. Barber MD, Ross JA, Voss AC, et al. The effect of an oral nutritional supplement enriched with fish oil on weight-loss in patients with pancreatic cancer. Br J Cancer 1999;81(1):80–6.

17. Moses AW, Slater C, Preston T, et al. Reduced total energy expenditure and physical activity in cachectic patients with pancreatic cancer can be modulated by an energy and protein dense oral supplement enriched with n-3 fatty acids. Br J Cancer 2004;90(5):996–1002.

18. Bye A, Jordhoy MS, Skjegstad G, et al. Symptoms in advanced pancreatic cancer are of importance for energy intake. Support Care Cancer 2013;21(1):219–27.

19. Fogelman DR, Morris J, Xiao L, et al. A predictive model of inflammatory markers and patient-reported symptoms for cachexia in newly diagnosed pancreatic cancer patients. Support Care Cancer 2017;25(6):1809–17.

20. Vujasinovic M, Valente R, Del Chiaro M, et al. Pancreatic exocrine insufficiency in pancreatic cancer. Nutrients 2017;9(3):183.

21. Carey S, Laws R, Ferrie S, et al. Struggling with food and eating-life after major upper gastrointestinal surgery. Support Care Cancer 2013;21(10):2749–57.

22. Gustavell T, Sundberg K, Frank C, et al. Symptoms and self-care following pancreaticoduodenectomy: Perspectives from patients and healthcare professionals - Foundation for an interactive ICT application. Eur J Oncol Nurs 2017;26:36–41.

23. Hendifar AE, Petzel MQB, Zimmers TA, et al. Pancreas cancer-associated weight loss. Oncologist 2019;24(5):691–701.

24. van Seventer EE, Fintelmann FJ, Roeland EJ, et al. Leveraging the potential synergy between patient-reported outcomes and body composition analysis in patients with cancer. Oncologist 2020;25(4):271–3.

25. Shen W, Punyanitya M, Wang Z, et al. Total body skeletal muscle and adipose tissue volumes: estimation from a single abdominal cross-sectional image. J Appl Physiol (1985) 2004;97(6):2333–8.

26. Williams GR, Dunne RF, Giri S, et al. Sarcopenia in the older adult with cancer. J Clin Oncol 2021;39(19):2068–78.

27. Pierobon ES, Moletta L, Zampieri S, et al. The prognostic value of low muscle mass in pancreatic cancer patients: a systematic review and meta-analysis. J Clin Med 2021;10(14):3033.

28. Pecorelli N, Carrara G, De Cobelli F, et al. Effect of sarcopenia and visceral obesity on mortality and pancreatic fistula following pancreatic cancer surgery. Br J Surg 2016;103(4):434–42.

29. Di Sebastiano KM, Yang L, Zbuk K, et al. Accelerated muscle and adipose tissue loss may predict survival in pancreatic cancer patients: the relationship with diabetes and anaemia. Br J Nutr 2013;109(2):302–12.

30. Sandini M, Bernasconi DP, Fior D, et al. A high visceral adipose tissue-to-skeletal muscle ratio as a determinant of major complications after pancreatoduodenectomy for cancer. Nutrition 2016;32(11–12):1231–7.

31. Ryu Y, Shin SH, Kim JH, et al. The effects of sarcopenia and sarcopenic obesity after pancreaticoduodenectomy in patients with pancreatic head cancer. HPB (Oxford) 2020;22(12):1782–92.
32. Tilg H, Moschen AR. Adipocytokines: mediators linking adipose tissue, inflammation and immunity. Nat Rev Immunol 2006;6(10):772–83.
33. Bundred JR, Kamarajah SK, Hammond JS, et al. Prehabilitation prior to surgery for pancreatic cancer: a systematic review. Pancreatology 2020;20(6):1243–50.
34. Rollins KE, Tewari N, Ackner A, et al. The impact of sarcopenia and myosteatosis on outcomes of unresectable pancreatic cancer or distal cholangiocarcinoma. Clin Nutr 2016;35(5):1103–9.
35. Choi Y, Oh DY, Kim TY, et al. Skeletal muscle depletion predicts the prognosis of patients with advanced pancreatic cancer undergoing palliative chemotherapy, independent of body mass index. PLoS One 2015;10(10):e0139749.
36. Emori T, Itonaga M, Ashida R, et al. Impact of sarcopenia on prediction of progression-free survival and overall survival of patients with pancreatic ductal adenocarcinoma receiving first-line gemcitabine and nab-paclitaxel chemotherapy. Pancreatology 2022;22(2):277–85.
37. Gilliam LA, St Clair DK. Chemotherapy-induced weakness and fatigue in skeletal muscle: the role of oxidative stress. Antioxid Redox Signal 2011;15(9):2543–63.
38. Babic A, Rosenthal MH, Bamlet WR, et al. Postdiagnosis loss of skeletal muscle, but not adipose tissue, is associated with shorter survival of patients with advanced pancreatic cancer. Cancer Epidemiol Biomarkers Prev 2019;28(12):2062–9.
39. Tan BH, Birdsell LA, Martin L, et al. Sarcopenia in an overweight or obese patient is an adverse prognostic factor in pancreatic cancer. Clin Cancer Res 2009;15(22):6973–9.
40. Prado CM, Baracos VE, McCargar LJ, et al. Sarcopenia as a determinant of chemotherapy toxicity and time to tumor progression in metastatic breast cancer patients receiving capecitabine treatment. Clin Cancer Res 2009;15(8):2920–6.
41. Kurita Y, Kobayashi N, Tokuhisa M, et al. Sarcopenia is a reliable prognostic factor in patients with advanced pancreatic cancer receiving FOLFIRINOX chemotherapy. Pancreatology 2019;19(1):127–35.
42. Prado CM, Lieffers JR, McCargar LJ, et al. Prevalence and clinical implications of sarcopenic obesity in patients with solid tumours of the respiratory and gastrointestinal tracts: a population-based study. Lancet Oncol 2008;9(7):629–35.
43. Dodds RM, Murray JC, Granic A, et al. Prevalence and factors associated with poor performance in the 5-chair stand test: findings from the Cognitive Function and Ageing Study II and proposed Newcastle protocol for use in the assessment of sarcopenia. J Cachexia Sarcopenia Muscle 2021;12(2):308–18.
44. Stolzenberg-Solomon RZ, Schairer C, Moore S, et al. Lifetime adiposity and risk of pancreatic cancer in the NIH-AARP Diet and Health Study cohort. Am J Clin Nutr 2013;98(4):1057–65.
45. Everhart J, Wright D. Diabetes mellitus as a risk factor for pancreatic cancer. A meta-analysis. JAMA 1995;273(20):1605–9.
46. Stolzenberg-Solomon RZ, Graubard BI, Chari S, et al. Insulin, glucose, insulin resistance, and pancreatic cancer in male smokers. JAMA 2005;294(22):2872–8.
47. Park J, Morley TS, Kim M, et al. Obesity and cancer–mechanisms underlying tumour progression and recurrence. Nat Rev Endocrinol 2014;10(8):455–65.
48. Abbruzzese JL, Andersen DK, Borrebaeck CAK, et al. The interface of pancreatic cancer with diabetes, obesity, and inflammation: research gaps and

opportunities: summary of a National Institute of Diabetes and Digestive and Kidney Diseases Workshop. Pancreas 2018;47(5):516–25.

49. Network NCC. NCCN Clinical Practice Guidelines in Oncology (NCCN Guidelines): cancer-related fatigue. Available at: https://www.nccn.org/professionals/physician_gls/pdf/fatigue.pdf. Accessed February 15, 2022.

50. Chari ST, Leibson CL, Rabe KG, et al. Probability of pancreatic cancer following diabetes: a population-based study. Gastroenterology 2005;129(2):504–11.

51. Pannala R, Leirness JB, Bamlet WR, et al. Prevalence and clinical profile of pancreatic cancer-associated diabetes mellitus. Gastroenterology 2008;134(4):981–7.

52. Chari ST, Leibson CL, Rabe KG, et al. Pancreatic cancer-associated diabetes mellitus: prevalence and temporal association with diagnosis of cancer. Gastroenterology 2008;134(1):95–101.

53. Sharma A, Kandlakunta H, Nagpal SJS, et al. Model to determine risk of pancreatic cancer in patients with new-onset diabetes. Gastroenterology 2018;155(3):730–9.e3.

54. Liao WC, Chen PR, Huang CC, et al. Relationship between pancreatic cancer-associated diabetes and cachexia. J Cachexia Sarcopenia Muscle 2020;11(4):899–908.

55. Garcia JM, Dunne RF, Santiago K, et al. Addressing unmet needs for people with cancer cachexia: recommendations from a multistakeholder workshop. J Cachexia Sarcopenia Muscle 2022;13(2):1418–25.

56. Basch E, Deal AM, Kris MG, et al. Symptom monitoring with patient-reported outcomes during routine cancer treatment: a randomized controlled trial. J Clin Oncol 2016;34(6):557–65.

57. Cella DF, Tulsky DS, Gray G, et al. The functional assessment of cancer therapy scale: development and validation of the general measure 1993;11(3):570–9.

58. Cella D, Butt Z, Kindler HL, et al. Validity of the FACT Hepatobiliary (FACT-Hep) questionnaire for assessing disease-related symptoms and health-related quality of life in patients with metastatic pancreatic cancer. Qual Life Res 2013;22(5):1105–12.

59. Abbott J, Teleni L, McKavanagh D, et al. Patient-Generated Subjective Global Assessment Short Form (PG-SGA SF) is a valid screening tool in chemotherapy outpatients. Support Care Cancer 2016;24(9):3883–7.

60. Kaiser MJ, Bauer JM, Ramsch C, et al. Validation of the Mini Nutritional Assessment Short-Form (MNA®-SF): a practical tool for identification of nutritional status. J Nutr Health Aging 2009;13(9):782–8.

61. Ferrell BR, Temel JS, Temin S, et al. Integration of palliative care into standard oncology care: American Society of Clinical Oncology Clinical Practice Guideline Update. J Clin Oncol 2016;35(1):96–112.

62. Roeland EJ, Bohlke K, Baracos VE, et al. Management of cancer cachexia: ASCO Guideline. J Clin Oncol 2020;38(21):2438–53.

63. Yavuzsen T, Davis MP, Walsh D, et al. Systematic review of the treatment of cancer-associated anorexia and weight loss. J Clin Oncol 2005;23(33):8500–11.

64. Loprinzi CL, Michalak JC, Schaid DJ, et al. Phase III evaluation of four doses of megestrol acetate as therapy for patients with cancer anorexia and/or cachexia. J Clin Oncol 1993;11(4):762–7.

65. Jatoi A, Windschitl HE, Loprinzi CL, et al. Dronabinol versus megestrol acetate versus combination therapy for cancer-associated anorexia: a North Central Cancer Treatment Group study. J Clin Oncol 2002;20(2):567–73.

66. Ruiz-García V, López-Briz E, Carbonell-Sanchis R, et al. Megestrol acetate for cachexia-anorexia syndrome. A systematic review. J Cachexia Sarcopenia Muscle 2018;9(3):444–452..

67. Dronabinol US Food and Drug Administration. Available at: https://www.accessdata.fda.gov/drugsatfda_docs/label/2017/018651s029lbl.pdf. Accessed February 21, 2022.

68. Temel JS, Abernethy AP, Currow DC, et al. Anamorelin in patients with non-small-cell lung cancer and cachexia (ROMANA 1 and ROMANA 2): results from two randomised, double-blind, phase 3 trials. Lancet Oncol 2016;17(4):519–31.

69. Katakami N, Uchino J, Yokoyama T, et al. Anamorelin (ONO-7643) for the treatment of patients with non-small cell lung cancer and cachexia: Results from a randomized, double-blind, placebo-controlled, multicenter study of Japanese patients (ONO-7643-04). Cancer 2018;124(3):606–16.

70. Hamauchi S, Furuse J, Takano T, et al. A multicenter, open-label, single-arm study of anamorelin (ONO-7643) in advanced gastrointestinal cancer patients with cancer cachexia. Cancer 2019;125(23):4294–302.

71. Henry DH, Viswanathan HN, Elkin EP, et al. Symptoms and treatment burden associated with cancer treatment: results from a cross-sectional national survey in the US. Support Care Cancer 2008;16(7):791–801.

72. Yennurajalingam S, Frisbee-Hume S, Palmer JL, et al. Reduction of cancer-related fatigue with dexamethasone: a double-blind, randomized, placebo-controlled trial in patients with advanced cancer. J Clin Oncol 2013;31(25):3076–82.

73. Mustian KM, Alfano CM, Heckler C, et al. Comparison of pharmaceutical, psychological, and exercise treatments for cancer-related fatigue: a meta-analysis. JAMA Oncol 2017;3(7):961–8.

74. Solheim TS, Laird BJA, Balstad TR, et al. A randomized phase II feasibility trial of a multimodal intervention for the management of cachexia in lung and pancreatic cancer. J Cachexia Sarcopenia Muscle 2017;8(5):778–88.

75. Dijksterhuis WPM, Latenstein AEJ, van Kleef JJ, et al. Cachexia and dietetic interventions in patients with esophagogastric cancer: a multicenter cohort study. J Natl Compr Canc Netw 2021;19(2):144–52.

76. Bargetzi L, Brack C, Herrmann J, et al. Nutritional support during the hospital stay reduces mortality in patients with different types of cancers: secondary analysis of a prospective randomized trial. Ann Oncol 2021;32(8):1025–33.

77. Lorton CM, Griffin O, Higgins K, et al. Late referral of cancer patients with malnutrition to dietitians: a prospective study of clinical practice. Support Care Cancer 2020;28(5):2351–60.

78. Trujillo EB, Claghorn K, Dixon SW, et al. Inadequate nutrition coverage in outpatient cancer centers: results of a national survey. J Oncol 2019;2019:7462940.

79. Rozga M, Handu D, Kelley K, et al. Telehealth during the COVID-19 pandemic: a cross-sectional survey of registered dietitian nutritionists. J Acad Nutr Diet 2021;121(12):2524–35.

80. Trapnell BC, Maguiness K, Graff GR, et al. Efficacy and safety of Creon 24,000 in subjects with exocrine pancreatic insufficiency due to cystic fibrosis. J Cyst Fibros 2009;8(6):370–7.

81. Zhao Z, Zhang J, Yin L, et al. Upregulated GDF-15 expression facilitates pancreatic ductal adenocarcinoma progression through orphan receptor GFRAL. Aging (Albany NY) 2020;12(22):22564–81.

82. Hurwitz HI, Uppal N, Wagner SA, et al. Randomized, double-blind, phase II study of ruxolitinib or placebo in combination with capecitabine in patients with

metastatic pancreatic cancer for whom therapy with gemcitabine has failed. J Clin Oncol 2015;33(34):4039–47.

83. Lainscak M, Laviano A. ACT-ONE - ACTION at last on cancer cachexia by adapting a novel action beta-blocker. J Cachexia Sarcopenia Muscle 2016;7(4):400–2.

84. Olson B, Zhu X, Norgard MA, et al. Lipocalin 2 mediates appetite suppression during pancreatic cancer cachexia. Nat Commun 2021;12(1):2057.

85. Solheim TS, Laird BJ, Balstad TR, et al. Cancer cachexia: rationale for the MENAC (Multimodal—Exercise, Nutrition and Anti-inflammatory medication for Cachexia) trial. BMJ Support Palliat Care 2018;8(3):258–65.

86. Dunne RF, Mustian KM, Garcia JM, et al. Research priorities in cancer cachexia: the university of Rochester Cancer Center NCI Community Oncology Research Program (NCORP) research base symposium on cancer cachexia and sarcopenia. Curr Opin Support Palliat Care 2017;11(4):278.

What Can We Learn About Pancreatic Adenocarcinoma from Imaging?

Michael Rosenthal, MD, PhD[a,b,c],*, Khoschy Schawkat, MD, PhD[b,c],
Mayssan Muftah, MD[b,c], Kunal Jajoo, MD[b,c]

KEYWORDS

- Pancreas • Imaging • Staging • Resectability • CT • MRI • Endoscopy • EUS

KEY POINTS

- High-quality anatomic imaging is required for accurate staging and assessment of resectability in pancreatic ductal adenocarcinoma.
- Computed tomography (CT) and endoscopic ultrasound play important and complementary roles in the diagnosis and primary staging of pancreatic cancer.
- MRI and fluorodeoxyglucose-positron emission tomography-PET-CT are useful modalities for problem-solving in complex or atypical cases.

INTRODUCTION

Pancreatic ductal adenocarcinoma (PDAC), the most common histologic type of pancreatic cancer, is the third most common cause of cancer-related death in the United States.[1] Clinically, PDAC exhibits aggressive behavior and typically presents at a late stage of the disease because of vascular invasion, perineural spread, locoregional or distant metastasis, including liver, lung, and peritoneal metastases.[2] On imaging, PDAC typically manifests as a poorly defined, hypoenhancing mass causing ductal obstruction and vascular involvement. Accurate pretreatment staging based on imaging characteristics is of utmost importance to guide oncologic therapy and surgical approach. Additional findings at initial stagings, such as pulmonary embolism, indeterminate liver lesions, and lung nodules, may dictate additional interventions.

IMAGING

In patients with PDAC, the assessment of tumor resectability is based on locoregional tumor extension, N staging, and M staging and is necessary to determine the treatment plan and predict prognosis. Imaging modalities used to assess the pancreas

[a] Department of Imaging, Dana-Farber Cancer Institute, 450 Brookline Avenue, Boston, MA 02215, USA; [b] Brigham and Women's Hospital, 75 Francis Street, Boston, MA 02115, USA; [c] Harvard Medical School, Boston, MA
* Corresponding author.
E-mail address: Michael_Rosenthal@dfci.harvard.edu

Hematol Oncol Clin N Am 36 (2022) 911–928
https://doi.org/10.1016/j.hoc.2022.06.003
0889-8588/22/© 2022 Elsevier Inc. All rights reserved.

include endoscopic ultrasound (EUS), computed tomography (CT), and MRI.[3] They play complementary roles because of the different advantages of each imaging modality. These techniques are widely available and allow visualization of anatomy, alteration of the normal anatomy because of underlying disease, and, depending on the modality used, image-guided interventions.[3] Endoscopic retrograde cholangiopancreaticography (ERCP) simultaneously provides anatomic and structural information and allows for interventions, such as the placement of biliary stents and endoscopic biopsies.[3,4] PET/CT serves as a problem-solving tool to distinguish metabolically active sites of disease from benign tissue. The following sections will examine the roles and importance of each of these modalities for pancreatic cancer.

Computed Tomography

- Primary method of abdominal imaging based on wide availability and moderate costs
- Uses ionizing X-rays to create images of thin sections of the body
- Typically performed using intravenous iodinated contrast when assessing the pancreas
- Routine studies are performed with a single scan acquired in the portal venous phase, approximately 70 s after the start of contrast injection
- Specialized pancreatic cancer protocols may involve two or three scans following contrast injection:
  ○ Early arterial phase for assessment of arterial anatomy for surgery (25 s after injection; optional at some centers)
  ○ Late arterial/pancreatic parenchymal phase for detection of pancreatic lesions and venous anatomy (at 40–45 s)
  ○ Portal venous phase for assessment of regional and metastatic disease, particularly in the liver (at 70 s)
  ○ Enteric water is preferred over high-attenuation barium or iodinated contrast to minimize streak artifacts through the pancreas

Magnetic Resonance Imaging

- Uses a combination of strong magnetic fields and nonionizing radio waves to produce images of the body
- Problem-solving modality: can detect and characterize lesions that may be occult or indeterminate on other modalities
- Each MRI sequence exploits a different combination of physical characteristics to produce contrast between tissue types
- MRI of the pancreas is typically performed with intravenous gadolinium contrast
  ○ Negative oral contrast media such as water, milk, or pineapple juice can be used to improve visualization of the gastric and duodenal margins near the pancreas
- A typical MRI of the pancreas will include T2-weighted, heavily T2-weighted magnetic resonance cholangiopancreatography (MRCP), T1 precontrast, in- and out-of-phase imaging, multiphase postcontrast, and diffusion-weighted sequences in at least two planes
- Secretin injection can be used to augment ductal dilatation in MRCP when strictures or main duct communication are questioned[5]

Fluorodeoxyglucose-Positron Emission Tomography-Computed Tomography and Fluorodeoxyglucose-Positron Emission Tomography-Magnetic Resonance Imaging

- PET uses positron-emitting radiotracers to localize tissues of interest

- Fluorodeoxyglucose (FDG), an analog of glucose and a marker of energy metabolism, is the most used radiotracer
- Often coupled with low-dose CT for correction of attenuation within the body
- Highly sensitive to sites of disease throughout the body, and often used for systemic staging in cancer care
- Relatively high dose of ionizing radiation
- In the context of PDAC, FDG-PET is typically used to evaluate lesions that are indeterminate on primary modalities, including atypical liver findings and marginally enlarged lymph nodes
- The FDG avidity of PDAC is variable, so the uptake of the primary site should be considered when evaluating for other potential sites of disease
- Very high costs and relatively restricted availability

Ultrasound

- Uses high-frequency sound waves to image the structure of tissues of interest
- Often used to assess for biliary or gallbladder pathology during the initial evaluation of symptoms
- Transabdominal ultrasound of the pancreas can be limited by gastric and duodenal air
- Relatively low cost and accessible, but performance and interpretation highly depend on the skill of the sonographer and radiologist
- Low cost and wide availability

Endoscopic Imaging and Intervention

Endoscopic ultrasound

EUS is an imaging modality that uses an ultrasound transducer on the tip of an endoscope. High-resolution images of the pancreas can be obtained without the disrupting effects of fat or gas since the probe is placed in the gastrointestinal lumen. Placement at the gastroesophageal junction and in the stomach allows for a view of the pancreatic body and tail, whereas placement in the duodenum allows for examination of the pancreatic head.

There are two basic EUS endoscopes—radial and linear. Linear EUS provides images that are in the same plane as/parallel to the shaft of the endoscope. Radial EUS provides images that are perpendicular to the shaft of the endoscope. Linear EUS is preferred for the evaluation of the pancreas. It has a higher sensitivity for the identification of pancreatic lesions and allows for tissue sampling and therapeutic intervention, whereas radial EUS does not.[6]

EUS is often used in tandem with cross-sectional imaging for the evaluation of pancreatic lesions and PDAC. The sensitivity of EUS for PDAC is higher than that of CT and MRI and is estimated at 92% to 100%.[7] It can often identify lesions missed on cross-sectional imaging, usually those measuring 2 cm or less, and can evaluate equivocal lesions seen on CT or MRI. It also allows for locoregional staging, though studies suggest it performs similarly to CT. Reported accuracy of EUS is 63% to 94% for T staging and 44% to 82% for N staging. Lastly, EUS facilitates tissue sampling of pancreatic lesions, regional lymph nodes (celiac, para-aortic, retroduodenopancreatic, and superior mesenteric), and hepatic metastases.[8]

EUS fine-needle aspiration (EUS-FNA) and fine-needle biopsy (EUS-FNB) allow for tissue acquisition and pathology diagnosis of PDAC. EUS-FNA was previously the gold standard.[8] However, EUS-FNB has emerged as the new standard over the last decade. Sensitivity and specificity of EUS-FNA and EUS-FNB for PDAC are quoted more than 90%, with similar technical success rates. Rapid on-site evaluation

(ROSE) by a pathologist improves the diagnostic yield of EUS-FNA by 10% to 15%,[9,10] whereas EUS-FNB has high diagnostic accuracy (above 96%) independent of the use of ROSE.[11] Clinical trials comparing the two methods suggest superior diagnostic accuracy and sample adequacy of EUS-FNB.[11,12] However, this has not been demonstrated in crossover trials where patients undergo both EUS-FNA and FNB for pancreatic lesions.[13] Studies have also consistently shown that EUS-FNB requires fewer passes with shorter procedure time.[12,13] Additionally, there is a potential benefit to having a core tissue specimen rather than cytology as histologic architecture can be examined and additional immunohistochemistry testing and molecular analysis can be performed. This may have implications on PDAC treatment in the era of precision medicine and with the emergence of newer targeted therapies, though this has yet to be demonstrated in cohort studies and clinical trials. In patients that do not need histologic confirmation before surgery for resectable lesions, providers may consider deferring evaluation with EUS.[8]

In some instances, EUS can be used for fiducial placement for external radiation therapy (XRT)[14] and fine-needle tattooing to assist with the detection of pancreatic body and tail lesions during surgery,[15] particularly small lesions with close relation to vessels or the pancreatic duct.[16]

Disadvantages to the use of EUS are related to its invasive nature as patients must undergo a procedure with moderate sedation or anesthesia, though the procedure is safe and well tolerated. There is a similar rate of adverse events associated with EUS-FNA and FNB, and these include pain, bleeding, and pancreatitis (0.5%–2%). There is a theoretic risk of tumor seeding, but this is exceedingly rare, and data is limited to case reports.[8]

Endoscopic retrograde cholangiopancreatography

With the emergence of EUS, endoscopic retrograde cholangiopancreatography (ERCP) has a limited role in the evaluation of pancreatic lesions and PDAC. In select cases, brush cytology or biopsy of suspicious pancreatic duct strictures can be done in the setting of a nondiagnostic EUS-FNA. The sensitivity of brush cytology is estimated at 15% to 50% and biopsy at 33% to 50%.[8,17] There is otherwise no role for ERCP in the staging of PDAC with the use of cross-sectional imaging and EUS.

ERCP primarily serves a therapeutic role in managing complications associated with adenocarcinoma of the pancreatic head such as biliary obstruction. It has little to no role in the management of adenocarcinoma in the body or tail. When to proceed with ERCP for biliary obstruction depends on tumor resectability. For resectable disease, ERCP should be reserved for patients with severe pruritis, cholangitis, or that need neoadjuvant chemoradiation as associated adverse events can delay, complicate, or preclude the possibility of undergoing surgery. Even in the absence of an adverse event, studies suggest preoperative ERCP can increase the rate of postoperative complications after pancreaticoduodenectomy.[18,19]

GUIDELINES
National Comprehensive Cancer Network

The National Comprehensive Cancer Network (NCCN) guidelines for pancreatic adenocarcinoma provide a detailed clinical framework for diagnosis and management.[20] They assist in clinical decision-making but are not intended to replace good clinical judgment or individualized treatment. The diagnosis and assessment of resectability in PDAC should be defined in multidisciplinary consultation at high-volume centers with aid of appropriate imaging studies.

The degree of tumor-vascular contract as assessed on CT or MRI is the primary determinant of resectability of PDAC.[21] The NCCN criteria for imaging-based

Table 1
Criteria defining resectability status according to NCCN version 2.2018

Resectability Status	Arterial	Venous
Resectable	No tumor contact with: • Celiac axis (CA); • Superior mesenteric artery (SMA); • Common hepatic artery (CHA).	No tumor contact with: • Superior mesenteric vein (SMV); • Portal vein (PV); Or • $\leq 180°$ contact without vein irregularity
Borderline resectable	Head/uncinate process: • Contact with CHA without extension to CA or hepatic artery allowing for resection; • Contact with SMA of $\leq 180°$; • Contact with variant arterial anatomy (eg, accessory right hepatic artery, replaced right hepatic artery, replaced CHA). Body/tail: • Contact with CA of $\leq 180°$; • Contact with CA of $>180°$ without involvement of aorta or gastroduodenal artery.	• Contact with SMV or PV of $>180°$ • Contact of $\leq 180°$ with SMV or PV with contour irregularity or thrombosis • Contact with inferior vena cava (IVC).
Unresectable	Distant metastasis including non-regional lymph node involvement Head/uncinate process: • Contact with SMA or CA $>180°$ Body/tail: • Contact with SMA or CA $>180°$; • Aortic involvement	Head/uncinate process: • Unreconstructable SMV/PV because of tumor involvement or occlusion (tumor or bland thrombus); • Contract with most proximal draining jejunal branch into SMV Body/tail: • Unreconstructable SMV/PV because of tumor involvement or occlusion (tumor or bland thrombus)

resectability of PDAC classify the tumor in absence of metastatic disease as resectable, borderline resectable, or unresectable (**Table 1**). The classification depends on tumor location within the pancreas and vessel involvement (arterial and venous).

Society of Abdominal Radiology

A consensus statement of the Society of Abdominal Radiology and the American Pancreatic Association describes a standardized reporting template to improve decision-making process for the management of PDAC.[22] Multidetector CT angiography using a dedicated dual-phase pancreatic protocol is the preferred method for initial staging.[23,24]

APPROACH
Primary Diagnosis

Noninvasive imaging

Owing to its high spatial resolution and rapid acquisition, multidetector-row CT (MDCT) systems have become the primary modality in pancreatic imaging, particularly for tumor detection and initial staging, resectability assessment, assessment of patients with symptomatic pancreatitis, evaluation of posttreatment complications, and surveillance.[22,25]

The detection of PDAC, a typically hypoattenuating hypovascular lesion, relies primarily on the post-contrast enhancement difference of the lesion compared with the surrounding pancreatic parenchyma.[25]

Most clinical CT devices use a single X-ray source with a single energy spectrum for imaging. Some modern instruments may use two X-ray sources, a single variable energy source, or spectrum-splitting detectors to acquire additional spectral absorption information, which is commonly known as dual-energy CT (DECT). In DECT, low-energy monochromic images (50 kiloelectron volts (keV)) provide the highest contrast-to-noise ratio for pancreatic lesions and increase the sensitivity of CT for the detection of small and isoattenuating pancreatic cancer, which account for approximately 10% of pancreatic tumors.[26,27]

Sensitivity of CT for detecting liver metastasis is lower compared with MRI.[28] In addition, subcentimeter focal liver lesions are often too small to fully characterize on CT and are one of the major limitations for initial cancer staging using CT.

MRI has gained an increasing role in pancreatic imaging for the detection and characterization of pancreatic lesions. MRI has been shown to be equally sensitive and specific in the staging of PDAC compared with CT and can be used interchangeably.[22,29] Compared with CT, MRI has better contrast resolution and is superior for the detection of tumors with little or no visibility on CT and for detecting liver metastases.[30] However, it is not usually used as a primary imaging tool in most centers, because of costs and availability.[22] It is also used as a problem-solving modality for the characterization of indeterminate focal liver lesions initially detected on CT.[31] The advantage of MRI over other imaging modalities is its ability to acquire high-quality images in patients nearly independent of body habitus and without the use of ionizing radiation. In addition, it provides high contrast-resolution and the ability to noninvasively image the biliary and pancreatic duct system with heavily T2-weighted MRI known as MR cholangiopancreatography (MRCP).[32] MRCP is commonly accepted as an alternative for endoscopic cholangiopancreatography for diagnostic evaluation of pancreaticobiliary abnormalities.[28] Diffusion-weighted imaging (DWI) of the pancreas is frequently used to detect small pancreatic lesions, lymph nodes, and distant metastases (REF). Disadvantages of MRI include cost, longer examination time, respiratory motion artifacts, limited compatibility with older implanted devices, and limited availability of the MRI slots.

PET/CT and PET/MR have no established role in the primary staging of pancreatic cancer but may be used for problem-solving in selected cases. It can be used after dedicated CT with pancreatic protocol in high-risk patients (markedly elevated CA 19–9, large primary tumor or locoregional lymph nodes) to detect extrapancreatic extension and metastasis.

Endoscopy

Endoscopy plays a key role in the diagnosis of PDAC. Patients are typically referred for endoscopic evaluation upon identification of a suspicious pancreatic lesion on cross-sectional imaging to confirm the diagnosis of PDAC, stage disease, and/or provide therapeutic intervention.

In general, patients undergo EUS-FNB for tissue sampling and confirmation of a suspected PDAC diagnosis. In select cases of patients with upfront resectable disease, pathology diagnosis may not be needed before proceeding with surgery. If EUS-FNB of a lesion is non-diagnostic and suspicion for PDAC persists, a repeat EUS-FNB vs EUS-FNA should be performed. ERCP with brush cytology or biopsy of pancreatic duct strictures can be also considered if EUS sampling continues to be non-diagnostic.

In patients with concomitant biliary obstruction that necessitates ERCP, EUS and ERCP are done concurrently. EUS is typically performed first as stent placement to relieve the obstruction may affect staging and determining disease resectability before ERCP may change the type of biliary stent placed.

A normal pancreas has a typical homogenous "salt and pepper" appearance on EUS.[33] When evaluating a solid lesion, hypoechoic hypovascular lesions with irregular margins are seen with malignancy. When evaluating cystic lesions, size > 3 cm, main pancreatic duct dilation, and thickened septal walls are suggestive.[34] ERCP findings suggestive of pancreatic head malignancy include pancreatic duct and bile duct strictures with upstream dilation (also referred to as "double duct" sign).[8]

Initial Staging and Assessment of Resectability

High-quality dedicated pancreatic protocol imaging at presentation should be performed even if standard CT imaging is available and should be done before stenting. Imaging should be done at initial diagnosis before surgical or chemotherapy. A multidisciplinary team should be involved in decisions about resectability with reference to high-quality imaging studies including complete staging for evaluation of disease extent.[20]

Preoperative Therapeutic Response

Approximately 85% to 90% of patients present with a disease that is not immediately resectable and therefore qualify for neoadjuvant or palliative chemotherapy treatment.[35] The complex effects of treatment regimens are currently a major challenge for radiologists as the diagnostic performance of standard morphologic criteria proved to be insufficient. Numerous studies have shown that the performance of CT in predicting resectability may diminish after neoadjuvant therapy and often the radiologic response underestimates the histologic response.[30,36,37] If successful, preoperative neoadjuvant treatment eliminates cancer cells in PDAC. Dense fibrous tissue and occasionally newly induced additional fibrosis may remain present and can mimic a lack of response or progression. In addition, radiation therapy may induce local and regional edema, which may mistakenly be interpreted as progression and new vascular involvement.[30,38] There are several strategies to overcome this challenge, such as using tumor markers (CA 19–9) for monitoring disease progression and clinical evaluation in addition to radiologic assessment. Surgical assessment remains the only means of definite evaluation for resectability after neoadjuvant therapy. Recognition and appreciation of posttreatment imaging pitfalls are therefore crucial to provide proper re-staging. Recently, novel functional imaging tools and postprocessing techniques such as radiomic analysis have shown some promise as predictors of disease status, but more work is needed to establish their role in a clinical workflow.[39–41]

Postoperative Surveillance

Following PDAC resection, local recurrence and/or distant metastasis occur in up to 80% of cases, but the impact of follow-up and early detection is not well established.[42,43] There is controversy regarding postoperative surveillance as current recommendations are based on mostly expert opinions and low-level evidence.[44] Elevation of serum tumor markers, such as carbohydrate antigen (CA) 19 to 9 typically raise suspicion for recurrence which prompts imaging. CT is commonly favored; however, MRI and PET-CT can be used and are relevant in specific cases.[42] Unfortunately, imaging evaluation for local recurrence is challenging, especially differentiation of postoperative fibrosis from the recurrent tumor at resection site can be difficult. A literature review showed moderate diagnostic value for contrast-enhanced CT with a sensitivity of 70% and specificity of 80%.[42] The highest accuracy was found for FDG PET-CT combined with contrast-enhanced CT with a sensitivity of 95% and specificity of 81%.[25]

Imaging for Complications

Management of biliary obstruction

Symptomatic biliary obstruction is typically managed with ERCP and stent placement. Stent size and type—plastic vs. self-expanding metal stent (SEMS)—depends on cancer resectability, patient prognosis, and biliary anatomy at the time of ERCP.[8] When choosing stent size, resectability must be considered as longer stents may preclude the ability to perform pancreaticoduodenectomy later. Plastic stents are less expensive and easier to place, although these require more frequent exchanges. They occlude after 3 to 6 months of placement because of the deposition of bacterial biofilms, leading to recurrent jaundice and cholangitis.[8] Although more expensive, SEMS remain patent longer and thus may be more cost-effective and less burdensome on patients by reducing the need for repeat ERCP and stent exchange.[45] SEMS can be covered or uncovered. Both types of stents have similar rates of cholecystitis and pancreatitis. Uncovered stents run the risk of occlusion because of tumor ingrowth, whereas covered stents are at higher risk of migration, particularly in patients still receiving chemotherapy. Despite the trade off, the overall complication rates for uncovered and covered stents are comparable[46] and choice of stent should be tailored to each individual patient.

Generally, for resectable disease, short metal stents placed distally are the intervention of choice. This alleviates biliary obstruction, remains patent longer preventing the need for stent exchange while awaiting surgery, and does not interfere with surgery later. For unresectable disease, metal stents are used without plans for further ERCP, though for those with poor prognosis, a plastic stent may be used for technically challenging cases.

In cases where the biliary tree is inaccessible via ERCP (as is the case with malignant duodenal obstruction), other options for relief of biliary obstruction include EUS-guided drainage, percutaneous transhepatic cholangiography with stent placement, and surgery. EUS-guided drainage facilitates transmural access to the biliary tree and is achieved either by creating a fistula between the gastrointestinal lumen and bile ducts (eg, cholecystoduodenostomy or hepaticogastrostomy) or by facilitating antegrade or transpapillary stenting. EUS-guided gallbladder drainage can also be considered to decompress the biliary tree if the cystic duct is patent.[47]

Management of gastric outlet obstruction

Adenocarcinoma of the pancreatic head can lead to duodenal and gastric outlet obstruction (GOO) associated with nausea, vomiting, and inability to get nutrition by mouth. Management options include enteral stenting, EUS-guided gastroenterostomy (EUS-GE), surgical gastrojejunostomy, or placement of a venting gastrostomy tube.

Enteral stenting is usually done by placing an SEMS under endoscopic and fluoroscopic guidance across the obstructed part of the small bowel.[48] Technical success ranges from 75% to 100%, whereas clinical success (relief of symptoms and/or improvement of oral intake) ranges from 63% to 97%. Complications occur at a rate of 7% to 18% and include stent dysfunction or migration (early), stent occlusion because of tumor ingrowth or food (late), perforation, fistula formation, hemorrhage, fever, and severe pain.[49]

EUS-GE has recently emerged as an option for malignant GOO with availability limited to high-volume tertiary care centers. EUS in the stomach is used to identify and access a part of the small bowel distal to the obstruction. A stent is then deployed across, creating a gastroenterostomy and bypassing the obstructed small bowel.[50] Technical success is estimated at around 90%, and clinical success is 85% to 90%.[51] A recent meta-analysis has shown that EUS-GE has higher clinical success with a decreased rate of adverse events and need for reintervention compared with enteral stenting,[52] though complications rates are still estimated approximately 18%.

Choice of endoscopic intervention depends on cancer resectability and patient prognosis. For patients with potentially resectable cancer, consultation with the hepatobiliary surgeon should be done regarding the preferred method, though enteral stenting is usually favored.

For patients with unresectable cancer, choice of therapy depends on prognosis. For patients with a life expectancy of 6 months or less, either is a viable option. Procedural considerations include:

- Usually, the major papilla cannot be accessed after enteral stenting. When the gastroduodenal obstruction is present while biliary obstruction is suspected or impending, metal biliary stent placement should be done before gastroduodenal stent placement.
- EUS-GE can manage more extensive or distal obstructions (that can be seen with peritoneal disease) that enteral stenting cannot.

For patients with a life expectancy greater than 6 months, EUS-GE is preferred as it is more durable. In patients that have already received treatment with chemotherapy, EUS-GE has similar clinical success to surgical gastrojejunostomy with shorter hospital length of stay and recovery.[51,52] For patients that are treatment naïve, there is controversy as to whether EUS-GE is equivalent to surgical gastrojejunostomy, and selection of patients for this procedure should be done on a case-by-case basis.

Diagnostic Dilemmas

Benign mimic of pancreatic ductal adenocarcinoma: autoimmune pancreatitis
Autoimmune pancreatitis is a rare fibroinflammatory form of chronic pancreatitis that may present with painless jaundice and a focal lesion in the pancreatic head, mimicking PDAC.[53,54] In most cases of AIP, histologic evaluation should be done to confirm the diagnosis and rule out malignancy, as distinguishing the two diagnoses can be difficult using clinical, imaging, and laboratory findings alone. The clinical presentation of AIP is like PDAC as it includes painless jaundice, weight loss, steatorrhea, and abdominal pain. There is a male predominance with most patients being over the age of 50 at diagnosis.[55]

Imaging findings that would be more typical of AIP include diffuse enlargement of the pancreas with a sausage-like appearance, presence of a hypoattenuating capsule rim, delayed parenchymal enhancement,[55] and penetrating duct sign (smooth narrowing of the pancreatic duct traversing a mass without abrupt obstruction).[56] However, there are focal mass-like presentations of AIP, which cannot be reliably distinguished from malignancy. Imaging findings that are suggestive of malignancy include pancreatic duct dilation (particularly if > 4 mm), double duct sign, hyperdense rim on non-contrast CT scan, hyperenhancement of the rim on CT portal venous phase, and persistent hypo-enhancement on delayed phase.[56]

Serologic markers such as IgG4 (twice the normal value is a diagnostic feature of type 1 AIP) and CA19 to 9 (can be elevated with PDAC) have been used to help differentiate the two; however, studies have shown more than 10% of patients with PDAC can have elevated IgG4 levels[54] and AIP can be associated with CA19 to 9 elevations. Other findings suggestive of AIP include concomitant manifestations of other IgG4-related disease (seen in 40%–50% of cases),[55] whereas the presence of metastases would only be seen with PDAC.

For patients with a strong suspicion for AIP, an empiric course of steroids can be trialed. Patients should respond to steroids within 2 to 4 weeks with complete resolution of symptoms and radiographic findings. A lack of response should raise concern for malignancy and warrant histologic evaluation.

Evaluation of potential metastases

Indeterminate lesions are frequently identified outside of the pancreas on initial staging studies and can warrant further evaluation to exclude metastatic disease. Benign liver lesions are present in at least 15% of patients, with the most common findings including focal fatty sparing, cysts, and hemangiomas.[57] In the National Lung Cancer Screening Trial, 28.7% of patients without cancer had a nodule at least 4 mm in size.[58] The high expected rate of benign observations can complicate the determination of metastasis staging with a high-risk disease like PDAC. F-18 FDG-PET-CT, liver MRI, and biopsy may be used for problem-solving in these situations. Lesions that are inaccessible for biopsy or are too small to further characterize with imaging may be observed.

Indeterminate liver lesions in PDAC include metastases, benign lesions like hemangiomas and cysts, infectious complications like cholangitic abscesses, and treatment-related complications like focal hepatopathy.[59] The diagnostic workflow for these lesions should be selected in consultation with a radiologist as part of a multidisciplinary care team in consideration of the radiologic appearance of the lesion and availability of prior imaging. This workflow often begins with a liver MRI with a standard extracellular contrast agent. These studies can definitively identify the most common benign lesions including hemangiomas, cysts, and focal fatty sparing. Lesions that may remain indeterminate after this phase include metastases, atypical hemangiomas, and cholangitic abscesses. Serum CA19 to 9, white blood cell count, and history of biliary obstruction and/or instrumentation should be considered in this circumstance, but biopsy is often necessary for definitive characterization.

Evaluation of local recurrence versus chronic inflammation after resection

There are little data to dictate the timing of postoperative surveillance imaging after PDAC resection, but empiric practice often includes CT imaging every 3 months for at least 2 years with subsequent widening of the scan intervals to 6 or 12 months. Margin-positive (R1 or R2) and node-positive resections carry an increased risk of local recurrence and may warrant more intensive surveillance. The purpose of surveillance in this setting is to optimize palliation rather than to attempt curative salvage interventions, which are generally not feasible in recurrent PDAC.

The detection of local recurrence requires differentiation of active tumor from postoperative scar, both of which have overlapping features on imaging. The acquisition of a postoperative baseline CT at 6 to 8 weeks after surgery can provide a useful upper limit for the extent of postoperative inflammation and scar. The development of a new

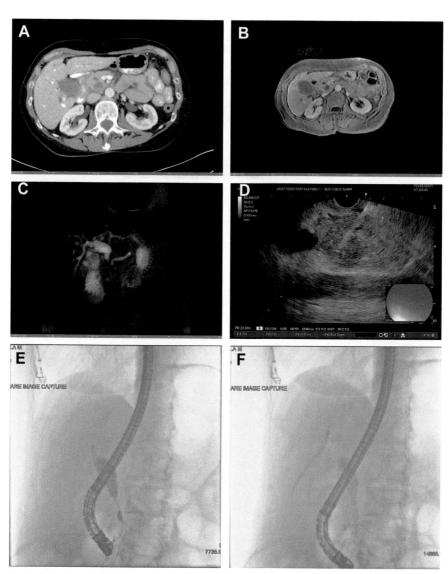

Fig. 1. (*A*) Late arterial phase CT of the pancreas shows a circumscribed hypodense mass in the pancreatic head. A rim of normal-appearing parenchyma remains present between the mass and the major vessels (SMA and SMV visible here). This lesion was staged as upfront resectable after a positive biopsy for PDAC. (*B*) Portal venous phase MRI with contrast also shows a well-circumscribed pancreatic head mass with a rim of preserved parenchyma separating the mass from the major vessels. (*C*) Coronal MRCP shows abrupt cutoffs of the common bile duct and pancreatic duct at the level of the pancreatic head mass, known as a "double duct" sign. (*D*) EUS image demonstrating hypoechoic mass in the head of the pancreas measuring 2.1 cm. A biopsy needle is visible as a bright linear structure extending into the mass. (*E*) ERCP demonstrating severe distal biliary stricture because of the pancreatic head mass and upstream common bile duct dilation (*F*) Placement of self-expanding metal stent for biliary decompression.

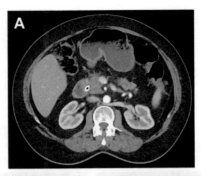

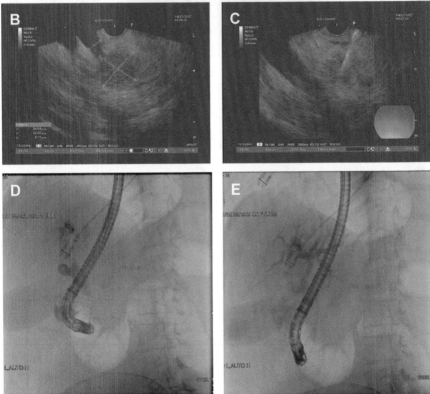

Fig. 2. (*A*) Late arterial phase CT of the pancreas shows an ill-defined hypoattenuating mass in the pancreatic head with extension to the right surface of the superior mesenteric vein. A metallic CBD stent is present. This lesion was staged as borderline resectable after a positive biopsy confirmed PDAC. (*B*) EUS demonstrating hypoechoic pancreatic head mass (2.0 cm × 2.5 cm) causing biliary obstruction with common bile duct dilation to 8.2 mm. (*C*) EUS guided FNBx of the hypoechoic mass. (*D*) ERCP demonstrating severe distal biliary stricture because of the pancreatic head mass and upstream diffuse biliary dilation and contrast filling a distended gall bladder. (*E*) Placement of self-expanding metal stent for biliary decompression.

or expanding area of soft tissue, particularly along an at-risk surgical margin, warrants careful evaluation for recurrence by a multidisciplinary care team. Serum CA19 to 9, patient symptoms, and, when feasible, percutaneous or EUS-guided biopsy may be useful in this workup.

Postsurgical anatomy can limit visualization and access to the pancreas for tissue sampling via EUS. This varies depending on the type of prior surgery a patient has undergone. In the case of PDAC, the most encountered scenario is sampling of recurrent lesions following pancreaticoduodenectomy. One study examined the performance of EUS in sampling a target pancreaticobiliary lesion and visualizing the pancreas. Technical success for EUS-guided tissue sampling for solid pancreatic lesions was 78.2% and for cystic lesions was 70.6%. For patients with prior pancreaticoduodenectomy, the pancreas was able to be visualized ~93% of the time. Visualization of the pancreatic head was limited in patients with prior total gastrectomy (6.7%), Billroth II (53.7%), Roux-en-Y gastric bypass (57.1%), and esophagectomy (72.2%). Visualization of the body and tail was more successful overall but was also limited in patients with prior total gastrectomy (71.4%) and esophagectomy (82.4%).[60]

Emerging Techniques

Emerging technique: endoscopic ultrasound elastography

EUS elastography (EUS-EG) couples EUS with strain elastography to provide real-time assessment of tissue elasticity at the time of EUS.[33] This can be particularly helpful in the assessment of suspicious lesions in patients with background chronic or autoimmune pancreatitis as standard EUS can have lower sensitivity (73.2%) and specificity (83.3%) in these cases, and EUS-FNA may have decreased sensitivity (54%–73%) as well because of associated sampling errors.[61] Unlike shear wave elastography, there is no numerical value associated with the elasticity assessment; rather it is done using a color map. Different colors represent levels of relative elasticity ranging from blue (hardest tissue) to green to yellow to red (softest tissue). PDAC appears as a heterogeneous blue on EUS-EG, whereas normal pancreas is a homogeneous green and inflammatory lesions are a heterogenous green.[62] EUS-EG is predominantly used in Europe with minimal use and availability in the United States as data on the benefits and cost-effectiveness of routine use for the evaluation of pancreatic lesions is limited. Limitations are associated with the subjective nature of elasticity assessments and variability in interpretation between endoscopists.

Emerging technique: contrast-enhanced endoscopic ultrasound

Contrast-enhanced EUS (CE-EUS) uses intravenous ultrasound contrast agents composed of microbubbles (2–5 μm) that allow for perfusion assessments without Doppler associated artifacts.[33] The small size of the contrast agent allows for the detection of slow flow and visualization of fine vessels.[62,63] This can allow for more accurate characterization of pancreatic lesions. Identification of hypo-enhancing, hypoechoic lesions has a sensitivity of 89% to 95% for PDAC. However, the presence of hyper-enhancing lesions essentially excludes the diagnosis.[63] The added assessment of lesion vascularity can help distinguish PDAC from neuroendocrine tumors (hypervascular with early arterial enhancement), lymphoma, autoimmune pancreatitis, and pseudo-papillary tumors. CE-EUS may also facilitate more targeted tissue sampling as necrotic parts of a lesion can be avoided when performing FNA.[62] Despite its perceived advantages, a recent randomized trial showed that the diagnostic sensitivity of CE-EUS is not superior to conventional EUS with tissue sampling.[64] Currently its use is limited to tertiary care centers for the evaluation of small indeterminate lesions.

Case Discussions

Case study 1—upfront resectable pancreatic ductal adenocarcinoma

This patient presented with a pancreatic head mass causing common bile duct obstruction. A pancreas protocol CT scan demonstrated a circumscribed 2 cm mass in the pancreatic head with an intact rim of normal pancreas between the mass and the major vessels (**Fig. 1**A). A subsequent MRI confirmed these findings (**Fig. 1**B) and also demonstrated the classic double-duct sign of a pancreatic head mass that obstructs the common bile duct (CBD) and pancreatic duct (**Fig. 1**C). EUS confirmed the presence of the mass and provided a diagnostic biopsy (**Fig. 1**D). Concurrent ERCP identified the CBD stricture and provided decompression via an SEMS (**Fig. 1**E, F). The case was subsequently referred for surgical resection.

Case study 2—borderline resectable pancreatic ductal adenocarcinoma
This patient presented with a pancreatic head mass causing common bile duct obstruction. A pancreas protocol CT scan demonstrated an ill-defined 2.5 cm mass in the pancreatic head with less than 180° of involvement of the superior mesenteric vein without stenosis (**Fig. 2**A). The other major vessels were not involved. EUS confirmed the presence of the mass and provided a diagnostic biopsy (**Fig. 2**B, C). ERCP had previously decompressed the CBD via placement of a metallic stent (**Fig. 2**D, E). A multidisciplinary tumor board recommended the patient for neoadjuvant chemotherapy based on the venous involvement to improve the likelihood of a margin-negative resection.

SUMMARY

PDAC is an aggressive and morbid disease that requires detailed assessments and timely interventions from the imaging members of a multidisciplinary care team. Although CT is the primary modality for detection, staging, and surveillance of PDAC, ERCP, and EUS serve an equally important role in diagnosis and in management of complications. The interpretation of these imaging studies to determine PDAC resectability and treatment pathways should be made as part of a multidisciplinary care discussion involving radiologists, gastroenterologists, surgeons, oncologists, and radiation oncologists.

CLINICS CARE POINTS

- Computed tomographic (CT) imaging with intravenous contrast using a pancreas-specific protocol is the primary modality for detection, staging, and surveillance of pancreatic ductal adenocarcinoma.

- Endoscopic ultrasound plays a complementary and vital role in the detection and characterization of pancreatic lesions and can provide minimally invasive diagnostic biopsies.

- Endoscopic retrograde cholangiopancreaticography can provide minimally invasive management of complications including decompression of biliary obstruction, acquisition of biliary brushings for occult disease, and stenting and bypass of small bowel and gastric obstruction.

- MRI and fluorodeoxyglucose-PET-CT are useful problem-solving tools that should be used in consideration of their strengths, limitations, and the clinical context of each case.

DISCLOSURE

M. Rosenthal receives research funding from the National Institutes of Health (U01 CA320272, U10 CA180821, and U01 CA200468), Stand Up to Cancer, Lustgarten Foundation, and the Hale Family Center for Pancreatic Cancer at Dana-Farber Cancer Institute.

REFERENCES

1. Siegel RL, Miller KD, Jemal A. Cancer Statistics. CA Cancer J Clin 2017; 67(1):7–30.
2. Chang ST, Jeffrey RB, Patel BN, et al. Preoperative Multidetector CT Diagnosis of Extrapancreatic Perineural or Duodenal Invasion Is Associated with Reduced Postoperative Survival after Pancreaticoduodenectomy for Pancreatic Adenocarcinoma: Preliminary Experience and Implications for Patient Care. Radiology 2016;281(3):816–25.
3. Dimastromatteo J, Brentnall T, Kelly KA. Imaging in pancreatic disease. Nat Rev Gastroenterol Hepatol 2017;14(2):97–109.
4. Cote GA, Smith J, Sherman S, et al. Technologies for imaging the normal and diseased pancreas. Gastroenterology 2013;144(6):1262–1271 e1.
5. Matos C, Metens T, Devière J, et al. Pancreatic duct: morphologic and functional evaluation with dynamic MR pancreatography after secretin stimulation. Radiology 1997;203(2):435–41.
6. Shin EJ, Topazian M, Goggins MG, et al. Linear-array EUS improves detection of pancreatic lesions in high-risk individuals: a randomized tandem study. Gastrointest Endosc 2015;82(5):812–8.
7. DeWitt J, Devereaux BM, Lehman GA, et al. Comparison of endoscopic ultrasound and computed tomography for the preoperative evaluation of pancreatic cancer: a systematic review. Clin Gastroenterol Hepatol 2006;4(6):717–25.
8. Committee ASoP, Eloubeidi MA, Decker GA, et al. The role of endoscopy in the evaluation and management of patients with solid pancreatic neoplasia. Gastrointest Endosc 2016;83(1):17–28.
9. Klapman JB, Logrono R, Dye CE, et al. Clinical impact of on-site cytopathology interpretation on endoscopic ultrasound-guided fine needle aspiration. Am J Gastroenterol 2003;98(6):1289–94.
10. Layfield LJ, Bentz JS, Gopez EV. Immediate on-site interpretation of fine-needle aspiration smears: a cost and compensation analysis. Cancer 2001;93(5): 319–22.
11. Crino SF, Di Mitri R, Nguyen NQ, et al. Endoscopic ultrasound-guided fine-needle biopsy with or without rapid on-site evaluation for diagnosis of solid pancreatic lesions: a randomized controlled non-inferiority trial. Gastroenterology 2021; 161(3):899–909 e5.
12. Li H, Li W, Zhou QY, et al. Fine needle biopsy is superior to fine needle aspiration in endoscopic ultrasound guided sampling of pancreatic masses: A meta-analysis of randomized controlled trials. Medicine (Baltimore) 2018;97(13):e0207.
13. Levine I, Trindade AJ. Endoscopic ultrasound fine needle aspiration vs fine needle biopsy for pancreatic masses, subepithelial lesions, and lymph nodes. World J Gastroenterol 2021;27(26):4194–207.
14. Luz LP, Al-Haddad MA, Sey MS, et al. Applications of endoscopic ultrasound in pancreatic cancer. World J Gastroenterol 2014;20(24):7808–18.
15. Lennon AM, Newman N, Makary MA, et al. EUS-guided tattooing before laparoscopic distal pancreatic resection (with video). Gastrointest Endosc 2010;72(5): 1089–94.
16. Rimbas M, Larghi A, Fusaroli P, et al. How to perform EUS-guided tattooing? Endosc Ultrasound 2020;9(5):291–7.
17. De Bellis M, Sherman S, Fogel EL, et al. Tissue sampling at ERCP in suspected malignant biliary strictures (Part 1). Gastrointest Endosc 2002;56(4):552–61.

18. van der Gaag NA, Rauws EA, van Eijck CH, et al. Preoperative biliary drainage for cancer of the head of the pancreas. N Engl J Med 2010;362(2):129–37.

19. Baron TH, Kozarek RA. Preoperative biliary stents in pancreatic cancer–proceed with caution. N Engl J Med 2010;362(2):170–2.

20. NCCN Guidelines, Pancreatic Adenocarcinoma. Version 2.2022.

21. Tempero MA, Malafa MP, Al-Hawary M, et al. Pancreatic Adenocarcinoma, Version 2.2017, NCCN Clinical Practice Guidelines in Oncology. J Natl Compr Canc Netw 2017;15(8):1028–61.

22. Al-Hawary MM, Francis IR, Chari ST, et al. Pancreatic ductal adenocarcinoma radiology reporting template: consensus statement of the society of abdominal radiology and the american pancreatic association. Gastroenterology 2014; 146(1):291–304 e1.

23. Tamm EP, Balachandran A, Bhosale PR, et al. Imaging of pancreatic adenocarcinoma: update on staging/resectability. Radiol Clin North Am 2012;50(3):407–28.

24. Sahani DV, Shah ZK, Catalano OA, et al. Radiology of pancreatic adenocarcinoma: current status of imaging. J Gastroenterol Hepatol 2008;23(1):23–33.

25. Almeida RR, Lo GC, Patino M, et al. Advances in Pancreatic CT Imaging. AJR Am J Roentgenol 2018;211(1):52–66.

26. Patel BN, Alexander L, Allen B, et al. Dual-energy CT workflow: multi-institutional consensus on standardization of abdominopelvic MDCT protocols. Abdom Radiol (Ny) 2017;42(3):676–87.

27. Agrawal MD, Pinho DF, Kulkarni NM, et al. Oncologic applications of dual-energy CT in the abdomen. Radiographics 2014;34(3):589–612.

28. Motosugi U, Ichikawa T, Morisaka H, et al. Detection of pancreatic carcinoma and liver metastases with gadoxetic acid-enhanced MR imaging: comparison with contrast-enhanced multi-detector row CT. Radiology 2011;260(2):446–53.

29. Bipat S, Phoa SS, van Delden OM, et al. Ultrasonography, computed tomography and magnetic resonance imaging for diagnosis and determining resectability of pancreatic adenocarcinoma: a meta-analysis. J Comput Assist Tomogr 2005; 29(4):438–45.

30. Zins M, Matos C, Cassinotto C. Pancreatic adenocarcinoma staging in the era of preoperative chemotherapy and radiation therapy. Radiology 2018;287(2): 374–90.

31. Hong SB, Choi SH, Kim KW, et al. Meta-analysis of MRI for the diagnosis of liver metastasis in patients with pancreatic adenocarcinoma. J Magn Reson Imaging 2020;51(6):1737–44.

32. Manfredi R, Pozzi Mucelli R. Secretin-enhanced MR Imaging of the Pancreas. Radiology 2016;279(1):29–43.

33. Kitano M, Yoshida T, Itonaga M, et al. Impact of endoscopic ultrasonography on diagnosis of pancreatic cancer. J Gastroenterol 2019;54(1):19–32.

34. Committee ASoP, Muthusamy VR, Chandrasekhara V, et al. The role of endoscopy in the diagnosis and treatment of cystic pancreatic neoplasms. Gastrointest Endosc 2016;84(1):1–9.

35. Hidalgo M. Pancreatic cancer. N Engl J Med 2010;362(17):1605–17.

36. Xia BT, Fu B, Wang J, et al. Does radiologic response correlate to pathologic response in patients undergoing neoadjuvant therapy for borderline resectable pancreatic malignancy? J Surg Oncol 2017;115(4):376–83.

37. Cassinotto C, Cortade J, Belleannee G, et al. An evaluation of the accuracy of CT when determining resectability of pancreatic head adenocarcinoma after neoadjuvant treatment. Eur J Radiol 2013;82(4):589–93.

38. Morgan DE, Waggoner CN, Canon CL, et al. Resectability of pancreatic adeno-carcinoma in patients with locally advanced disease downstaged by preoperative therapy: a challenge for MDCT. AJR Am J roentgenology 2010;194(3): 615–22.

39. Rigiroli F, Hoye J, Lerebours R, et al. CT radiomic features of superior mesenteric artery involvement in pancreatic ductal adenocarcinoma: a pilot study. Radiology 2021;301(3):610–22.

40. Chen X, Oshima K, Schott D, et al. Assessment of treatment response during chemoradiation therapy for pancreatic cancer based on quantitative radiomic analysis of daily CTs: An exploratory study. PLoS One 2017;12(6):e0178961.

41. Chakraborty J, Langdon-Embry L, Cunanan KM, et al. Preliminary study of tumor heterogeneity in imaging predicts two year survival in pancreatic cancer patients. PLoS One 2017;12(12):e0188022.

42. Daamen LA, Groot VP, Goense L, et al. The diagnostic performance of CT versus FDG PET-CT for the detection of recurrent pancreatic cancer: a systematic review and meta-analysis. Eur J Radiol 2018;106:128–36.

43. Groot VP, Rezaee N, Wu W, et al. Patterns, timing, and predictors of recurrence following pancreatectomy for pancreatic ductal adenocarcinoma. Ann Surg 2018;267(5):936–45.

44. Groot VP, Daamen LA, Hagendoorn J, et al. Current strategies for detection and treatment of recurrence of pancreatic ductal adenocarcinoma after resection: a nationwide survey. Pancreas 2017;46(9):e73–5.

45. Davids PH, Groen AK, Rauws EA, et al. Randomised trial of self-expanding metal stents versus polyethylene stents for distal malignant biliary obstruction. Lancet 1992;340(8834–8835):1488–92.

46. Nakai Y, Isayama H, Wang HP, et al. International consensus statements for endoscopic management of distal biliary stricture. J Gastroenterol Hepatol 2020;35(6): 967–79.

47. Isayama H, Nakai Y, Itoi T, et al. Clinical practice guidelines for safe performance of endoscopic ultrasound/ultrasonography-guided biliary drainage: 2018. J Hepatobiliary Pancreat Sci 2019;26(7):249–69.

48. Ge PS, Young JY, Dong W, et al. EUS-guided gastroenterostomy versus enteral stent placement for palliation of malignant gastric outlet obstruction. Surg Endosc 2019;33(10):3404–11.

49. Brimhall B, Adler DG. Enteral stents for malignant gastric outlet obstruction. Gastrointest Endosc Clin N Am 2011;21(3):389–403, vii-viii.

50. Committee ASoP, Jue TL, Storm AC, et al. ASGE guideline on the role of endoscopy in the management of benign and malignant gastroduodenal obstruction. Gastrointest Endosc 2021;93(2):309–322 e4.

51. Carbajo AY, Kahaleh M, Tyberg A. Clinical review of EUS-guided gastroenterostomy (EUS-GE). J Clin Gastroenterol 2020;54(1):1–7.

52. Boghossian MB, Funari MP, De Moura DTH, et al. EUS-guided gastroenterostomy versus duodenal stent placement and surgical gastrojejunostomy for the palliation of malignant gastric outlet obstruction: a systematic review and meta-analysis. Langenbecks Arch Surg 2021;406(6):1803–17.

53. Committee ASoP, Chandrasekhara V, Chathadi KV, et al. The role of endoscopy in benign pancreatic disease. Gastrointest Endosc 2015;82(2):203–14.

54. Dite P, Novotny I, Dvorackova J, et al. Pancreatic solid focal lesions: differential diagnosis between autoimmune pancreatitis and pancreatic cancer. Dig Dis 2019;37(5):416–21.

55. Raina A, Yadav D, Krasinskas AM, et al. Evaluation and management of autoimmune pancreatitis: experience at a large US center. Am J Gastroenterol 2009; 104(9):2295–306.
56. Schima W, Bohm G, Rosch CS, et al. Mass-forming pancreatitis versus pancreatic ductal adenocarcinoma: CT and MR imaging for differentiation. Cancer Imaging 2020;20(1):52.
57. Kaltenbach TE-M, Engler P, Kratzer W, et al. Prevalence of benign focal liver lesions: ultrasound investigation of 45,319 hospital patients. Abdom Radiol 2016; 41(1):25–32.
58. Pinsky PF, Gierada DS, Nath PH, et al. National lung screening trial: variability in nodule detection rates in chest CT studies. Radiology 2013;268(3):865–73.
59. Han NY, Park BJ, Sung DJ, et al. Chemotherapy-induced focal hepatopathy in patients with gastrointestinal malignancy: gadoxetic acid–enhanced and diffusion-weighted MR imaging with clinical-pathologic correlation. Radiology 2014;271(2):416–25.
60. Brozzi L, Petrone MC, Poley JW, et al. Outcomes of biliopancreatic EUS in patients with surgically altered upper gastrointestinal anatomy: a multicenter study. Endosc Int Open 2020;8(7):E869–76.
61. Mondal U, Henkes N, Patel S, et al. Endoscopic ultrasound elastography: current clinical use in pancreas. Pancreas 2016;45(7):929–33.
62. Zhang L, Sanagapalli S, Stoita A. Challenges in diagnosis of pancreatic cancer. World J Gastroenterol 2018;24(19):2047–60.
63. Kitano M, Sakamoto H, Kudo M. Contrast-enhanced endoscopic ultrasound. Dig Endosc 2014;26(Suppl 1):79–85.
64. Cho IR, Jeong SH, Kang H, et al. Comparison of contrast-enhanced versus conventional EUS-guided FNA/fine-needle biopsy in diagnosis of solid pancreatic lesions: a randomized controlled trial. Gastrointest Endosc 2021;94(2):303–10.

Screening and Surveillance for Pancreatic Adenocarcinoma in High-Risk Individuals

Arielle J. Labiner, MHS, Anne Aronson, MPH,
Aimee L. Lucas, MD, MS*

KEYWORDS

- High-risk • Familial pancreatic cancer • Pancreatic surveillance • Cancer screening
- Pancreatic ductal adenocarcinoma • Consensus guidelines

KEY POINTS

- Individuals with a family history of pancreatic ductal adenocarcinoma (PDAC) and/or a genetic predisposition have an increased risk of developing PDAC and may benefit from pancreas surveillance for early detection.
- Individuals with PDAC and their first-degree relatives are candidates for germline genetic testing, which may guide surveillance intervals and recommendations.
- Pancreas surveillance is currently achieved through imaging, with preference for endoscopic ultrasound and magnetic resonance imaging, while refinements in risk stratification, novel biomarkers, and imaging strategies are being developed.

INTRODUCTION

Pancreatic ductal adenocarcinoma (PDAC) has a 5-year survival of 11%, largely due to late stage at diagnosis.[1] Although outcomes from other cancers, such as breast, lung, and colorectal, have improved due to screening, surveillance, and interventions such as tobacco cessation, PDAC is projected to become the second cause of cancer death in the United States by 2030.[2] About 10% to 15% of individuals with PDAC have a familial aggregation or inherited predisposition.[3] Patients with stage I PDAC have a 5-year survival greater than 80%, demonstrating that one mechanism of improving PDAC outcomes may be identification of high-risk individuals (HRIs) for enrollment in surveillance programs and early detection.[4] The primary goals of HRI surveillance are detection and treatment of advanced precursor lesions and early PDAC.[5,6]

Henry D. Janowitz Division of Gastroenterology, Icahn School of Medicine at Mount Sinai, One
Gustave L. Levy Place, New York, NY 10029, USA
* Corresponding author.
E-mail address: aimee.lucas@mssm.edu

Hematol Oncol Clin N Am 36 (2022) 929–942
https://doi.org/10.1016/j.hoc.2022.06.004
0889-8588/22/© 2022 Elsevier Inc. All rights reserved.
hemonc.theclinics.com

Because the incidence of PDAC in the general population is low (~1.7% lifetime risk), population-based PDAC screening would not be cost-effective due to false positives and potential harms even with near-perfect screening test characteristics.[7,8] In 2019, the US Preventive Services Task Force reaffirmed its previous Grade D "do not screen" recommendation on pancreatic cancer screening in the general population.[9] In 2010, the International Cancer of the Pancreas Screening (CAPS) Consortium assembled a multidisciplinary panel of experts to develop consensus guidelines for PDAC surveillance in HRIs.[10] Since that time, additional guidance has been published by the American Gastroenterology Association (AGA), American College of Gastroenterology (ACG), American Society of Clinical Oncology (ASCO), National Comprehensive Cancer Network (NCCN), and others.[5,6,11–13]

ASSESSMENT OF PANCREATIC DUCTAL ADENOCARCINOMA RISK
Germline Variants in Pancreatic Ductal Adenocarcinoma Cohorts

Several well-established cancer predisposition syndromes contribute to PDAC risk, including the hereditary breast-ovarian cancer (HBOC) syndrome (*BRCA1*, *BRCA2*), Partner and Localizer of *BRCA2* (*PALB2*), ataxia-telangiectasia mutated (*ATM*), familial atypical multiple mole melanoma or FAMMM syndrome (*CDKN2A/p16*), Peutz-Jeghers syndrome (*STK11*), Lynch syndrome (mismatch repair genes), hereditary pancreatitis (*PRSS1*), and Li-Fraumeni syndrome (*TP53*).[12] Several recent studies have found pathogenic germline variants (PGVs) in up to 10.4% of sporadic PDACs.[14–19]

The proportion of patients harboring PGVs differs by study population and number of genes analyzed. For example, Grant and colleagues analyzed 13 genes in a cohort of Canadian PDAC patients and found 11/290 (3.8%, 95% CI 2.1–5.6) with pathogenic variants, including *ATM*, *BRCA1*, *BRCA2*, *MLH1*, *MSH2*, *MSH6*, and *TP53*.[17] Similarly, Shindo and colleagues studied 854 patients who underwent PDAC resection and found 33/854 (3.9%, 95% CI 3.0–5.8) carried a pathogenic germline variant. Variants again included known PDAC susceptibility genes, such as *ATM*, *BRCA1*, *BRCA2*, *MLH1*, *CDKN2A*, and *TP53* but also included 1 patient with *BUB1B* and another with *BUB3*.[15]

Other studies have reported more frequent detection of PGVs in PDAC. For example, a study from New York demonstrated 21.6% of Ashkenazi Jewish PDAC patients who underwent surgical resection carried a founder variant in *BRCA1* or *BRCA2*, suggesting that germline testing in this population may be of higher yield.[13,20] Another analysis from Pittsburgh found 29/298 (9.7%) patients with PDAC with clinically actionable variants, including 23 (7.7%) in established PDAC susceptibility genes, most commonly *ATM*, *BRCA1*, and *BRCA2* variants but also *BARD1* and *CHEK2*.[18] Additionally, an analysis of 274 unselected patients with PDAC found 10.4% (95% CI 6.5–14.9) with a clinically actionable PGV.[19] Once again, variants in PDAC susceptibility genes were described, as well as in *BARD1*, *CHEK2*, and *NBN*. These studies provide evidence that germline testing in patients with PDAC detects clinically actionable PGVs in both PDAC susceptibility genes and genes that may increase the risk of nonpancreatic malignancies.[21]

Other groups analyzed the impact of a family history (FH) or personal history (PH) of malignancy on yield of genetic testing in PDAC. Yurgelun and colleagues studied 289 patients with PDAC who underwent surgical resection and found that 28 patients (9.7%, 95% CI 6.5–13.7) harbored a PGV in PDAC susceptibility genes, of whom 21.4% had an FH of PDAC and 57.1% had a prior malignancy.[14] In another study, where 85.5% of the cohort had a PH of prior malignancy or ≥1 first-degree or second-degree relative (FDR/SDR) with breast, ovarian, colorectal, or pancreatic cancer, 24/159

(15.1%, 95% CI 9.5–20.7) had a pathogenic variant in a PDAC susceptibility gene.[22] Another large study of 21 predisposition genes in 3030 unselected patients with PDAC identified 249/3030 (8.2%, 95% CI 7.3–9.3) with PGVs.[16] This proportion was enriched to 65/513 patients (12.3%, 95% CI 9.9–15.9) in the setting of a PH of malignancy and 43/143 patients (12.9%, 95% CI 9.2–16.5) when at least one FDR or SDR was affected by PDAC.[16] However, multiple studies have found that many patients with PGVs lack an FH or PH of cancer; therefore, requiring these more stringent criteria before genetic testing will fail to identify those with PGVs and, as a result, their at-risk relatives.[14,15,17,22] Additionally, studies have demonstrated that when unaffected individuals enrolled in surveillance programs undergo genetic testing, their PDAC risk stratification and candidacy for pancreatic and extrapancreatic surveillance can change when PGVs are identified.[23] For example, one study of unaffected presumed familial pancreatic cancer (FPC) kindreds demonstrated 4.3% harbored a PGV, including *ATM*, *BRCA1*, *BRCA2*, *PALB2*, and *TP53*.[24] As a result of these and other data, the NCCN and others recommend genetic testing for all individuals with PDAC; FDRs of individuals affected with PDAC are candidates for germline testing, with the caveat that negative genetic testing in unaffected relatives may be uninformative.[6,13]

Risk of Pancreatic Ductal Adenocarcinoma with Germline Variants

Early studies of PDAC risk with PGVs were limited by ascertainment and other biases. One of the largest studies of PDAC risk compared 3030 unselected PDAC cases to controls and found that several PDAC susceptibility genes provide an increased risk of PDAC, including *BRCA1* (odds ratio [OR], 2.58; 95% CI, 1.54 to 4.05), *BRCA2* (OR, 6.20; 95% CI 4.62–8.17), *ATM* (OR, 5.71; 95% CI 4.38–7.33), *MLH1* (OR, 6.66; 95% CI 1.94–17.53), *TP53* (OR, 6.70; 95% CI, 2.52–14.95), and *CDKN2A* (OR, 12.33; 95% CI 5.43–25.61).[16] Other genes, including *PMS2* (OR, 0.70; 95% CI 0.12–2.22), *MSH2* (OR, 1.58; 95% CI 0.09–7.54), *MSH6* (OR, 1.98; 95% CI 0.77–4.14), and *PALB2* (OR, 2.33; 95% CI 1.23–4.01, not significant after Bonferroni correction) did not confer excess PDAC risk. Earlier studies have demonstrated that *STK11* (relative risk, 132; 95% CI 44 to 261) and *PRSS1* (standard incidence ratio [SIR], 87; 95% CI 25 to 150) confer a greater lifetime risk of PDAC, although the broad confidence intervals suggest uncertainty on degree of risk.[25,26]

Familial Pancreatic Cancer

FPC kindreds are defined as families with at least 2 affected FDRs in the absence of a PGV associated with PDAC.[3,12,27] Although PGVs may be found in approximately 10 to 20% of families with multiple affected blood relatives, the cause of increased PDAC susceptibility is unknown in most FPC kindreds.[3,6] It is likely that additional genetic, epigenetic, and/or environmental factors predispose these kindreds to PDAC.[6] PDAC risk increases with the number of affected relatives: those with a single affected FDR have a PDAC SIR 4.5 (95% CI 0.5–16.3), whereas SIR increased to 6.4 (95% CI 1.8–16.4) with 2 affected FDRs, and SIR 32.0 (95% CI 10.4–74.7) with 3 or greater affected FDRs.[3]

CANDIDATES FOR PANCREATIC DUCTAL ADENOCARCINOMA SURVEILLANCE

Guidance on pancreatic surveillance of HRIs has been published by the CAPS consortium, AGA, ACG, NCCN, and others (**Table 1**).[5,6,10–13] All recommend that surveillance should be performed at centers that have appropriate expertise in the care of HRIs, when possible.

Table 1
Summary of pancreatic ductal adenocarcinoma surveillance strategies

Gene	ACG	CAPS	NCCN
ATM, BRCA1[c], BRCA2[d], PALB2, Lynch Syndrome[a]	≥2 affected relatives (≥1 FDR) at 50[b]	≥1 FDR at 45 or 50[b]	≥1 FDR/SDR at 50[b,h]
Peutz-Jeghers Syndrome (STK11)	35	40	30–35[b]
FAMMM (CDKN2A)	50[b]	≥1 FDR[e] at 40	40[b]
TP53			≥1 FDR/SDR at 50[b,h]
PRSS1	50[b]		20 y after onset of pancreatitis or 40, whichever is earlier[f]
Member of FPC kindred with ≥1 affected FDR	50[b]	50 or 55[b,g]	
≥2 affected FDRs from same side of family[i]			yes
≥3 affected FDRs/SDRs relatives from same side of family			yes

[a] Encompassing MLH1, MSH2, and MSH6 (no age recommendation for MSH6) (CAPS); MLH1, MSH2, MSH6, and EPCAM (NCCN).
[b] Or initiate surveillance at 10 y younger than earliest PDAC case in family, whichever is earlier.
[c] 69.6% agreement + 20.3% somewhat agreed, total 89.9% (CAPS).
[d] Mutation carriers with 2 affected blood family members relatives considered for surveillance (CAPS).
[e] Only CDKN2A mutations leading to changes in p16 protein; ≥ 1 FDR (99% agreement) or regardless of family history (77% agreement).
[f] Only if clinical phenotype consistent with hereditary pancreatitis.
[g] Consensus of age to initiate surveillance was not reached.
[h] FDR/SDR from (presumably) same lineage as pathogenic variant.
[i] Many centers will accept individuals with 1 FDR and 1 SDR.

The CAPS Consortium gathered a team of 50 international experts in PDAC surveillance to reach consensus (≥75% concordance) on initial guidance for pancreatic surveillance of HRIs.[10] Individuals with lifetime PDAC risk greater than 5% were candidates for surveillance, including those with BRCA2, PALB2, p16, and Lynch syndrome in the setting of an FDR with PDAC, as well as FDRs of FPC kindreds. Individuals with Peutz-Jeghers syndrome were also candidates for surveillance irrespective of their FH. BRCA2 PGV carriers with 2 affected family members, even in the absence of an FDR, were also considered for surveillance. Consensus was not reached on surveillance of BRCA1 carriers.

In 2015, the ACG published clinical guidelines on the management of hereditary gastrointestinal cancers including PDAC.[12] One notable difference from the initial CAPS recommendations was the inclusion of individuals with ATM PGVs in the setting of an FDR or SDR with PDAC. The ACG also determined that individuals with BRCA1, BRCA2, PALB2, and Lynch syndrome were candidates for surveillance when there was an affected FDR or SDR. Individuals with FAMMM syndrome (CDKN2A/p16) were also candidates for surveillance, irrespective of FH.

The CAPS Consortium reconvened in 2018 to update its initial guidance, using a modified Delphi approach to vote on consensus statements; consensus was again reached if 75% or greater of experts agreed.[5] In the new guidance, consensus was reached for individuals with Lynch syndrome and *ATM* PGV carriers with $\geq$1 affected FDRs. However, *PMS2* was excluded. Additionally, the experts reached consensus on the recommendation that *BRCA1* carriers undergo surveillance but were unable to reach consensus on FH criteria; among experts, 69.6% agreed on surveillance for *BRCA1* carriers with $\geq$1 affected FDR and an additional 20.3% somewhat agreed. Surveillance of patients with *CDKN2A/p16* and Peutz-Jeghers syndrome was also recommended, even in the absence of FH PDAC.

The NCCN also incorporated PDAC in their assessment of Genetic/Familial High-Risk Assessment.[13] These guidelines additionally recommended surveillance for individuals with a *TP53* PGV and $\geq$1 FDR or SDR with PDAC. Surveillance was also recommended for hereditary pancreatitis patients who present with a clinical phenotype. ASCO's provisional clinical opinion and AGA's clinical practice update provide similar surveillance recommendations.[6,11]

TARGETS AND GOALS OF SURVEILLANCE

The ultimate goal of pancreatic surveillance is to prevent PDAC by the detection and successful management of high-grade dysplasia (HGD).[6] Successful surveillance includes detection and treatment of resectable PDAC confined in the pancreas with negative margins at baseline or follow-up, high-grade multifocal pancreatic intraepithelial neoplasm (PanIN-3), unifocal PanIN-3, intraductal papillary mucosal neoplasms (IPMNs) with HGD, as well as pancreatic neuroendocrine tumors $\geq$10 mm.[5] One limitation is the challenge of detecting high-grade PanINs using current techniques, although some studies have suggested a correlation with lobular parenchymal atrophy on endoscopic ultrasound (EUS).[28]

CURRENT APPROACHES TO PANCREATIC CANCER SURVEILLANCE
Imaging

Currently, the preferred surveillance strategies include use imaging with magnetic resonance imaging (MRI) with cholangiopancreatography (MRCP) or EUS (**Fig. 1**).[6] A study of 216 HRIs (2 Peutz-Jeghers, 19 *BRCA2* with FH, and 195 FPC) who underwent blinded sequential gadolinium and secretin-enhanced MRI, pancreatic protocol computed tomography (CT), and EUS found pancreatic abnormalities on at least one modality in 92/216 (42.6%).[29] Most of these lesions were sub-CM presumed branch-duct IPMNs, which were often multifocal (defined as $\geq$ 3 cysts). However, the incidence of pancreatic abnormalities differed based on imaging modality: 11, 33.3, and 42.6% of HRIs had lesions detected on CT, MRI, and EUS, respectively. EUS and MRI demonstrated the highest level of agreement (91%). CT detected fewer cystic lesions than EUS and MRI, and a combination of CT and EUS failed to detect 6.9% of cystic lesions detected on MRI. Furthermore, both CT and MRI missed 22.3% of lesions detected on EUS, including 3 solid nodules ultimately determined to be pancreatic neuroendocrine tumors. The authors concluded that MRI and EUS are preferred methods for PDAC surveillance of HRIs.

Several studies have compared EUS and MRI in the detection of clinically important pancreatic lesions in HRIs. A European study of 139 asymptomatic HRIs (49% FPC, 27% *CDKN2A*, 16% HBOC, 5% Peutz-Jeghers, and 2% Li-Fraumeni) who underwent both EUS and MRI in a blinded fashion demonstrated 11 clinically relevant pancreatic lesions (solid lesions, main duct IPMNs, and cysts $\geq$10 mm) in 9 (6%) HRIs.[30] Only 6/11 (55%) of these clinically relevant lesions were detected by both EUS and MRI. Importantly, 2 solid lesions, one of which was a stage I PDAC, were detected by EUS alone. All 9 cystic lesions were detected with MRI, whereas only 6 were detected

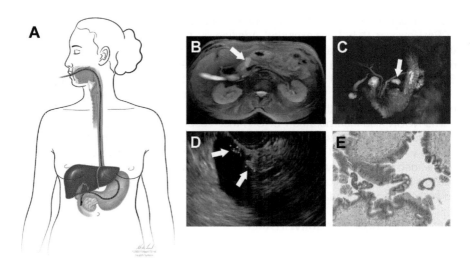

Fig. 1. Surveillance of high-risk individuals using EUS or MRI with MRCP (A) EUS involves the insertion of an endoscope with an ultrasound probe through the oropharynx into the stomach and small intestine (image from Ni-ka Ford, printed with permission from Mount Sinai Health System). This allows pancreatic lesions to be visualized and sampled. (B and C) MRI and MRCP images from a FPC patient, arrows indicate a 3 cm pancreatic cyst. (D) A representative EUS image from the same patient, arrows indicate two mural nodules within the cyst (with permission from Christopher DiMaio). (E) The patient underwent surgical resection, which ultimately identified an IPMN lined by gastric foveolar-type epithelium with HGD (hematoxylin and eosin staining; printed with permission from Hongfa Zhu). Original magnification, x100.

by EUS. Similar findings were reported from the Dutch Familial Pancreatic Cancer Surveillance Study group, where EUS had improved ability to detect solid lesions (100% vs 22%, $P<.001$) but MRI was better able to detect cystic lesions (42% vs 83%, $P<.001$), although a combination of the 2 modalities resulted in the best sensitivity for most pancreatic lesions.[31]

A recent meta-analysis evaluated the ability of EUS and MRI to detect pancreatic abnormalities on initial imaging of 2112 HRIs in 24 studies.[32] Although EUS detected more focal pancreatic abnormalities (34%, 95% CI 30-37%) than MRI (31%, 95% CI 28-33%, $P = .006$), there was no difference in detection of HGD or T1N0M0 PDAC by EUS (1.1%, 95% CI 0.28-2.0%) compared with MRI (0.78%, 95% CI 0.0-1.6%, $P = .47$). There was also no difference between detection of any stage PDAC by EUS (0.89%, 95% CI 0.0-1.8%) compared with MRI (0.29%, 95% CI 0.0-1.1%, $P = .41$). These findings support the use of EUS or MRI in surveillance programs, depending on patient preference, cost, availability, and local expertise.

Although transabdominal ultrasound is an attractive imaging modality due to its low cost, lack of ionizing radiation and noninvasive nature, its diagnostic performance for pancreatic imaging is highly dependent on both the operator's experience as well as patient factors.[33] Current guidelines for PDAC surveillance do not recommend transabdominal ultrasound.[5]

When to Initiate Surveillance

Several studies have evaluated the age of PDAC diagnosis in FPC cases, as well as the age at which to initiate surveillance. The Pancreatic Cancer Genetic Epidemiology

Consortium reported the average age of onset of PDAC in FPC kindreds was 65.4 years, the National Familial Pancreas Tumor Registry reported 69.7 years, whereas the German national case collection for FPC reported a median age of 63 years.[34–36] Several groups have noted anticipation, or earlier age at diagnosis, in FPC kindreds in subsequent generations.[34,37]

Since earlier studies had reported increased PDAC risk in the setting of BRCA2, FAMMM syndrome, Lynch syndrome, and in FPC kindreds, McWilliams and colleagues evaluated the age of PDAC onset in the setting of an FH of breast, ovarian, colorectal, melanoma, pancreatic, as well as other cancers.[38] The authors found a younger age of PDAC onset in the setting of an FH of these malignancies (P≤.001 for all), although the median age of PDAC diagnosis ranged from 57.9 to 65.6 years. Interestingly, those with an FH of PDAC had a similar age of onset to those without an FH (−0.61 years, P = .65).

Another study from the National Familial Pancreas Tumor Registry sought to understand the impact of age of PDAC onset and PDAC risk in family members.[36] The authors found an increased PDAC risk among family members of FPC kindreds when the affected member was diagnosed under the age of 50 years compared with 50 years or greater (SIR 9.31 vs 6.34, P<.001). However, cumulative PDAC risk did not typically begin to increase until after the age of 50.

A European study of 253 HRIs (including FPC kindreds, BRCA1, BRCA2, PALB2 but excluding those with CDKN2A) under surveillance evaluated the prevalence of significant lesions (PDAC, PanIN-3, high-grade IPMN) according to age.[39] The authors divided the cohort by age at first pancreatic imaging (≤40 vs ≥40, <45 vs ≤45, ≤50 vs ≥50, and so forth) and found that no significant lesions were detected in HRIs before the age of 50.[39] Similarly, Canto and colleagues found that pancreatic lesions, including cysts, pancreatic neuroendocrine tumors, and dilated pancreatic ducts, increase in prevalence with age; 14% of HRIs less than 50 years had pancreatic abnormalities compared with 34% of 50 to 59 years and 53% of those between 60 and 69 years.[29]

In a meta-analysis of PDAC surveillance programs, Kogekar and colleagues found that the number-needed-to-screen to detect one HGD or T1N0M0 PDAC was 111 HRIs.[32] However, the mean/median age of HRIs was 50 to 56 years; therefore, many HRIs included in previous surveillance cohorts were younger than 50 years. It is likely that if surveillance were limited to those 50 or greater to 55 years, the number-needed-to-screen would decrease. Surveillance of HRIs should typically begin around the age of 50 to 55 years, or 10 years before the age of the youngest affected blood relative (see **Table 1**). Exceptions include Peutz-Jeghers syndrome and individuals with pathogenic mutations in CDKN2A or PRSS1.

Risk Factors for Progression

Certain imaging features have been associated with increased neoplastic progression. In a study of 354 HRIs (97% FPC kindred, 16% with PGV) with a mean time under surveillance of 5.6 years, 24/345 (7%) of participants had neoplastic progression (14 PDACs and 10 high-grade IPMNs and/or PanINs).[40] Risk factors for progression included multifocal (≥3) cysts, the presence of a solid mass, rapid cyst growth, thickened cyst wall, the presence of a mural nodule and a main pancreatic duct (MPD) 5 mm or greater. Interestingly, in this analysis a PGV was not associated with neoplastic progression (hazard ratio (HR) .66, 95% CI .18–2.14). The rate of progression was 1.6% per year and median time to development of PDAC was 4.8 years, with a shorter timeline for individuals who began screening at ≥60 years (median 1.7 years). Importantly, the median survival for those who developed PDAC or a high-grade neoplasm while adhering to surveillance was longer than those who discontinued or had delayed surveillance (5.3 vs 1.4 years, $P<.0001$). The 3-year survival was also improved for those detected during surveillance (85% vs 25%, $P<.0001$).

Analyses including a larger proportion of HRIs with PGVs have suggested that these patients may be more likely to progress to PDAC. In a comparison of HRIs with and without PGVs, Abe and colleagues found that those with a PGV are more likely to progress to HGD and PDAC than individuals from FPC kindreds (HR 2.81; 95% CI 1.17–6.76) with a greater cumulative incidence of PDAC in those with a PGV (HR 2.85, 95% CI 1.0–8.18).[24] Similarly, a European study found patients with PGVs had a higher incidence of PDAC (9.3% at 10 years of follow-up) compared with FPC kindreds (0%).[31] Importantly, 58% of this cohort had *CKDN2A/p16* and 6% had Peutz-Jeghers syndrome. Most (9/10) PDACs in the PGV group were found in these higher-penetrance variants, whereas 1 PDAC was in a *BRCA2* carrier. Risk factors for progression included dilated MPD (5–9 mm) and a solid lesion on imaging. Overall, 60% of detected PDAC cases were resectable, and 30% met the definition for CAPS successful targets.

Interval for Surveillance

Further investigation is required to determine the optimal surveillance interval for HRIs. In a retrospective study of HRIs who were diagnosed with PDAC and/or underwent pancreatic surgery, 1% developed PDAC or HGD within a median of 29 months under surveillance.[41] Of those who progressed, 13 (46%) had a new lesion detected after a median of 11 months from a previous visit and 15 (54%) progressed from an existing lesion (mostly cystic) with a median of 19 months after the first detection. Concerningly, only 7/28 (25%) of neoplastic progressors had successful outcomes (HGD or localized PDAC).

A recent meta-analysis of 2169 HRIs in 13 studies highlighted some challenges with PDAC surveillance.[42] Authors reported 1.7 per 1000 patient-years (95% CI 0.2–4.0) cumulative incidence of surveillance-detected late-stage PDAC, whereas the incidence of successful surveillance was 0.8 per 1000 patient-years (95% CI 0.2–3.1). The time period between preceding imaging and late-stage PDAC presentation ranged from 1 to 24 months. Of 39 PDAC cases detected at late-stages, 10 HRIs had a normal prior imaging, 4 had imaging ≤12 months of presentation, and 6 had imaging >12 months prior. Authors were unable to identify predictive factors for neoplastic progression or advanced PDAC diagnosis.

Annual surveillance is recommended in the absence of concerning features.[5] EUS may be considered at a more frequent interval when a lesion is detected that is of low-risk (6–12 months), intermediate-risk (3–6 months), or high-risk (≤3 months).[11] CAPS recommends shortening the interval of surveillance on detection of concerning abnormalities such as a cyst with worrisome features, a solid lesion, or MPD stricture and/or dilation ≥6 mm.[5] A follow-up interval of 6 months is recommended for cystic lesions with lymphadenopathy, growth rate ≥5 mm/2 years, size ≥3 cm, elevated serum carbohydrate antigen 19-9 (CA19-9), or MPD dilation of 5 to 9 mm. An interval of 3 months is recommended for solid lesions less than 5 mm, MPD dilation of 5 to 9 mm, or MPD stricture and/or dilation ≥6 mm without the presence of a mass.

Surgical Intervention

Surgical resection is recommended for localized PDAC and precursor neoplasms with HGD.[5] CAPS recommends that a solid lesion ≥5 mm or a solid lesion with MPD stricture and/or dilation ≥10 mm warrants resection.[5] Cystic lesions with a mural nodule, enhanced solid component, symptoms (including pancreatitis, jaundice, pain), thickened/enhanced cyst walls, abrupt MPD caliber change with distal atrophy, MPD $\geq$10 mm (97%), and growth of $\geq$5 mm/2 years should also prompt surgical evaluation.[5]

ADDITIONAL RECOMMENDATIONS FOR HIGH-RISK INDIVIDUALS
Tobacco Cessation

Smoking accounts for approximately 20% to 30% of all PDAC cases and is the primary modifiable risk factor, even in the hereditary setting.[43] For example, Klein and colleagues found higher incidence of PDAC in smokers ($\geq$100 lifetime cigarettes) with an FH of PDAC (SIR 19.2; 95% CI 7.7–39.5) compared with nonsmokers (SIR 6.25; 95% CI 1.7–16.0).[3] Similarly, Molina-Montes and colleagues found that among those with an FH of PDAC, ever-smokers had greater odds of developing PDAC when compared with never-smokers (OR 3.16; 95% CI 2.56–5.78).[44]

McWilliams and colleagues reported cumulative PDAC incidence of 57.6% by age 80 with CDKN2A, compared with 3.2% in noncarriers.[45] However, PDAC risk with a CDKN2A PGV was attributable to tobacco exposure. When the analyses were limited to who smoked $\geq$100 lifetime cigarettes, an HR 25.8 ($P = 2.1 \times 10^{-13}$) was noted for those with CDKN2A compared with those without. For nonsmokers, no significant increased risk was noted for CDKN2A (HR 4.9, $P = .27$). A study of 217 PRSS1 PGV carriers reported PDAC SIR 59 (95% CI 19–138) with a cumulative risk of 7.2% by the age of 70 years, markedly decreased from previous reports.[46] One proposed mechanism includes lower tobacco exposure in recent years.

Monitor Hyperglycemia and Diabetes

Multiple studies have identified an association between PDAC, hyperglycemia, and new onset diabetes, typically within 3 years before PDAC diagnosis.[47–49] These data have been preliminarily replicated in a cohort of patients with PDAC with an affected FDR.[50] In HRIs, Bar-Mashiah and colleagues found that a hemoglobin A1c level above the prediabetes cutoff was associated with the presence of pancreatic cysts on the initial surveillance imaging.[51] Guidance now suggests that new-onset of diabetes in HRIs should prompt further evaluation.[5,11]

POTENTIAL HARMS

A crucial component of a successful pancreatic surveillance program is ensuring that the benefits outweigh the risks. Overdiagnosis and overtreatment of benign or low-risk lesions is a major concern. In a meta-analysis, Kogekar and colleagues reported that the proportion of HRIs who underwent surgery did not differ between those who underwent baseline imaging with EUS (4.1%, 95% CI 3.0-5.2%) compared with MRI baseline imaging (4.4%, 95% CI 3.2-5.5%, $P = .64$), although 5.4% of HRIs underwent surgical resection.[32] Reported 30-day and 90-day mortality for pancreatectomy is 3.7% and 7.4%, respectively, although in a small cohort of 48 HRIs who underwent surgery 35% experienced complications with zero mortality at 90 days.[52,53]

Another potential harm is the potential increased anxiety that may be associated with PDAC surveillance. One study using the Cancer Worry and Hospital Anxiety scales to assess patient-reported burden of HRIs undergoing surveillance at intensified intervals found that intensified surveillance intervals temporarily increased cancer worry but did not affect overall anxiety or depression.[54] Another study of HRIs in surveillance found consistently low anxiety and depression scores during 3-years of follow-up.[55]

FUTURE DIRECTIONS
Risk Stratification

Current estimates of PDAC risk with PGVs are imprecise, and risk varies with affected gene and possibly specific variant within the gene. However, current guidance applies a uniform surveillance approach in the setting of varied risk. For example, those with *BRCA1* or *PALB2* variants likely have lower PDAC risk than those with *CDKN2A* or *ATM*, and yet annual surveillance is recommended for both. More precise PDAC risk estimates for those with PGVs and FPC, which may incorporate environmental exposures and polygenic risk scores, may allow for a more tailored approach.[56,57]

Biomarkers

The development of novel biomarkers has the potential to be an indispensable tool for pancreatic surveillance in HRIs. The most established biomarker for PDAC is CA19-9; however, test characteristics limit its ability to be used as a surveillance tool and 10% of the population does not produce CA19-9.[5,6] Several biomarkers and combinations of biomarkers are in development, and show promise for early detection of PDAC.[58–62] Additional studies have evaluated unique genetic signatures of pancreatic secretions from the ductal epithelium, whereas others have evaluated methylated DNA markers in pancreatic juice as well as stool samples.[63–66] It is possible that biomarker-based tests may complement already established surveillance modalities and allow for improved early detection in HRIs.

Imaging Techniques

Optimization of existing imaging techniques, development of novel imaging strategies, and evaluation of metabolic changes during PDAC development may aid in early detection. For example, deep learning algorithms and computer-assisted diagnostic systems have the potential to distinguish PDAC from benign disease on cross-sectional imaging and EUS.[67,68] Additional studies are ongoing using enhanced molecular imaging agents.[69,70] Imaging alterations in subcutaneous and visceral abdominal fat and muscle wasting have also been associated with PDAC and periodic cross-sectional imaging to measure metabolic changes may detect early disease in HRIs.[71]

SUMMARY

Pancreatic surveillance of HRIs may improve survival by identification and treatment of precancerous lesions and early stage PDAC. Refinements in risk stratification and novel screening methods to complement imaging-based modalities may allow for improved outcomes.

CLINICS CARE POINTS

- Pancreatic surveillance may be considered in individuals with lifetime risk greater than 5%.
- Evaluation for a hereditary cause is recommended for all patients with pancreatic ductal adenocarcinoma and if not available, their first-degree relatives.
- Pancreatic surveillance of high-risk individuals typically begins at 50 years of age or 10 years younger than the earliest pancreatic cancer diagnosis in the family. Exceptions include *CDKN2A*, *PRSS1*, and *STK11*.
- Endoscopic ultrasound and magnetic resonance imaging are the current preferred imaging modalities for pancreatic surveillance.

- In the absence of worrisome features, surveillance is performed annually.

REFERENCES

1. American Cancer Society. Cancer Facts & Figures 2022. Available at: https://www.cancer.org/research/cancer-facts-statistics/all-cancer-facts-figures/cancer-facts-figures-2022.html. Accessed January 10, 2022.
2. Rahib L, Smith BD, Aizenberg R, et al. Projecting cancer incidence and deaths to 2030: the unexpected burden of thyroid, liver, and pancreas cancers in the United States. Cancer Res 2014;74:2913–21.
3. Klein AP, Brune KA, Petersen GM, et al. Prospective risk of pancreatic cancer in familial pancreatic cancer kindreds. Cancer Res 2004;64:2634–8.
4. Blackford AL, Canto MI, Klein AP, et al. Recent Trends in the Incidence and Survival of Stage 1A Pancreatic Cancer: A Surveillance, Epidemiology, and End Results Analysis. J Natl Cancer Inst 2020;112:1162–9.
5. Goggins M, Overbeek KA, Brand R, et al. Management of patients with increased risk for familial pancreatic cancer: updated recommendations from the International Cancer of the Pancreas Screening (CAPS) Consortium. Gut 2020;69:7–17.
6. Stoffel EM, McKernin SE, Brand R, et al. Evaluating Susceptibility to Pancreatic Cancer: ASCO Provisional Clinical Opinion. J Clin Oncol 2019;37:153–64.
7. National Cancer Institute. Surveillance, Epidemiology, and End Results Program. Cancer Stat Facts: Pancreatic Cancer. 2022. Available at: https://seer.cancer.gov/statfacts/html/pancreas.html. Accessed January 14, 2022.
8. Lucas AL, Kastrinos F. Screening for Pancreatic Cancer. Jama 2019;322:407–8.
9. US Preventive Services Task Force. Screening for pancreatic cancer: US Preventive Services Task Force reaffirmation recommendation statement. Jama 2019;322(5):438–44.
10. Canto MI, Harinck F, Hruban RH, et al. International Cancer of the Pancreas Screening (CAPS) Consortium summit on the management of patients with increased risk for familial pancreatic cancer. Gut 2013;62:339–47.
11. Aslanian HR, Lee JH, Canto MI. AGA Clinical Practice Update on Pancreas Cancer Screening in High-Risk Individuals: Expert Review. Gastroenterology 2020;159:358–62.
12. Syngal S, Brand RE, Church JM, et al. ACG clinical guideline: Genetic testing and management of hereditary gastrointestinal cancer syndromes. Am J Gastroenterol 2015;110:223–62.
13. National Comprehensive Cancer Network. Genetic/Familial High-Risk Assessment: Breast, Ovarian, and Pancreatic. In: Clinical Practice Guidelines in Oncology Version 1.2022. 2021. Available at: https://www.nccn.org/professionals/physician_gls/pdf/genetics_bop.pdf. Accessed: January 2, 2022.
14. Yurgelun MB, Chittenden AB, Morales-Oyarvide V, et al. Germline cancer susceptibility gene variants, somatic second hits, and survival outcomes in patients with resected pancreatic cancer. Genet Med 2019;21:213–23.
15. Shindo K, Yu J, Suenaga M, et al. Deleterious Germline Mutations in Patients With Apparently Sporadic Pancreatic Adenocarcinoma. J Clin Oncol 2017;35:3382–90.
16. Hu C, Hart SN, Polley EC, et al. Association Between Inherited Germline Mutations in Cancer Predisposition Genes and Risk of Pancreatic Cancer. Jama 2018;319:2401–9.

17. Grant RC, Selander I, Connor AA, et al. Prevalence of germline mutations in cancer predisposition genes in patients with pancreatic cancer. Gastroenterology 2015;148:556–64.

18. Brand R, Borazanci E, Speare V, et al. Prospective study of germline genetic testing in incident cases of pancreatic adenocarcinoma. Cancer 2018;124:3520–7.

19. Young EL, Thompson BA, Neklason DW, et al. Pancreatic cancer as a sentinel for hereditary cancer predisposition. BMC Cancer 2018;18:697.

20. Lucas AL, Shakya R, Lipsyc MD, et al. High prevalence of BRCA1 and BRCA2 germline mutations with loss of heterozygosity in a series of resected pancreatic adenocarcinoma and other neoplastic lesions. Clin Cancer Res 2013;19:3396–403.

21. Cybulski C, Wokołorczyk D, Kładny J, et al. Germline CHEK2 mutations and colorectal cancer risk: different effects of a missense and truncating mutations? Eur J Hum Genet 2007;15:237–41.

22. Salo-Mullen EE, O'Reilly EM, Kelsen DP, et al. Identification of germline genetic mutations in patients with pancreatic cancer. Cancer 2015;121:4382–8.

23. Lucas AL, Frado LE, Hwang C, et al. BRCA1 and BRCA2 germline mutations are frequently demonstrated in both high-risk pancreatic cancer screening and pancreatic cancer cohorts. Cancer 2014;120:1960–7.

24. Abe T, Blackford AL, Tamura K, et al. Deleterious Germline Mutations Are a Risk Factor for Neoplastic Progression Among High-Risk Individuals Undergoing Pancreatic Surveillance. J Clin Oncol 2019;37:1070–80.

25. Giardiello FM, Brensinger JD, Tersmette AC, et al. Very high risk of cancer in familial Peutz-Jeghers syndrome. Gastroenterology 2000;119:1447–53.

26. Rebours V, Boutron-Ruault MC, Schnee M, et al. Risk of pancreatic adenocarcinoma in patients with hereditary pancreatitis: a national exhaustive series. Am J Gastroenterol 2008;103:111–9.

27. Brand RE, Lerch MM, Rubinstein WS, et al. Advances in counselling and surveillance of patients at risk for pancreatic cancer. Gut 2007;56:1460–9.

28. Brune K, Abe T, Canto M, et al. Multifocal neoplastic precursor lesions associated with lobular atrophy of the pancreas in patients having a strong family history of pancreatic cancer. Am J Surg Pathol 2006;30:1067–76.

29. Canto MI, Hruban RH, Fishman EK, et al. Frequent detection of pancreatic lesions in asymptomatic high-risk individuals. Gastroenterology 2012;142:796–804.

30. Harinck F, Konings IC, Kluijt I, et al. A multicentre comparative prospective blinded analysis of EUS and MRI for screening of pancreatic cancer in high-risk individuals. Gut 2016;65:1505–13.

31. Overbeek KA, Levink IJM, Koopmann BDM, et al. Long-term yield of pancreatic cancer surveillance in high-risk individuals. Gut 2021;0:1–9.

32. Kogekar N, Diaz KE, Weinberg AD, et al. Surveillance of high-risk individuals for pancreatic cancer with EUS and MRI: A meta-analysis. Pancreatology 2020;20:1739–46.

33. Ashida R, Tanaka S, Yamanaka H, et al. The Role of Transabdominal Ultrasound in the Diagnosis of Early Stage Pancreatic Cancer: Review and Single-Center Experience. Diagnostics (Basel) 2018;9:2.

34. Schneider R, Slater EP, Sina M, et al. German national case collection for familial pancreatic cancer (FaPaCa): ten years experience. Fam Cancer 2011;10:323–30.

35. Petersen GM, de Andrade M, Goggins M, et al. Pancreatic cancer genetic epidemiology consortium. Cancer Epidemiol Biomarkers Prev 2006;15:704–10.

36. Brune KA, Lau B, Palmisano E, et al. Importance of age of onset in pancreatic cancer kindreds. J Natl Cancer Inst 2010;102:119–26.
37. McFaul CD, Greenhalf W, Earl J, et al. Anticipation in familial pancreatic cancer. Gut 2006;55:252–8.
38. McWilliams RR, Bamlet WR, Rabe KG, et al. Association of family history of specific cancers with a younger age of onset of pancreatic adenocarcinoma. Clin Gastroenterol Hepatol 2006;4:1143–7.
39. Bartsch DK, Slater EP, Carrato A, et al. Refinement of screening for familial pancreatic cancer. Gut 2016;65:1314–21.
40. Canto MI, Almario JA, Schulick RD, et al. Risk of Neoplastic Progression in Individuals at High Risk for Pancreatic Cancer Undergoing Long-term Surveillance. Gastroenterology 2018;155:740–51.
41. Overbeek KA, Goggins MG, Dbouk M, et al. Timeline of development of pancreatic cancer and implications for successful early detection in high-risk individuals. Gastroenterology 2022;162(3):772–85.e4.
42. Chhoda A, Vodusek Z, Wattamwar K, et al. Late-Stage Pancreatic Cancer Detected During High-Risk Individual Surveillance: A Systematic Review and Meta-Analysis. Gastroenterology 2022;162(3):786–98.
43. Iodice S, Gandini S, Maisonneuve P, et al. Tobacco and the risk of pancreatic cancer: a review and meta-analysis. Langenbecks Arch Surg 2008;393:535–45.
44. Molina-Montes E, Gomez-Rubio P, Márquez M, et al. Risk of pancreatic cancer associated with family history of cancer and other medical conditions by accounting for smoking among relatives. Int J Epidemiol 2018;47:473–83.
45. McWilliams RR, Wieben ED, Rabe KG, et al. Prevalence of CDKN2A mutations in pancreatic cancer patients: implications for genetic counseling. Eur J Hum Genet 2011;19:472–8.
46. Shelton CA, Umapathy C, Stello K, et al. Hereditary Pancreatitis in the United States: Survival and Rates of Pancreatic Cancer. Am J Gastroenterol 2018;113:1376.
47. Sharma A, Smyrk TC, Levy MJ, et al. Fasting Blood Glucose Levels Provide Estimate of Duration and Progression of Pancreatic Cancer Before Diagnosis. Gastroenterology 2018;155:490–500.e2.
48. Huang BZ, Pandol SJ, Jeon CY, et al. New-Onset Diabetes, Longitudinal Trends in Metabolic Markers, and Risk of Pancreatic Cancer in a Heterogeneous Population. Clin Gastroenterol Hepatol 2020;18:1812–21.e7.
49. Brewer MJ, Doucette JT, Bar-Mashiah A, et al. Glycemic Changes and Weight Loss Precede Pancreatic Ductal Adenocarcinoma by up to 3 Years in a Diverse Population. Clin Gastroenterol Hepatol 2022;20(5):1105–11.e2.
50. Garg SK, Singh DP, Sharma A, et al. Glycemic Profile of Subjects with Familial Pancreatic Cancer: Mayo Clinic Experience from 2000-2018. Gastroenterology 2019;152:S–38.
51. Bar-Mashiah A, Aronson A, Naparst M, et al. Elevated hemoglobin A1c is associated with the presence of pancreatic cysts in a high-risk pancreatic surveillance program. BMC Gastroenterol 2020;20:161.
52. Canto MI, Kerdsirichairat T, Yeo CJ, et al. Surgical Outcomes After Pancreatic Resection of Screening-Detected Lesions in Individuals at High Risk for Developing Pancreatic Cancer. J Gastrointest Surg 2020;24:1101–10.
53. Swanson RS, Pezzi CM, Mallin K, et al. The 90-day mortality after pancreatectomy for cancer is double the 30-day mortality: more than 20,000 resections from the national cancer data base. Ann Surg Oncol 2014;21:4059–67.

54. Overbeek KA, Cahen DL, Kamps A, et al. Patient-reported burden of intensified surveillance and surgery in high-risk individuals under pancreatic cancer surveillance. Fam Cancer 2020;19:247–58.

55. Konings IC, Sidharta GN, Harinck F, et al. Repeated participation in pancreatic cancer surveillance by high-risk individuals imposes low psychological burden. Psychooncology 2016;25:971–8.

56. Galeotti AA, Gentiluomo M, Rizzato C, et al. Polygenic and multifactorial scores for pancreatic ductal adenocarcinoma risk prediction. J Med Genet 2021;58:369–77.

57. Zhong J, Jermusyk A, Wu L, et al. A Transcriptome-Wide Association Study Identifies Novel Candidate Susceptibility Genes for Pancreatic Cancer. J Natl Cancer Inst 2020;112:1003–12.

58. Mellby LD, Nyberg AP, Johansen JS, et al. Serum Biomarker Signature-Based Liquid Biopsy for Diagnosis of Early-Stage Pancreatic Cancer. J Clin Oncol 2018;36:2887–94.

59. Cohen JD, Li L, Wang Y, et al. Detection and localization of surgically resectable cancers with a multi-analyte blood test. Science 2018;359:926–30.

60. Cohen JD, Javed AA, Thoburn C, et al. Combined circulating tumor DNA and protein biomarker-based liquid biopsy for the earlier detection of pancreatic cancers. Proc Natl Acad Sci U S A 2017;114:10202–7.

61. Klein EA, Richards D, Cohn A, et al. Clinical validation of a targeted methylation-based multi-cancer early detection test using an independent validation set. Ann Oncol 2021;32:1167–77.

62. Guler GD, Ning Y, Ku CJ, et al. Detection of early stage pancreatic cancer using 5-hydroxymethylcytosine signatures in circulating cell free DNA. Nat Commun 2020;11:5270.

63. Chen R, Pan S, Cooke K, et al. Comparison of pancreas juice proteins from cancer versus pancreatitis using quantitative proteomic analysis. Pancreas 2007;34:70–9.

64. Majumder S, Raimondo M, Taylor WR, et al. Methylated DNA in Pancreatic Juice Distinguishes Patients With Pancreatic Cancer From Controls. Clin Gastroenterol Hepatol 2020;18:676–83.e3.

65. Kisiel JB, Yab TC, Taylor WR, et al. Stool DNA testing for the detection of pancreatic cancer: assessment of methylation marker candidates. Cancer 2012;118:2623–31.

66. Sadakari Y, Kanda M, Maitani K, et al. Mutant KRAS and GNAS DNA Concentrations in Secretin-Stimulated Pancreatic Fluid Collected from the Pancreatic Duct and the Duodenal Lumen. Clin Transl Gastroenterol 2014;5:e62.

67. Gao X, Wang X. Performance of deep learning for differentiating pancreatic diseases on contrast-enhanced magnetic resonance imaging: A preliminary study. Diagn Interv Imaging 2020;101:91–100.

68. Tonozuka R, Itoi T, Nagata N, et al. Deep learning analysis for the detection of pancreatic cancer on endosonographic images: a pilot study. J Hepatobiliary Pancreat Sci 2021;28:95–104.

69. Alauddin MM, De Palatis L. Current and Future Trends in Early Detection of Pancreatic Cancer: Molecular Targets and PET Probes. Curr Med Chem 2015;22:3370–89.

70. England CG, Hernandez R, Eddine SB, et al. Molecular Imaging of Pancreatic Cancer with Antibodies. Mol Pharm 2016;13:8–24.

71. Zaid M, Elganainy D, Dogra P, et al. Imaging-Based Subtypes of Pancreatic Ductal Adenocarcinoma Exhibit Differential Growth and Metabolic Patterns in the Pre-Diagnostic Period: Implications for Early Detection. Front Oncol 2020;10:596931.

Germline Testing for Individuals with Pancreatic Adenocarcinoma and Novel Genetic Risk Factors

Anu Chittenden, MS, LGC[a], Sigurdis Haraldsdottir, MD, PhD[b],
Ethan Chen[c], Sahar Nissim, MD, PhD[d],*

KEYWORDS

• Genetic testing • Germline mutations • Pancreatic ductal adenocarcinoma

KEY POINTS

• Germline mutations can increase risk of pancreatic cancer.
• Genetic testing for these germline mutations can guide risk assessment.
• Genetic testing for these germline mutations can inform precision medicine strategies.

Advances in our understanding of the genetic basis of pancreatic ductal adenocarcinoma (PDAC) have uncovered new strategies for interception and treatment. Alongside somatic mutation drivers such as oncogenic activation of *KRAS* and inactivation of tumor suppressors *CDKN2A*, *TP53*, and *SMAD4*, germline variants have been implicated in modulating risk of PDAC. Recent studies have identified germline variants associated with cancer predisposition in ~4% to 10% of PDAC cases.[1–6] Importantly, clinical features such as family history have poor sensitivity in identifying carriers of these risk variants, motivating universal germline genetic testing.[2,3,5,6] Genetic testing for these germline variants has potential to guide risk assessment and surveillance recommendations in high-risk individuals to promote prevention and early detection measures. Moreover, identification of novel germline

The authors have no commercial or financial conflicts of interest to disclose.

Funding sources: S. Nissim: NIH, Burroughs Wellcome Fund, Hale Center for Pancreatic Cancer Research.

[a] Dana-Farber Cancer Institute, Center for Cancer Genetics and Prevention, 450 Brookline Avenue, Mail Stop DA10, Boston, MA 02215, USA; [b] Landspitali University Hospital, University of Iceland, Eiriksgata 21, 101 Reykjavik, Iceland; [c] Brigham and Women's Hospital, New Research Building Room 458, 77 Ave Louis Pasteur, Boston, MA 02115, USA; [d] Dana-Farber Cancer Institute, Brigham and Women's Hospital, Harvard Medical School, New Research Building Room 458, 77 Ave Louis Pasteur, Boston, MA 02115, USA
* Corresponding author.
E-mail address: snissim@bwh.harvard.edu

variants can offer insights into pathogenesis that may inform precision medicine approaches. This review summarizes current understanding of germline mutations associated with PDAC risk, recently discovered genetic variants that have been implicated in PDAC risk, and the implications of genetic testing for risk assessment and tailored therapy in PDAC.

Initial evidence for a hereditary basis of PDAC came from reports of family clusters.[7–11] Subsequent case-control and cohort analyses have shown elevated risk of PDAC with a family history.[12] Furthermore, a segregation analysis on 287 families incorporating smoking data as a covariate has suggested that a rare autosomal dominant germline causal variant is the most parsimonious model for family clusters.[13] Compared with the general population, individuals from families harboring at least one pair of first-degree relatives with PDAC have an approximately 4.5-, 6.4-, or 32-fold increased lifetime risk of developing PDAC with 1, 2, or 3 affected first-degree relatives, respectively.[13] Although shared environmental factors such as heavy smoking or alcohol use may contribute to family clusters, these epidemiologic observations support a heritable contribution to PDAC risk. Indeed, increased lifetime risk of PDAC has been identified with several germline mutations linked to hereditary cancer susceptibility syndromes (**Table 1**).

Although the causal germline mutations listed in **Table 1** result in loss of function of associated protein activity, the mutations clinically manifest with an autosomal dominant mode of inheritance. For some of these genes, biallelic germline mutations have been associated with a distinct autosomal recessive syndrome for which PDAC predisposition has not been demonstrated, including ataxia-telangiectasia (*ATM*), Fanconi anemia (*BRCA1*, *BRCA2*), and constitutional mismatch repair (MMR) deficiency syndrome (*MLH1*, *MSH2*, *MSH6*, *PMS2*, or *EPCAM*). The causal genes listed in **Table 1** are estimated to account for ~10% to 20% of PDAC family clusters,[2,14,15] suggesting that other causes remain to be discovered. New candidate genes with preliminary evidence of associated PDAC risk are discussed later.

To more rigorously define the prevalence of these mutations, several recent studies have used next-generation sequencing panels to detect these mutations among patients with PDAC. In a cohort of 290 probands with PDAC, 11 pathogenic mutations (prevalence of 3.8%) were detected in *ATM*, *BRCA1*, *BRCA2*, *MLH1*, *MSH2*, *MSH6*, and *TP53*.[2] Carrier status was associated significantly with breast cancer and colorectal cancer in the proband or first-degree relative, but not with a family history of PDAC or age of diagnosis.[2] In another study of 159 patients with PDAC who pursued germline genetic testing, 24 pathogenic mutations (prevalence of 15.1%) were

Table 1
Hereditary cancer susceptibility syndromes

Syndrome	Genes with Causal Germline Mutations	Estimated Lifetime Risk of PDAC
HBOC	dsDDR genes: *BRCA1*, *BRCA2*, *ATM*, or *PALB2*	2%–10%
FAMMM	*CDKN2A*	> 15%
PJS	*STK11/LKB1*	> 15%
LFS	*TP53*	5%–10%
Lynch syndrome	*MLH1*, *MSH2*, *MSH6*, *PMS2*, or *EPCAM*	< 5–10%

Abbreviations: dsDDR, double-strand DNA damage repair; FAMMM, familial atypical multiple mole/melanoma; HBOC, hereditary breast and ovarian cancer; LFS, Li-Fraumeni syndrome; PJS, Peutz-Jeghers syndrome.

identified in *BRCA1*, *BRCA2*, *CDKN2A*, *PALB2*, or Lynch syndrome (LS) genes, with these mutations enriched among patients with early-onset (age $\leq$ 50 years) disease.[6] In a study of 96 patients with PDAC not selected for family history, pathogenic mutations were identified in 9 patients (9.4%) in *ATM*, *BRCA1*, *BRCA2*, and *MSH6*.[4] Germline mutations were also identified in *CHEK2*, *BARD1*, *FANCM*, and *NBN* genes, although the association of these mutations with PDAC susceptibility is not well established.[4] In another cohort of 854 patients with PDAC, 31 (3.6%) were found to carry a deleterious germline mutation in known PDAC susceptibility genes including *ATM*, *BRCA1*, *BRCA2*, *CDKN2A*, *MLH1*, *PALB2*, and *TP53*, only 3 (9.7%) of whom had a family history of PDAC.[5] An additional 5 patients had mutations in cancer susceptibility genes *BUB1B*, *BUB3*, *CDH1*, *RAD51B*, and *RAD51D*, for which evidence linking to PDAC is limited.[5] Finally, in a study of 289 patients with resected PDAC, 28 (9.7%) patients carried pathogenic or likely pathogenic germline variants in double-strand DNA damage repair (dsDDR) genes (*BRCA1*, *BRCA2*, *ATM*, *PALB2*, *CHEK2*, *NBN*, *RAD50*, *RAD51 C*), LS genes, *APC*, *CDKN2A*, or *TP53*.[16] Supporting the pathogenicity of these loss-of-function germline variants, a second hit mutation was identified by somatic sequencing and immunohistochemistry in the tumor of 12 of 27 (44.4%) patients.[16] This last study again found that many patients with PDAC with the germline variants did not have a family history or prior personal history of cancer.

These collective findings, summarized in **Fig. 1**, convincingly reveal an ~4% to 10% prevalence of pathogenic germline mutations in known cancer susceptibility genes among all cases of PDAC, and importantly, that classical clinical features alone such as family history or age of onset are insufficient to identify carriers.

CURRENT GUIDELINES FOR GERMLINE GENETIC TESTING OF PANCREATIC DUCTAL ADENOCARCINOMA SUSCEPTIBILITY GENES

Motivated by these findings as well as by the aggressive course of PDAC that may preclude genetic evaluation in advanced stages, the standard of care in the past few years has evolved to testing all individuals with PDAC at the time of initial diagnosis, regardless of family history, to identify patients and families with inherited risk.[17-19]

For unaffected individuals, germline genetic testing may be performed in unaffected first-degree relatives if it is impossible to test the patient with PDAC.[19] Furthermore, germline genetic testing can be considered in any unaffected individual who has a family history of PDAC as well as a known cancer predisposition gene mutation on the same side of the family.

There are 2 primary rationales for germline genetic testing. First, for individuals affected with PDAC, personalized treatment options are emerging for PDAC associated with some germline risk genes. Specifically, as discussed later, PDAC associated with dsDDR gene mutations may be more vulnerable to treatment with poly(ADP-ribose) polymerase (PARP) inhibitors, and PDAC associated with LS mutations may be more vulnerable to immune checkpoint blockade (ICB) strategies. Second, identification of a germline genetic basis for PDAC susceptibility can guide risk assessment and surveillance recommendations in unaffected relatives. Specifically, carriers of a germline mutation associated with a family history of PDAC may consider pancreas surveillance with annual alternating magnetic resonance cholangiopancreatography (MRCP) and endoscopic ultrasonography (EUS). Given the high lifetime risk of PDAC (see **Table 1**), surveillance is also indicated in carriers of *CDKN2A* or *STK11/ LKB1* germline mutations regardless of family history. With the exception of genes associated with hereditary pancreatitis, germline predisposition genes are typically associated with risk of cancer in other organs including breast, ovarian, and colorectal

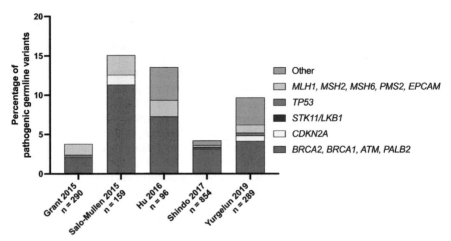

Fig. 1. Prevalence of pathogenic germline mutations among pancreatic cancer cases.

cancers, and thus identification of a risk mutation can guide surveillance and prophylactic measures of these other cancers as well.

Genes Associated with Hereditary Pancreatic Ductal Adenocarcinoma Predisposition

Hereditary breast and ovarian cancer syndrome

Syndrome presentation, epidemiology, and absolute lifetime risk. Mutations in the genes BRCA1/2 (breast cancer type 1/2), PALB2 (partner and localizer of BRCA2), and ATM (Ataxia telangiectasia mutated) have been associated with the hereditary breast and ovarian cancer syndrome.

BRCA1 and BRCA2 mutations increase the risk of breast and ovarian cancer, fallopian tube cancer, male breast cancer, and prostate cancer. Furthermore, BRCA2 mutations are associated with PDAC and melanoma risk, whereas those associations are not as strong for BRCA1 mutations.[20] BRCA2 mutations are the single most common germline genetic finding in patients with PDAC, contributing to 10% to 20% of all PDAC cases in familial PDAC[21-24] and to 1% to 8% of unselected PDAC cases.[2,3,25,26] The population-based prevalence of BRCA1 or BRCA2 mutations is estimated around 1 in 400,[27] although founder mutations lead to a higher prevalence in some populations such as the Ashkenazi Jews.[28] The relative risk of PDAC ranges from 3- to 6-fold in BRCA2 mutation carriers with a lifetime risk estimated at 4% to 8%.[20,29] In BRCA1 mutation carriers the relative risk ranges from 1 to 3.5 times with an estimated lifetime risk of 2% to 5%.[30,31]

PALB2 germline mutations have also been implicated in PDAC risk.[32,33] The population-based prevalence of PALB2 mutations is estimated around 0.2%. PALB2 mutations are found in 3% to 4% of familial PDAC cases.[34] The largest study to date and the first study to quantify PDAC risk in PALB2 mutation carriers included 524 families from 21 countries[35] and found a relative risk of 2.37 (95% confidence interval [CI], 1.24–4.50) for PDAC and an estimated lifetime risk to age 80 years of 2% to 3% (95% CI, 1%–4%) for females and 1% to 4% for males (95% CI, 2%–5%). Risk of female breast cancer, ovarian cancer, and male breast cancer were all increased as well.[35]

Biallelic germline mutations in *BRCA1, BRCA2,* or *PALB2* cause Fanconi anemia, a severe condition with a shortened lifespan, short stature, bone marrow failure, and childhood malignancies among others.[36]

Similarly, heterozygous *ATM* mutations are associated with increased cancer risk, whereas biallelic germline mutations cause ataxia-telangiectasia. The prevalence of *ATM* mutations is estimated to range from 1:100 to 1:300. Risk of breast cancer, gastric cancer, colorectal cancer, and PDAC are elevated[37,38] with an odds ratio of 3.81 for PDAC (95% CI, 1.98–7.34) and an estimated lifetime risk of 3% to 5% in a population-based study.[39] *ATM* mutations are found in 3% of patients with familial PDAC[37] and 2.3% of unselected PDAC cases.[40] More recent studies have estimated the risk to be higher with a 9.5% lifetime risk until age 80 years.[41,42]

Mechanism. *BRCA1/2, PALB2*, and *ATM* encode for proteins that are part of the homologous recombination pathway responsible for repairing DNA after it suffers double-strand breaks. Double-strand DNA (dsDNA) breaks are recognized by protein complexes containing BRCA1 and ATM. ATM is a serine/threonine kinase that, upon activation by dsDNA breaks, delays cell cycle progression and promotes DNA repair through homologous recombination.[43] BRCA1 recruits PALB2 and BRCA2, and this in turn promotes DNA strand invasion into homologous sequences that serve as templates for repair.[44]

Given the critical role of these genes in repair of dsDNA damage, mutations in these genes create a vulnerability that can be exploited for treatment of associated cancers. Repair of single-strand DNA (ssDNA) breaks requires the enzyme PARP. When the activity of PARP is inhibited, ssDNA breaks become dsDNA breaks in dividing cells, and these dsDNA breaks can ordinarily fall back to repair by homologous recombination. However, cells defective in dsDNA repair machinery, such as cancers associated with mutations in dsDDR genes, do not have this option and therefore undergo apoptosis with PARP inhibition.[45] This selective vulnerability is the basis for use of PARP inhibitors as a therapeutic strategy for cancers associated with dsDDR gene mutations. Indeed, the PARP inhibitor olaparib has shown efficacy and is approved by the US Food and Drug Administration in the management of advanced PDAC with a *BRCA1/2* germline mutation after disease control for greater than 4 months on platinum-based therapy.[46]

Familial atypical multiple mole/melanoma: CDKN2A

Syndrome presentation. *CDKN2A* (formerly known as *p16*) mutations are associated with familial atypical multiple mole/melanoma (FAMMM) syndrome[47] and are thought to account for 10% to 40% of familial melanoma. This syndrome was originally characterized by the presence of multiple nevi (including some with atypia), certain features within the nevi, and family history of melanoma.[48]

A case report in 1995 described the first melanoma-PDAC family found to have a *p16* mutation.[49] Multiple studies since have showed that the combination of both melanoma and PDAC in a single individual had a higher chance of being related to *CDKN2A* mutation, and that *CDKN2A* mutations are responsible for a small but measurable fraction (<1%) of PDAC and thus should be included in any genetic testing for patients with PDAC.[5,14,16,25,26,40]

Researchers proposed that certain families have higher risk for PDAC than others, leading to a distinction between the 2 types, FAMMM-PC versus FAMMM.[50] There are also clearly PDAC families with *CDKN2A* mutations who do not have a history of melanoma, leading to the question of modifying factors.[51] It is widely known that environmental factors such as sun exposure can modify the risk of melanoma in families with FAMMM.[52] Similarly, specific genotypes may interact with environmental exposures such as tobacco to increase the risk of PDAC in families.[53]

Many additional types of cancers and tumors have been reported in families with FAMMM including astrocytomas, sarcomas, breast cancer, head and neck squamous cell cancer, lung cancer, neurofibroma, uveal melanoma, non-Hodgkin lymphoma, and glioblastoma multiforme.[54–57] For some of these, such as astrocytomas, there is a defined link, but most are less clearly related.

The mode of inheritance is autosomal dominant with incomplete penetrance and variable expressivity.

Mechanism. CDKN2A is a cyclin-dependent kinase inhibitor located on 9p21.3 considered to be a tumor suppressor gene. The gene has 4 exons: 1α, 1β, 2, and 3 and encodes 2 different isoforms known as p16 or p16-INK4a (encoded by exons 1α, 2, and 3) and p14ARF (encoded by exons 1β, 2, and 3).

The p16 isoform inhibits the ability of the CDK4/6-cyclin D complex to phosphorylate pRb, preventing the transition from G1 to S phase.[58,59] The p14ARF isoform inhibits human MDM2, which prevents ubiquitination and subsequent degradation of p53.[56,60,61]

Germline mutations of CDKN2A are often missense or nonsense mutations that impair the inhibitory functions of p16 and/or p14ARF, but all types of mutations have been described.[62] Moderate penetrance variants as well as common polymorphisms have been identified.[63]

Epidemiology. The prevalence of CDKN2A mutations is low in the general population, extrapolated to be about 1 in 10,000 in one population.[64] CDKN2A mutations are seen in about 2% of unselected melanoma cohorts and less than 1% of unselected PDAC cohorts but in much higher fractions of familial melanoma (10%–40%) and a small fraction (<5%) of familial PDAC cohorts.[56,65,66]

CDKN2A founder mutations have been described in multiple different ancestries.[67–73] The idea of specific genotype-phenotype correlations for PDAC risk has been postulated to involve variants affecting p16INK4A (with or without an effect on p14ARF).[62] Genetic modifiers of PDAC risk in these families are likely and warrant further research.

De novo mutations have been reported, but it is likely that most individuals with apparently sporadic PDAC found to have CDKN2A mutations inherited the mutation from a parent.[66,74]

Absolute lifetime risk. The most widely quoted absolute lifetime risk for PDAC is based on one older study of the p16-Leiden mutation (c.225_243del p.Ala76 fs) and is estimated to be 17% by age 75 years.[71] Whether this is truly representative of the general risk with CDKN2A mutations deserves further study. Pathogenic variants that affect only the p14ARF isoform may not confer an increased risk for PDAC.[62]

Peutz-Jeghers syndrome: STK11/LKB1
Syndrome presentation. STK11 (also known as LKB1) is associated with Peutz-Jeghers syndrome (PJS). A clinical diagnosis of PJS is made by a personal and family history of PJS-type hamartomatous polyps, characteristic mucocutaneous pigmentation, or a mutation in STK11 as delineated in a European consensus statement.[75]

Individuals and families with STK11 mutations have some of the highest risks for PDAC of any known genetic syndrome.[76–78]

The mode of inheritance is autosomal dominant with incomplete penetrance and variable expressivity.

Mechanism. *STK11* is a serine threonine kinase located on 19p13.3. *STK11* is ubiquitously expressed throughout the body, containing 433 amino acids and 9 coding exons as well as 1 noncoding exon. *STK11* is part of the mammalian target of rapamycin pathway; it acts as a tumor suppressor by regulating cell growth, metabolism, autophagy, and polarity.[79]

Epidemiology. Mutations in the *STK11* gene are responsible for the preponderance of people with PJS, but approximately 5% of families or individuals who meet clinical criteria remain unexplained.[80] Large rearrangements of this gene are present in approximately 15% to 30% of *STK11* mutation carriers.[81]

Genotype-phenotype correlations have been studied in relatively small cohorts with limited significance. Preliminary correlations include the following[80]:

- Truncating variants may have earlier onset of symptoms than missense variants.
- Exon 3 variants showed a trend toward a higher risk of malignancy, particularly for gastrointestinal cancer.
- Splice site variants may have a lower risk of malignancy.

The exact prevalence of de novo *STK11* mutations is unknown. In one study, de novo variants were found in ~24% of patients.[81] This rate may be higher in the pediatric population because children who present with intussusception may not have been followed due to family history.[82] Germline mosaicism has also been reported.[83]

Absolute lifetime risk. The absolute lifetime risk of PDAC is estimated to be in the range of 11% to 36% based on 2 studies. It is important to note that *STK11* was not analyzed in the large PDAC cohort described by Hu and colleagues.[40]

Li-Fraumeni syndrome: TP53
Syndrome presentation. *TP53* pmutations are associated with Li-Fraumeni syndrome (LFS). Originally described by Frederick Li and Joseph Fraumeni in 1969 as a "family cancer syndrome,"[84] it is characterized by high risk of pediatric and early-adult cancers.

A diagnosis of LFS and performing *TP53* gene mutation testing is considered for anyone with a personal and family history of tumors delineated by the Chompret, Birch, or Eeles criteria.[85–88]

The finding of a pathogenic TP53 variant in the absence of a strong personal and family history has been added to the criteria for a diagnosis of LFS, although there is debate about whether this should be given a different name.[89] PDAC has been reported in families with LFS and is part of Birch criteria for LFS.[87,90]

The mode of inheritance is autosomal dominant with incomplete penetrance and variable expressivity.

Mechanism. *TP53* was implicated in LFS in 1990.[91,92] *TP53* is a tumor suppressor gene located on 17p13.1; it has multiple roles in DNA repair, controlling cell growth and apoptosis, regulating metabolism, aging, homeostasis, immune function, and other processes.[93] More than half of all malignancies harbor *TP53* mutations.

The spectrum of pathogenic variants in *TP53* includes classic loss of function mutations, missense mutations that can have a dominant negative effect, as well as certain missense mutations with gain-of-function-like properties, knocking out DNA-binding capacity as well as favoring oncogenic activity.[94] Certain polymorphisms within and outside of *TP53* may also modify cancer risks and age at diagnosis.[95] There are moderate-penetrance variants as well as variants that seem to confer higher susceptibility to specific cancer types such as the R337H variant in Southern Brazil and its association with pediatric adrenocortical carcinomas.[96,97]

Epidemiology. The prevalence of *TP53* mutations in a gnomAD-based cohort is estimated to be between 1:3000 and 1:5000, but this may not be reflective of "clinical LFS," given the presence of low- and moderate-penetrance variants.[98–102] The de novo mutation rate is thought to be from 7% to 20%.[103]

Absolute lifetime risk. Increased risks for PDAC were noted in families with LFS with a relative risk of 7.3.[104] Different temporal phases in LFS have been postulated including a late adulthood phase (age 51–80 years) in which prostate and PDAC may be more prevalent.[105] PDAC occurs at a median age of 53 years versus 72 years in the Surveillance, Epidemiology, and End Results (SEER) data.[106] Hu and colleagues[40] in their 2018 pancreatic cohort described an odds ratio of 6.70. The absolute lifetime risk of PDAC is not well known in LFS. However, a recent presentation by Hatton and colleagues (PMID 35366121) at the Collaborative Group of the Americas on an NCI LFS cohort of 510 individuals estimated the lifetime risk as 7.3% by age 70 years.

Lynch syndrome: MLH1, MSH2, MSH6, PMS2, EPCAM
Syndrome presentation. LS (formerly called hereditary nonpolyposis colorectal cancer) is the most common inherited form of colorectal and endometrial cancer. Tumors in patients with LS show characteristic MMR deficiency and microsatellite instability (MSI). Assessment for MSI is standard in somatic analysis for the purposes of targeted therapies. LS-related cancers include colorectal, endometrial, gastric, ovarian, pancreas, urothelial, brain (usually glioblastoma), biliary tract, small intestine, sebaceous tumors, and keratoacanthomas.

Current NCCN (National Comprehensive Cancer Network) criteria (v1.2021) for the evaluation of LS include personal or family history of a tumor with MMR deficiency and early-onset colorectal or endometrial cancer.[107]

The mode of inheritance is autosomal dominant with incomplete penetrance and variable expressivity.

Mechanism. There are 5 causative genes established as LS genes: *MLH1* (3p22.2), *MSH2* (2p21-p.16.3), *MSH6* (2p16.3), *PMS2* (7p22.1), and *EPCAM* (2p21). Four of the five (all but *EPCAM*) are directly involved in DNA MMR. This process is a proofreading system that consists of multiple parts including recognition of mismatched bases, excision, resynthesis of the appropriate bases, and ligation of the DNA. Deletions at the end of *EPCAM* are thought to cause transcriptional read-through of *MSH2* leading to methylation and silencing. Another rare cause of LS is through germline methylation of the *MLH1* gene.

Tumor development in LS is believed to follow the 2-hit model, where loss of the remaining normal copy of the gene through somatic changes can lead to MMR deficiency, MSI, and high mutational burden. Importantly, the accumulation of mutation-associated neoantigens in MMR-deficient PDAC may promote immune cell infiltration and thus create a unique vulnerability to ICB. Indeed, colorectal cancer contains 10 to 100 times the mutation burden when associated with MSI,[108] and early evidence supports a benefit of ICB for MMR-deficient cancers.[109] Ongoing studies are evaluating the response of MMR-deficient PDAC to ICB.[110]

Epidemiology. The prevalence of LS is estimated to about 1 in 279 in the general population: 0.051% (1:1946) for *MLH1* mutations, 0.035% (1:2841) for *MSH2* mutations, 0.132% (1:758) for *MSH6* mutations, and 0.140% (1:714) for *PMS2* mutations.

Of these genes, *MLH1* and *MSH2* mutations are associated with the highest risks for colonic and extracolonic cancers. *MSH6* pathogenic variants are associated with a higher risk for gynecologic cancers and later ages of diagnosis, and *PMS2* pathogenic variants are associated with the lowest risks for cancer. Founder mutations are described in multiple ancestries, and de novo pathogenic variants have been reported in up to 1 in 45 individuals ($\sim$2.2%).

Absolute lifetime risk. The lifetime risk of PDAC is not well established in families with LS. One study estimated a lifetime risk of 3.68% by age 70 years for all carriers of *MLH1*, *MSH2*, and *MSH6* mutations (vs 0.52% by age 70 years in SEER) but the number of *MSH6*-associated PDACs was small.[111] The largest PDAC cohort to date[40] showed a statistically significant increased risk for *MLH1* mutation carriers and increased risks for *MSH2* and *MSH6* carriers that were not statistically significant compared with gnomAD controls. Unaffected individuals are estimated to have a 0.95% 10-year cumulative risk of PDAC.[112] Although data on *PMS2* families are limited, carriers do not seem to have an increased risk for PDAC.

Germline Genetic Risk Factors for Pancreatitis

Pancreatitis is a well-established risk factor for PDAC. Not surprisingly, germline mutations associated with hereditary pancreatitis also confer an increased lifetime risk of PDAC. In particular, mutations in genes that dysregulate trypsinogen activity and degradation (*PRSS1*, *SPINK1*), cause misfolding of digestive enzymes and endoplasmic reticulum (ER) stress in acinar cells (*CPA1*, *CPB1*, *CTRC*), dysregulate calcium signaling in exocrine pancreas cells (*CASR*), and disrupt pancreatic duct secretions (*CFTR*) have been associated with risk of pancreatitis.[113–116] In a cohort of 200 patients with a clinical history of hereditary pancreatitis or a known mutation in *PRSS1*, PDAC occurred with a standardized incidence ratio of 87 (95% CI, 42–114).[117] In another study, approximately 1% of PDAC cases were found to have otherwise rare germline mutations in the genes *CPA1* and *CPB1* resulting in misfolding of the digestive enzyme carboxypeptidase and ER stress in acinar cells,[118] consistent with these mutations contributing to PDAC risk. However, the penetrance of these mutations for pancreatitis is variable and thought to have significant genetic and environmental modifiers.[119] Furthermore, the significance of these mutations to lifetime PDAC risk in the absence of a clinical history of pancreatitis remains unclear. Therefore, germline testing of these genes associated with pancreatitis is considered only when there is a history suggestive of hereditary pancreatitis.[19] Likewise, if these germline mutations are found incidentally, pancreas surveillance with MRCP and EUS is generally recommended if there is a history suggestive of hereditary pancreatitis.[19]

Counseling on Genetic Testing

Genetic counseling and testing for PDAC predisposition are important in providing hope for affected families. Knowledge of a genetic mutation in the family can help define risk in family members and allow for earlier detection of PDAC as well as improved screening and prevention for associated cancers.[17,120] Patients with PDAC who are tested and found to have high-risk mutations share this information with family members, but uptake of genetic testing in relatives ("cascade testing") is still low.[121,122] In families that meet the definition of familial PDAC without a defined mutation, it is still important for close relatives of patients with PDAC to be aware of increased risks and the availability of screening.

Families with PDAC face special psychosocial issues, including the feeling that the diagnosis is inevitable and unchangeable.[123] There are, however, important interventions that can be made, and with the support of all providers involved in the care of patients with PDAC and their families, the discovery of hereditary and familial risk can empower them to change the course of this disease.

Future Directions

Current germline genetic testing for PDAC predisposition focuses on the causes listed in **Table 1**. These known causal genes are estimated to account for only ~10% to 20% of PDAC family clusters.[2,14,15] Although not yet demonstrated, it is likely that rare undiscovered high-effect germline mutations, polygenic variants that may be more common and low-effect size, and shared environmental causes may explain other PDAC family clusters.

Discovery of novel germline causes has several challenges. Often, by the time a PDAC family syndrome is recognized, affected relatives have deceased before samples can be collected for genome analysis. Moreover, rare or even private variants can cosegregate with PDAC within a family by chance, and so mechanistic and functional analysis may be required to validate causality. To identify novel candidate monogenic germline causes, a genomic survey of 638 patients with familial PDAC (defined as families with at least 2 affected first-degree relatives) revealed an average of hundreds of thousands of insertions and deletions per individual, including 6114 premature truncating variants in 4553 genes,[14] illustrating the challenges of novel causal gene discovery without family segregation analysis and functional validation. A recent genomic analysis of 2 affected individuals in a family with 5 cases uncovered a rare gain-of-function mutation in the gene RABL3 p.Ser36* not previously associated with cancer predisposition. The heterozygous mutation results in premature truncation of RABL3 and cosegregated with cancer in the family. Consistent with a robust impact on cancer risk, the gain-of-function p.Ser36* RABL3 mutation has a very rare allele frequency 0.00001591 on the GnomAD database and has not been detected in other PDAC cohorts.[124,125] Furthermore, recapitulating the heterozygous mutation in zebrafish resulted in cancer predisposition in adult populations, supporting the causality of the mutation. The RABL3 protein accelerates intracellular trafficking of KRAS, the most common oncogenic driver in PDAC,[126] and somatic overexpression of RABL3 has been associated with PDAC[127] and other cancers including hepatocellular cancer[128] and non–small cell lung cancer.[129] Thus, although rare, discovery of this and other germline causes in familial PDAC has potential to uncover important and broadly relevant insights in cancer biology.

Familial clustering of PDAC may also result from shared cumulative effects of multiple germline variants, each of which may have small effect size and be more common in the general population. Indeed, genome-wide association studies (GWAS) have demonstrated that polygenic variants account for much of the heritable risk of diseases such as myocardial infarction.[130,131] For several diseases including breast cancer, genome-wide polygenic risk scores (PRS) have been generated to provide a single, normally distributed quantification of disease risk based on the cumulative impact of these common variants.[132] GWAS for PDAC have implicated several loci in modulating risk,[133–136] but this polygenic architecture has yet to be translated into a PRS with clinical utility comparable to monogenic germline testing.

Discovery of new pathways that modulate PDAC risk, both high-effect monogenic causes identified in PDAC families and more common low-effect variants implicated by GWAS, will continue to enhance our risk stratification in the clinic. The application of this information will also critically require integration with environmental risk factors, ethnicity differences, and other nongenetic modifiers. Finally, as best illustrated with the use of PARP inhibition for treatment of PDAC associated with DDR mutations or the use of ICB for treatment of PDAC associated with LS, a deep mechanistic understanding of how germline causes modulate PDAC risk has the potential to unveil new strategies for personalized medicine.

REFERENCES

1. Cancer Genome Atlas Research Network. Electronic address aadhe, Cancer Genome Atlas Research N. Integrated Genomic Characterization of Pancreatic Ductal Adenocarcinoma. Cancer cell 2017;32(2):185–203.e13.
2. Grant RC, Selander I, Connor AA, et al. Prevalence of germline mutations in cancer predisposition genes in patients with pancreatic cancer. Gastroenterology 2015;148(3):556–64.
3. Holter S, Borgida A, Dodd A, et al. Germline BRCA Mutations in a Large Clinic-Based Cohort of Patients With Pancreatic Adenocarcinoma. J Clin Oncol 2015; 33(28):3124–9.
4. Hu C, Hart SN, Bamlet WR, et al. Prevalence of Pathogenic Mutations in Cancer Predisposition Genes among Pancreatic Cancer Patients. Cancer Epidemiol Biomarkers Prev 2016;25(1):207–11.
5. Shindo K, Yu J, Suenaga M, et al. Deleterious Germline Mutations in Patients With Apparently Sporadic Pancreatic Adenocarcinoma. J Clin Oncol 2017; 35(30):3382–90.
6. Salo-Mullen EE, O'Reilly EM, Kelsen DP, et al. Identification of germline genetic mutations in patients with pancreatic cancer. Cancer 2015;121(24):4382–8.
7. Dat NM, Sontag SJ. Pancreatic carcinoma in brothers. Ann Intern Med 1982; 97(2):282.
8. Ehrenthal D, Haeger L, Griffin T, et al. Familial pancreatic adenocarcinoma in three generations. A case report and a review of the literature. Cancer 1987; 59(9):1661–4.
9. Friedman JM, Fialkow PJ. Familial carcinoma of the pancreas. Clin Genet 1976; 9(5):463–9.
10. Ghadirian P, Simard A, Baillargeon J. Cancer of the pancreas in two brothers and one sister. Int J Pancreatol 1987;2(5–6):383–91.
11. MacDermott RP, Kramer P. Adenocarcinoma of the pancreas in four siblings. Gastroenterology 1973;65(1):137–9.
12. Petersen GM. Familial Pancreatic Adenocarcinoma. Hematol Oncol Clin North Am 2015;29(4):641–53.
13. Klein AP, Brune KA, Petersen GM, et al. Prospective risk of pancreatic cancer in familial pancreatic cancer kindreds. Cancer Res 2004;64(7):2634–8.
14. Roberts NJ, Norris AL, Petersen G, et al. Whole genome sequencing defines the genetic heterogeneity of familial pancreatic cancer. Cancer Discov 2015. https://doi.org/10.1158/2159-8290.CD-15-0402.
15. Chaffee KG, Oberg AL, McWilliams RR, et al. Prevalence of germ-line mutations in cancer genes among pancreatic cancer patients with a positive family history. Genet Med 2018;20(1):119–27.
16. Yurgelun MB, Chittenden AB, Morales-Oyarvide V, et al. Germline cancer susceptibility gene variants, somatic second hits, and survival outcomes in patients with resected pancreatic cancer. Genet Med 2019;21(1):213–23.
17. Goggins M, Overbeek KA, Brand R, et al. Management of patients with increased risk for familial pancreatic cancer: updated recommendations from the International Cancer of the Pancreas Screening (CAPS) Consortium. Gut 2020;69(1):7–17.

18. Stoffel EM, McKernin SE, Brand R, et al. Evaluating Susceptibility to Pancreatic Cancer: ASCO Provisional Clinical Opinion. J Clin Oncol 2019;37(2):153–64.

19. NCCN Genetic/Familial High-Risk Assessment: Breast, Ovarian, and Pancreatic Cancer. 2021. Available at: https://www.nccn.org/professionals/physician_gls/pdf/genetics_bop.pdf. Accessed December 1, 2021.

20. Breast Cancer Linkage C. Cancer risks in BRCA2 mutation carriers. J Natl Cancer Inst 1999;91(15):1310–6.

21. Murphy KM, Brune KA, Griffin C, et al. Evaluation of candidate genes MAP2K4, MADH4, ACVR1B, and BRCA2 in familial pancreatic cancer: deleterious BRCA2 mutations in 17. Cancer Res 2002;62(13):3789–93.

22. Hahn SA, Greenhalf B, Ellis I, et al. BRCA2 germline mutations in familial pancreatic carcinoma. J Natl Cancer Inst 2003;95(3):214–21.

23. Zhen DB, Rabe KG, Gallinger S, et al. BRCA1, BRCA2, PALB2, and CDKN2A mutations in familial pancreatic cancer: a PACGENE study. Genet Med 2015;17(7):569–77.

24. Couch FJ, Johnson MR, Rabe KG, et al. The prevalence of BRCA2 mutations in familial pancreatic cancer. Cancer Epidemiol Biomarkers Prev 2007;16(2):342–6.

25. Brand R, Borazanci E, Speare V, et al. Prospective study of germline genetic testing in incident cases of pancreatic adenocarcinoma. Cancer 2018;124(17):3520–7.

26. Lowery MA, Wong W, Jordan EJ, et al. Prospective Evaluation of Germline Alterations in Patients With Exocrine Pancreatic Neoplasms. J Natl Cancer Inst 2018;110(10):1067–74.

27. Prevalence and penetrance of BRCA1 and BRCA2 mutations in a population-based series of breast cancer cases. Anglian Breast Cancer Study Group. Br J Cancer 2000;83(10):1301–8.

28. Offit K, Gilewski T, McGuire P, et al. Germline BRCA1 185delAG mutations in Jewish women with breast cancer. Lancet 1996;347(9016):1643–5.

29. van Dijk S, Otten W, Timmermans DR, et al. What's the message? Interpretation of an uninformative BRCA1/2 test result for women at risk of familial breast cancer. Genet Med 2005;7(4):239–45.

30. Brose MS, Rebbeck TR, Calzone KA, et al. Cancer risk estimates for BRCA1 mutation carriers identified in a risk evaluation program. J Natl Cancer Inst 2002;94(18):1365–72.

31. Thompson D, Easton DF, Breast Cancer Linkage C. Cancer Incidence in BRCA1 mutation carriers. J Natl Cancer Inst 2002;94(18):1358–65.

32. Tischkowitz MD, Sabbaghian N, Hamel N, et al. Analysis of the gene coding for the BRCA2-interacting protein PALB2 in familial and sporadic pancreatic cancer. Gastroenterology 2009;137(3):1183–6.

33. Slater EP, Langer P, Niemczyk E, et al. PALB2 mutations in European familial pancreatic cancer families. Clin Genet 2010;78(5):490–4.

34. Hofstatter EW, Domchek SM, Miron A, et al. PALB2 mutations in familial breast and pancreatic cancer. Fam Cancer 2011;10(2):225–31.

35. Yang X, Leslie G, Doroszuk A, et al. Cancer Risks Associated With Germline PALB2 Pathogenic Variants: An International Study of 524 Families. J Clin Oncol 2020;38(7):674–85.

36. Kutler DI, Singh B, Satagopan J, et al. A 20-year perspective on the International Fanconi Anemia Registry (IFAR). Blood 2003;101(4):1249–56.

37. Roberts NJ, Jiao Y, Yu J, et al. ATM mutations in patients with hereditary pancreatic cancer. Cancer Discov 2012;2(1):41–6.

38. Marabelli M, Cheng SC, Parmigiani G. Penetrance of ATM Gene Mutations in Breast Cancer: A Meta-Analysis of Different Measures of Risk. Genet Epidemiol 2016;40(5):425–31.

39. Helgason H, Rafnar T, Olafsdottir HS, et al. Loss-of-function variants in ATM confer risk of gastric cancer. Nat Genet 2015;47(8):906–10.

40. Hu C, Hart SN, Polley EC, et al. Association Between Inherited Germline Mutations in Cancer Predisposition Genes and Risk of Pancreatic Cancer. Jama 2018;319(23):2401–9.

41. Hall MJ, Bernhisel R, Hughes E, et al. Germline Pathogenic Variants in the Ataxia Telangiectasia Mutated (ATM) Gene are Associated with High and Moderate Risks for Multiple Cancers. Cancer Prev Res (Phila) 2021;14(4):433–40.

42. Hsu FC, Roberts NJ, Childs E, et al. Risk of Pancreatic Cancer Among Individuals With Pathogenic Variants in the ATM Gene. JAMA Oncol 2021;7(11):1664–8.

43. Rustgi AK. Familial pancreatic cancer: genetic advances. Genes Dev 2014;28(1):1–7.

44. Lord CJ, Ashworth A. BRCAness revisited. Nat Rev Cancer 2016;16(2):110–20.

45. O'Connor MJ. Targeting the DNA Damage Response in Cancer. Mol Cell 2015;60(4):547–60.

46. Golan T, Locker GY, Kindler HL. Maintenance Olaparib for Metastatic Pancreatic Cancer. Reply. N Engl J Med 2019;381(15):1492–3.

47. Hussussian CJ, Struewing JP, Goldstein AM, et al. Germline p16 mutations in familial melanoma. Nat Genet 1994;8(1):15–21.

48. Goldstein AM, Chan M, Harland M, et al. Features associated with germline CDKN2A mutations: a GenoMEL study of melanoma-prone families from three continents. J Med Genet 2007;44(2):99–106.

49. Whelan AJ, Bartsch D, Goodfellow PJ. Brief report: a familial syndrome of pancreatic cancer and melanoma with a mutation in the CDKN2 tumor-suppressor gene. N Engl J Med 1995;333(15):975–7.

50. Lynch HT, Brand RE, Hogg D, et al. Phenotypic variation in eight extended CDKN2A germline mutation familial atypical multiple mole melanoma-pancreatic carcinoma-prone families: the familial atypical mole melanoma-pancreatic carcinoma syndrome. Cancer 2002;94(1):84–96.

51. Cremin C, Howard S, Le L, et al. CDKN2A founder mutation in pancreatic ductal adenocarcinoma patients without cutaneous features of Familial Atypical Multiple Mole Melanoma (FAMMM) syndrome. Hered Cancer Clin Pract 2018;16:7.

52. Chaudru V, Chompret A, Bressac-de Paillerets B, et al. Influence of genes, nevi, and sun sensitivity on melanoma risk in a family sample unselected by family history and in melanoma-prone families. J Natl Cancer Inst 2004;96(10):785–95.

53. Helgadottir H, Hoiom V, Jonsson G, et al. High risk of tobacco-related cancers in CDKN2A mutation-positive melanoma families. J Med Genet 2014;51(8):545–52.

54. Kaufman DK, Kimmel DW, Parisi JE, et al. A familial syndrome with cutaneous malignant melanoma and cerebral astrocytoma. Neurology 1993;43(9):1728–31.

55. Bahuau M, Vidaud D, Jenkins RB, et al. Germ-line deletion involving the INK4 locus in familial proneness to melanoma and nervous system tumors. Cancer Res 1998;58(11):2298–303.

56. Soura E, Eliades PJ, Shannon K, et al. Hereditary melanoma: Update on syndromes and management: Genetics of familial atypical multiple mole melanoma syndrome. J Am Acad Dermatol 2016;74(3):395–407 [quiz: 408-10].

57. Goldstein AM, Chan M, Harland M, et al. High-risk melanoma susceptibility genes and pancreatic cancer, neural system tumors, and uveal melanoma across GenoMEL. Cancer Res 2006;66(20):9818–28.

58. Rayess H, Wang MB, Srivatsan ES. Cellular senescence and tumor suppressor gene p16. Int J Cancer 2012;130(8):1715–25.

59. Li Y, Nichols MA, Shay JW, et al. Transcriptional repression of the D-type cyclin-dependent kinase inhibitor p16 by the retinoblastoma susceptibility gene product pRb. Cancer Res 1994;54(23):6078–82.

60. Foulkes WD, Flanders TY, Pollock PM, et al. The CDKN2A (p16) gene and human cancer. Mol Med 1997;3(1):5–20.

61. Stott FJ, Bates S, James MC, et al. The alternative product from the human CDKN2A locus, p14(ARF), participates in a regulatory feedback loop with p53 and MDM2. EMBO J 1998;17(17):5001–14.

62. Chan SH, Chiang J, Ngeow J. CDKN2A germline alterations and the relevance of genotype-phenotype associations in cancer predisposition. Hered Cancer Clin Pract 2021;19(1):21.

63. McWilliams RR, Wieben ED, Chaffee KG, et al. CDKN2A Germline Rare Coding Variants and Risk of Pancreatic Cancer in Minority Populations. Cancer Epidemiol Biomarkers Prev 2018;27(11):1364–70.

64. Aoude LG, Gartside M, Johansson P, et al. Prevalence of Germline BAP1, CDKN2A, and CDK4 Mutations in an Australian Population-Based Sample of Cutaneous Melanoma Cases. Twin Res Hum Genet 2015;18(2):126–33.

65. Harland M, Cust AE, Badenas C, et al. Prevalence and predictors of germline CDKN2A mutations for melanoma cases from Australia, Spain and the United Kingdom. Hered Cancer Clin Pract 2014;12(1):20.

66. Kimura H, Klein AP, Hruban RH, et al. The Role of Inherited Pathogenic CDKN2A Variants in Susceptibility to Pancreatic Cancer. Pancreas 2021;50(8):1123–30.

67. Lang J, Hayward N, Goldgar D, et al. The M53I mutation in CDKN2A is a founder mutation that predominates in melanoma patients with Scottish ancestry. Genes Chromosomes Cancer 2007;46(3):277–87.

68. Gensini F, Sestini R, Piazzini M, et al. The p.G23S CDKN2A founder mutation in high-risk melanoma families from Central Italy. Melanoma Res 2007;17(6):387–92.

69. Goldstein AM, Liu L, Shennan MG, et al. A common founder for the V126D CDKN2A mutation in seven North American melanoma-prone families. Br J Cancer 2001;85(4):527–30.

70. Hashemi J, Bendahl PO, Sandberg T, et al. Haplotype analysis and age estimation of the 113insR CDKN2A founder mutation in Swedish melanoma families. Genes Chromosomes Cancer 2001;31(2):107–16.

71. Vasen HF, Gruis NA, Frants RR, et al. Risk of developing pancreatic cancer in families with familial atypical multiple mole melanoma associated with a specific 19 deletion of p16 (p16-Leiden). Int J Cancer 2000;87(6):809–11.

72. Ciotti P, Struewing JP, Mantelli M, et al. A single genetic origin for the G101W CDKN2A mutation in 20 melanoma-prone families. Am J Hum Genet 2000;67(2):311–9.

73. Goldstein AM, Stacey SN, Olafsson JH, et al. CDKN2A mutations and melanoma risk in the Icelandic population. J Med Genet 2008;45(5):284–9.

74. Frigerio S, Disciglio V, Manoukian S, et al. A large de novo 9p21.3 deletion in a girl affected by astrocytoma and multiple melanoma. BMC Med Genet 2014;15:59.

75. Beggs AD, Latchford AR, Vasen HF, et al. Peutz-Jeghers syndrome: a systematic review and recommendations for management. Gut 2010;59(7):975–86.
76. van Lier MG, Wagner A, Mathus-Vliegen EM, et al. High cancer risk in Peutz-Jeghers syndrome: a systematic review and surveillance recommendations. Am J Gastroenterol 2010;105(6):1258–64 [author reply: 1265].
77. Giardiello FM, Brensinger JD, Tersmette AC, et al. Very high risk of cancer in familial Peutz-Jeghers syndrome. Gastroenterology 2000;119(6):1447–53.
78. Hearle N, Schumacher V, Menko FH, et al. Frequency and spectrum of cancers in the Peutz-Jeghers syndrome. Clin Cancer Res 2006;12(10):3209–15.
79. Momcilovic M, Shackelford DB. Targeting LKB1 in cancer - exposing and exploiting vulnerabilities. Br J Cancer 2015;113(4):574–84.
80. Daniell J, Plazzer JP, Perera A, et al. An exploration of genotype-phenotype link between Peutz-Jeghers syndrome and STK11: a review. Fam Cancer 2018; 17(3):421–7.
81. Aretz S, Stienen D, Uhlhaas S, et al. High proportion of large genomic STK11 deletions in Peutz-Jeghers syndrome. Hum Mutat 2005;26(6):513–9.
82. Zhao HM, Yang YJ, Duan JQ, et al. Clinical and Genetic Study of Children With Peutz-Jeghers Syndrome Identifies a High Frequency of STK11 De Novo Mutation. J Pediatr Gastroenterol Nutr 2019;68(2):199–206.
83. Butel-Simoes GI, Spigelman AD, Scott RJ, et al. Low-level parental mosaicism in an apparent de novo case of Peutz-Jeghers syndrome. Fam Cancer 2019;18(1): 109–12.
84. Li FP, Fraumeni JF Jr. Soft-tissue sarcomas, breast cancer, and other neoplasms. A familial syndrome? Ann Intern Med 1969;71(4):747–52.
85. Chompret A, Abel A, Stoppa-Lyonnet D, et al. Sensitivity and predictive value of criteria for p53 germline mutation screening. J Med Genet 2001;38(1):43–7.
86. Tinat J, Bougeard G, Baert-Desurmont S, et al. 2009 version of the Chompret criteria for Li Fraumeni syndrome. J Clin Oncol 2009;27(26):e108–9 [author reply: e110].
87. Birch JM, Alston RD, McNally RJ, et al. Relative frequency and morphology of cancers in carriers of germline TP53 mutations. Oncogene 2001;20(34):4621–8.
88. Eeles RA. Germline mutations in the TP53 gene. Cancer Surv 1995;25:101–24.
89. Frebourg T, Bajalica Lagercrantz S, Oliveira C, et al. European Reference Network G. Guidelines for the Li-Fraumeni and heritable TP53-related cancer syndromes. Eur J Hum Genet 2020;28(10):1379–86.
90. Mai PL, Best AF, Peters JA, et al. Risks of first and subsequent cancers among TP53 mutation carriers in the National Cancer Institute Li-Fraumeni syndrome cohort. Cancer 2016;122(23):3673–81.
91. Malkin D, Li FP, Strong LC, et al. Germ line p53 mutations in a familial syndrome of breast cancer, sarcomas, and other neoplasms. Science 1990;250(4985): 1233–8.
92. Srivastava S, Zou ZQ, Pirollo K, et al. Germ-line transmission of a mutated p53 gene in a cancer-prone family with Li-Fraumeni syndrome. Nature 1990; 348(6303):747–9.
93. Kastenhuber ER, Lowe SW. Putting p53 in Context. Cell 2017;170(6):1062–78.
94. Gargallo P, Yanez Y, Segura V, et al. Li-Fraumeni syndrome heterogeneity. Clin Transl Oncol 2020;22(7):978–88.
95. Guha T, Malkin D. Inherited TP53 Mutations and the Li-Fraumeni Syndrome. Cold Spring Harb Perspect Med 2017;7(4). https://doi.org/10.1101/cshperspect.a026187.

96. Kratz CP, Freycon C, Maxwell KN, et al. Analysis of the Li-Fraumeni Spectrum Based on an International Germline TP53 Variant Data Set: An International Agency for Research on Cancer TP53 Database Analysis. JAMA Oncol 2021; 7(12):1800–5.

97. Ferreira AM, Brondani VB, Helena VP, et al. Clinical spectrum of Li-Fraumeni syndrome/Li-Fraumeni-like syndrome in Brazilian individuals with the TP53 p.R337H mutation. J Steroid Biochem Mol Biol 2019;190:250–5.

98. de Andrade KC, Frone MN, Wegman-Ostrosky T, et al. Variable population prevalence estimates of germline TP53 variants: A gnomAD-based analysis. Hum Mutat 2019;40(1):97–105.

99. Bougeard G, Renaux-Petel M, Flaman JM, et al. Revisiting Li-Fraumeni Syndrome From TP53 Mutation Carriers. J Clin Oncol 2015;33(21):2345–52.

100. Hanson H, Brady AF, Crawford G, et al. UKCGG Consensus Group guidelines for the management of patients with constitutional TP53 pathogenic variants. J Med Genet 2020. https://doi.org/10.1136/jmedgenet-2020-106876.

101. Batalini F, Peacock EG, Stobie L, et al. Li-Fraumeni syndrome: not a straightforward diagnosis anymore-the interpretation of pathogenic variants of low allele frequency and the differences between germline PVs, mosaicism, and clonal hematopoiesis. Breast Cancer Res 2019;21(1):107.

102. Leroy B, Anderson M, Soussi T. TP53 mutations in human cancer: database reassessment and prospects for the next decade. Hum Mutat 2014;35(6):672–88.

103. Gonzalez KD, Buzin CH, Noltner KA, et al. High frequency of de novo mutations in Li-Fraumeni syndrome. J Med Genet 2009;46(10):689–93.

104. Ruijs MW, Verhoef S, Rookus MA, et al. TP53 germline mutation testing in 180 families suspected of Li-Fraumeni syndrome: mutation detection rate and relative frequency of cancers in different familial phenotypes. J Med Genet 2010; 47(6):421–8.

105. Amadou A, Achatz MIW, Hainaut P. Revisiting tumor patterns and penetrance in germline TP53 mutation carriers: temporal phases of Li-Fraumeni syndrome. Curr Opin Oncol 2018;30(1):23–9.

106. Cancer Stat Facts: Pancreatic Cancer. National Cancer Institute. 2020. Available at: https://seer.cancer.gov/statfacts/html/pancreas.html. Accessed November 20, 2021.

107. NCCN Genetic/Familial High-Risk Assessment: Colorectal Cancer. 2021. Available at: https://www.nccn.org/professionals/physician_gls/pdf/genetics_colon. pdf. Accessed December 1, 2021.

108. Cancer Genome Atlas N. Comprehensive molecular characterization of human colon and rectal cancer. Nature 2012;487(7407):330–7.

109. Le DT, Durham JN, Smith KN, et al. Mismatch repair deficiency predicts response of solid tumors to PD-1 blockade. Science 2017;357(6349):409–13.

110. Ghidini M, Lampis A, Mirchev MB, et al. Immune-Based Therapies and the Role of Microsatellite Instability in Pancreatic Cancer. Genes (Basel) 2020;12(1).

111. Kastrinos F, Mukherjee B, Tayob N, et al. Risk of pancreatic cancer in families with Lynch syndrome. Jama 2009;302(16):1790–5.

112. Win AK, Young JP, Lindor NM, et al. Colorectal and other cancer risks for carriers and noncarriers from families with a DNA mismatch repair gene mutation: a prospective cohort study. J Clin Oncol 2012;30(9):958–64.

113. Whitcomb DC. Genetic risk factors for pancreatic disorders. Gastroenterology 2013;144(6):1292–302.

114. Rosendahl J, Witt H, Szmola R, et al. Chymotrypsin C (CTRC) variants that diminish activity or secretion are associated with chronic pancreatitis. Nat Genet 2008;40(1):78–82.
115. Witt H, Beer S, Rosendahl J, et al. Variants in CPA1 are strongly associated with early onset chronic pancreatitis. Nat Genet 2013;45(10):1216–20.
116. Lowenfels AB, Maisonneuve P, DiMagno EP, et al. Hereditary pancreatitis and the risk of pancreatic cancer. International Hereditary Pancreatitis Study Group. J Natl Cancer Inst 1997;89(6):442–6.
117. Rebours V, Boutron-Ruault MC, Schnee M, et al. Risk of pancreatic adenocarcinoma in patients with hereditary pancreatitis: a national exhaustive series. Am J Gastroenterol 2008;103(1):111–9.
118. Tamura K, Yu J, Hata T, et al. Mutations in the pancreatic secretory enzymes CPA1 and CPB1 are associated with pancreatic cancer. Proc Natl Acad Sci U S A 2018;115(18):4767–72.
119. Hasan A, Moscoso DI, Kastrinos F. The Role of Genetics in Pancreatitis. Gastrointest Endosc Clin N Am 2018;28(4):587–603.
120. Biller LH, Wolpin BM, Goggins M. Inherited Pancreatic Cancer Syndromes and High-Risk Screening. Surg Oncol Clin N Am 2021;30(4):773–86.
121. Peters MLB, Stobie L, Dudley B, et al. Family communication and patient distress after germline genetic testing in individuals with pancreatic ductal adenocarcinoma. Cancer 2019;125(14):2488–96.
122. Wang Y, Golesworthy B, Cuggia A, et al. Oncology clinic-based germline genetic testing for exocrine pancreatic cancer enables timely return of results and unveils low uptake of cascade testing. J Med Genet 2021. https://doi.org/10.1136/jmedgenet-2021-108054.
123. Underhill M, Berry D, Dalton E, et al. Patient experiences living with pancreatic cancer risk. Hered Cancer Clin Pract 2015;13(1):13.
124. Puzzono M, Crippa S, Zuppardo RA, et al. Low-frequency of RABL3 pathogenetic variants in hereditary and familial pancreatic cancer. Dig Liver Dis 2021;53(4):519–21.
125. Roberts NJ, Grant RC, Gallinger S, et al. Familial Pancreatic Cancer Genome Sequencing P. Germline sequence analysis of RABL3 in a large series of pancreatic ductal adenocarcinoma patients reveals no evidence of deleterious variants. Genes Chromosomes Cancer 2021;60(8):559–64.
126. Nissim S, Leshchiner I, Mancias JD, et al. Mutations in RABL3 alter KRAS prenylation and are associated with hereditary pancreatic cancer. Nat Genet 2019;51(9):1308–14.
127. 2021. Available at: http://gepia.cancer-pku.cn/detail.php?gene=RABL3. Accessed December 20, 2021.
128. An J, Liu Z, Liang Q, et al. Overexpression of Rabl3 and Cullin7 is associated with pathogenesis and poor prognosis in hepatocellular carcinoma. Hum Pathol 2017;67:146–51.
129. Zhang W, Sun J, Luo J. High Expression of Rab-like 3 (Rabl3) is Associated with Poor Survival of Patients with Non-Small Cell Lung Cancer via Repression of MAPK8/9/10-Mediated Autophagy. Med Sci Monit 2016;22:1582–8.
130. Golan D, Lander ES, Rosset S. Measuring missing heritability: inferring the contribution of common variants. Proc Natl Acad Sci U S A 2014;111(49):E5272–81.
131. Gibson G. Rare and common variants: twenty arguments. Nat Rev Genet 2012;13(2):135–45.

132. Khera AV, Chaffin M, Aragam KG, et al. Genome-wide polygenic scores for common diseases identify individuals with risk equivalent to monogenic mutations. Nat Genet 2018;50(9):1219–24.

133. Amundadottir L, Kraft P, Stolzenberg-Solomon RZ, et al. Genome-wide association study identifies variants in the ABO locus associated with susceptibility to pancreatic cancer. Nat Genet 2009;41(9):986–90.

134. Petersen GM, Amundadottir L, Fuchs CS, et al. A genome-wide association study identifies pancreatic cancer susceptibility loci on chromosomes 13q22.1, 1q32.1 and 5p15.33. Nat Genet 2010;42(3):224–8.

135. Wolpin BM, Rizzato C, Kraft P, et al. Genome-wide association study identifies multiple susceptibility loci for pancreatic cancer. Nat Genet 2014;46(9):994-1000.

136. Wu C, Kraft P, Stolzenberg-Solomon R, et al. Genome-wide association study of survival in patients with pancreatic adenocarcinoma. Gut 2014;63(1):152–60.

Decision-Making Regarding Perioperative Therapy in Individuals with Localized Pancreatic Adenocarcinoma

Malvi Savani, MD, Rachna T. Shroff, MD, MS*

KEYWORDS

• Pancreatic adenocarcinoma • Perioperative therapy • Systemic therapy

KEY POINTS

- With the rising annual incidence of pancreatic cancer, the need to strategize multimodality treatment methods to improve clinical outcomes is crucial.
- Enhancement of imaging modality, surgical techniques, and biomarker analysis is crucial in optimizing and individualizing the treatment of localized pancreatic cancer.
- Innovative therapeutic approaches including novel combination chemotherapy, immunotherapies, hyperthermic therapies, vaccines, small compound drugs, and tumor treating fields are essential in delivering improved outcomes for localized pancreatic cancer.

INTRODUCTION

In 2021, the estimated incidence of pancreatic cancer was an estimated 60,430 with the projected death toll of 48,220 and a 1% rise in incidence per year.[1] Pancreatic cancer remains a fatal malignancy with a 5-year survival rate of 10%. Based on individuals diagnosed between 2010 and 2016, the 5-year relative survival rate for localized pancreatic cancer is approximately 39%.[2,3] Nearly 30% of patients initially present with locally advanced malignancy at the time of diagnosis, whereas 20% present with localized resectable disease. Pancreatic cancer is projected to be the second leading cause of cancer-related death by 2040 in the United States compelling rapid developments in treatment.[4]

In 1962, fluorouracil (5-FU) claimed the first US Food and Drug Administration (FDA) approval for pancreatic adenocarcinoma. Since that time, in 1996, Buris and colleagues[5] demonstrated a significant clinical benefit response of 23.8% in patients treated with gemcitabine with a median survival duration of 5.65 months compared

Division of Hematology/Oncology, Department of Medicine, University of Arizona Cancer Center, 1515 N. Campbell Avenue, Tucson, AZ 85724-5024, USA
* Corresponding author.
E-mail address: rshroff@arizona.edu

Hematol Oncol Clin N Am 36 (2022) 961–978
https://doi.org/10.1016/j.hoc.2022.07.003
0889-8588/22/© 2022 Elsevier Inc. All rights reserved.

hemonc.theclinics.com

with 4.8% and 4.41 months, respectively, in those treated with 5-FU. The trial revolutionized the care of advanced pancreatic cancer by demonstrating the survival advantage of gemcitabine over 5-FU leading to the FDA approval of gemcitabine for pancreatic cancer in 1997. Leucovorin, 5-FU, irinotecan, oxaliplatin (FOLFIRINOX) and gemcitabine with nap-paclitaxel were approved in the first-line setting in 2011 and 2013, respectively.[6,7] In 2015, irinotecan liposome injection was subsequently approved for those previously treated with gemcitabine.[8] With the introduction of comprehensive germline and somatic genomic sequencing as standard of care, targeted treatment opportunities have emerged for select cases of pancreatic cancer. In 2019, olaparib was approved by the FDA for maintenance therapy for patients with germline BReast CAncer gene 1 (BRCA)-mutated metastatic pancreatic cancer whose disease had not progressed on at least 16 weeks of the first-line platinum-based regimen based on the progression-free survival advantage demonstrated in the POLO trial.[9]

The role of clinical research in halting this alarming rising trajectory of pancreatic cancer deaths is effectively highlighted by the National Comprehensive Cancer Network (NCCN) guidelines that emphasize clinical trials as the preferred treatment modality at any stage of pancreatic cancer.[10] Although there have been incremental advances in the treatment of pancreatic cancer thus far with progresses in diagnostic approaches, surgical and radiotherapy techniques, and systemic therapy, there remains a dire need for the development of innovative therapeutic approaches within pancreatic cancer. In this article, the authors aim to focus on the advances and current therapeutic approaches in the perioperative management of individuals with localized pancreatic adenocarcinoma.

HISTORY OF ADJUVANT CARE

Surgical resection with negative margins remains the only potentially curative approach for pancreatic adenocarcinoma at this time. However, only 10% to 20% of individuals are diagnosed with resectable disease at the time of diagnosis.[11] In most cases, initial diagnosis is obtained during advanced stages of the disease course with vascular invasion and/or distant metastasis obscured with multiple genetic/epigenetic alterations and complex tumor microenvironment leading to incurred resistance to conventional chemoradiation.[12–15] In addition, treatment failures including local recurrence or hepatic metastasis usually occur within 1 to 2 years following the surgical resection which led to the investigation of the role of adjuvant therapy.

In 2004, the European Study Group for Pancreatic Cancer (ESPAC) conducted a multicenter trial (ESPAC-1) that investigated the utility of adjuvant chemoradiation and maintenance chemotherapy in pancreatic cancer.[16] The study found a significant 5-year survival benefit of 21% with adjuvant chemotherapy consisting of 5-FU compared with 8% among patients who did not receive chemotherapy. The almost doubling of survival rates with adjuvant chemotherapy shifted the paradigm in the treatment of pancreatic cancer following surgical resection. In 2013, the long-term outcomes of patients enrolled in the CONKO-001 trial evaluating the disease-free survival (DFS) of adjuvant gemcitabine among patients with resected pancreatic cancer found a 5-year overall survival (OS) of 20.7% compared with 10.4% in the observation arm and a median DFS of 13.4 months compared with 6.7 months in the observation arm.[17] In 2017, ESPAC-4 compared adjuvant gemcitabine and capecitabine with gemcitabine monotherapy in patients with resected pancreatic adenocarcinoma.[18] The study established adjuvant combination gemcitabine and capecitabine as the new standard of care following the surgical resection of pancreatic cancer with a significant OS benefit. The estimated 5-year OS was notably slightly better in the CONKO-001 trial compared with ESPAC-4 which has been attributed to the stringent inclusion criteria of CONKO-001 which excluded patients with a Carbohydrate antigen 19-9 (CA19-9) concentration of 2.5 times the upper limit of normal or above. In addition, higher tumor grade and lymph node positivity were noted in ESPAC-4 compared with CONKO-001. The compelling survival benefit of ESPAC-4 is particularly impressive as the patients enrolled did remarkably well with adjuvant gemcitabine and capecitabine despite worse independent prognostic measures.

Although considering advances in clinical outcomes with the introduction of adjuvant chemotherapy, the recurrence rates remain as high as 69% to 75% with relapses occurring predominantly within the first 2 years. With the FDA approval of FOLFIRINOX in 2011 which showed superior OS compared with gemcitabine in the first-line metastatic setting in the PRODIGE trial, FOLFIRINOX was subsequently evaluated in the adjuvant setting.[6] In 2018, 493 patients with resected pancreatic adenocarcinoma were randomized to receive modified FOLFIRINOX or gemcitabine for 24 weeks with DFS as the primary end point.[19] Adjuvant modified FOLFIRINOX demonstrated a significantly longer survival (median OS of 54.4 months in the modified FOLFIRINOX cohort compared with 35 months in the gemcitabine cohort). Moreover, the 3-year OS was 63.4% and 48.6% in the FOLFIRINOX and gemcitabine groups, respectively. However, the survival benefit was notably at the expense of higher levels of toxicity with FOLFIRINOX. More recently, the phase III, multicenter APACT trial evaluated adjuvant nab-paclitaxel plus gemcitabine (nab-P/G) versus gemcitabine alone for surgically resected pancreatic adenocarcinoma The updated 5-year OS demonstrated a median OS of 41.8 vs 37.7 months (HR 0.82; 95% CI, 0.687-0.973) favoring nab-paclitaxel and gemcitabine. Median DFS of 16.6 months vs 13.7 months also favored the nab-paclitaxel plus gemcitabine over gemcitabine.20 As such adjuvant nab-paclitaxel plus gemcitabine may be a consideration for patients deemed ineligible for FOLFIRINOX.

ROLE OF SURGICAL RESECTION

Although surgical resection presents a window of opportunity for cure in this highly lethal disease, with recent advances in systemic therapy and radiotherapy, optimization of this multimodality treatment algorithm becomes crucial. Historically, borderline resectable and locally advanced pancreatic cancer was often described to be unresectable.[20] With evolving consensus definitions of resectability including those provided by the MD Anderson Cancer Center, NCCN, and the American Society of Surgical Oncology, the delineation of tumor to its surrounding major blood vessels chiefly the celiac artery, common hepatic artery, superior mesenteric artery, superior mesenteric vein, and portal vein become crucial.[21–23]

In addition, multidetector computed tomography (CT) imaging-based resectability proposed by the NCCN guidelines has been extensively used to stratify the possibility of margin-negative resection of pancreatic cancer.[22,24] The preferred imaging tool for dedicated pancreatic imaging is a multidetector CT angiography that can acquire thin, submillimeter, axial sections with images obtained in the arterial, pancreatic and portal venous phase of contrast enhancement. An estimated 70% to 85% of patients with resectable pancreatic tumor noted in dedicated pancreatic imaging were able to undergo resection.[25–28] Consensus definition for resectable tumor includes absence of tumor–artery interface, less than 180° tumor–vein interface, and no abnormal lymph nodes outside the surgical basin.[29] Based on these stringent criteria, only 15%,

15%, and 20% of all cases of pancreatic cancer are classified as resectable, border-line resectable, and locally advanced (unresectable) disease, respectively.[30,31]

Although the standard of care for early-stage pancreatic cancer remains surgical resection to achieve a potential cure and prolong survival, a recent population-based study revealed that surgical resection remains underutilized globally[32,33]; over 150,000 records analyzed across six different European population-based cancer registries, and the US Surveillance, Epidemiology, and End Results Program database from 2012 to 2014 found that for early-stage I–II tumors, resection rates ranged from 34.8% to 68.7%.[34] In earlier years, 2003 to 2014, resection rates increased only in the United States, the Netherlands, and Denmark. Another population-based study in the United States found a 5-year survival of 24.6% for patients with stage I pancreatic cancer who had undergone a resection. Of note, only 38.2% of patients with stage I disease underwent surgical resection despite the lack of identifiable contraindications.[32]

[35,36] Racial disparity also exerts a crucial role in surgical resection for resectable localized pancreatic cancer. In a retrospective cohort study evaluating over 35,000 patients of which 87.6% were white from 1988 to 2009, pancreatic cancer resection was less often recommended and performed in blacks compared with white adjusting for tumor stage.[37] Moreover, in multivariate adjusted analyses, blacks declined surgery more often than whites when it was recommended. Acknowledging and minimizing potential racial bias while factoring in patient- and physician-related biases is essential in eliminating such disparity.

LOCALIZED PANCREATIC ADENOCARCINOMA

With considerations of adjuvant and neoadjuvant therapy coupled with improvement tin surgical expertise, the indications for resection have expanded to encompass locally advanced tumors.[38] Techniques including multivisceral resections with or without major mesenteric vessel resection are now increasingly being performed with notable improvement in clinical outcomes while limiting postoperative morbidity.[20] For patients with locally advanced and unresectable pancreatic cancers, neoadjuvant strategies including chemotherapy and combination radiation therapy (RT) and consecutive surgical resection are increasingly being explored, whereas adjuvant therapy has been extensively investigated for localized tumors. Ongoing clinical trials are in dire need and continue to enrich our understanding in improving patient selection and outcomes for an ideal multimodality treatment approach.

Adjuvant Chemoradiation

Currently, the adjuvant approaches are increasingly under investigation for resectable local pancreatic cancer. In 1985, the Gastrointestinal Tumor Study Group (GITSG) first evaluated the potential for DFS with combined radiation and chemotherapy with 5-FU following surgical resection in 41 patients. Unfortunately, the trial was terminated prematurely due to unacceptably low accrual along with large differences in study arms with the patients randomized to the treatment arm achieving a significantly longer median survival of 20 months versus 11 months in the observation cohort.[39] Subsequently, the EORTC gastrointestinal tract cancer cooperative group conducted a large phase III trial reexamining the role of adjuvant radiotherapy and 5-FU after curative resection of pancreatic and periampullary region cancer in 218 patients with T1-2N0-1aM0 pancreatic head or T1-3N0-1aM0 periampullary adenocarcinoma.[40]

Although combination chemoradiation following surgical resection was safe and well-tolerated, there was minimal nonsignificant benefit in survival.

In an interim follow-up of the clinical impact of the ESPAC-1 trial in shifting the treatment paradigm of pancreatic cancer treatment, the group noted that 6 years after the publication of ESPAC-1 results in 2004, the use of adjuvant chemotherapy superseded the use of adjuvant chemoradiation.[41] Following 2010, R1 disease remained a significant predictor of chemoradiation use.[41] The addition of gemcitabine to adjuvant 5-FU chemoradiation was investigated in a large randomized phase III trial of 451 patients with resected pancreatic adenocarcinoma.[42] The study found the addition of gemcitabine to adjuvant 5-FU-based chemoradiation derived an improved but not statistically significant survival in resected pancreatic cancer. In addition, another randomized phase III trial (LAP07) did not demonstrate any statistically significant difference in OS with chemoradiation compared with chemotherapy alone, nor was there a significant difference in OS with gemcitabine compared with gemcitabine plus erlotinib in the maintenance treatment setting for locally advanced pancreatic cancer.[43] Given the current data, further prospective studies are required to define the role of adjuvant chemoradiation in resectable localized pancreatic cancer.

Adjuvant Chemotherapy

Although adjuvant chemoradiation has not validated a survival benefit for resectable pancreatic cancer, adjuvant systemic chemotherapy has shown promising results. CONKO-001 was the first trial to demonstrate a significant improvement in DFS with the addition of gemcitabine after surgery. Sinn and colleagues[44] recently evaluated tissue samples from 101 patients that were enrolled in the CONKO-001 phase III trial. The samples were sent for the next-generation sequencing for 37 genes to identify clinically relevant prognostic and predictive mutations. The most common mutations identified were KRAS (75%), TP53 (60%), SMAD4 (10%), CDKNA2 (9%), and SWI/SNF (12%) complex alterations. Patients with identified TP53 mutations derived the most benefit from adjuvant gemcitabine. Further prospective studies need to be conducted to further evaluate the role of other such prognostic variables that can better delineate which patients may derive the most benefit from adjuvant systemic therapy following resection.

ESPAC-3 also evaluated the use of gemcitabine versus 5-FU in the adjuvant setting for resected pancreatic cancer.[45] Thirty-nine percent of the patients in the 5-FU arm and 37% in the gemcitabine arm had stage I–II disease. Interestingly, resection margin status was not statistically significant on multivariate analysis as noted in ESPAC-1 as well.[16] However, tumor grade, nodal status, tumor size, and postoperative CA19-9 levels were among the independent prognostic factors of OS. Given less toxicity and similar survival rates as 5-FU, gemcitabine was accepted as the standard of care in the adjuvant setting in resected pancreatic cancer. ESPAC-4 was subsequently conducted and demonstrated survival advantage of combination gemcitabine and capecitabine compared with gemcitabine monotherapy in resected pancreatic adenocarcinoma.[18] Of note, 89% of patients enrolled in ESPAC-4 had stage III disease. Patients with R0 resections in this trial had superior survival to those with R1 resection margins. However, both achieved a substantially significant survival benefit with adjuvant chemotherapy.

PERIOPERATIVE MANAGEMENT

Although adjuvant chemotherapy has demonstrated an improvement in survival outcomes, upfront surgery may render a significant number of patients incapable of tolerating systemic therapy. The role of neoadjuvant therapy may allow control of systemic disease earlier in the course and may identify individuals who develop progressive disease despite systemic therapy which may spare these individuals from undergoing extensive surgery that ultimately may not improve their outcome.[46–48] Although data exist for the role of neoadjuvant therapy in borderline resectable and unresectable pancreatic cancer, the current use of neoadjuvant therapy as a therapeutic approach in resectable pancreatic cancer remains controversial particularly in cases of high-risk disease.[46]

Neoadjuvant Chemotherapy

In a recent phase II trial evaluating the 2-year OS of perioperative chemotherapy for resectable pancreatic cancer, investigators noted that perioperative chemotherapy with modified FOLFIRINOX or gemcitabine did not improve OS compared with historical data.[48] Two-year OS was 47% with modified FOLFIRINOX and 48% with gemcitabine/nab-paclitaxel for all eligible patients starting treatment of resectable pancreatic cancer. The Alliance for Clinical Trials in Oncology (A021101 trial) also evaluated the feasibility of preoperative modified FOLFIRINOX followed by capecitabine-based chemoradiation for borderline resectable pancreatic cancer[49,50] Of the 22 patients enrolled, 15 underwent a pancreatectomy of which 12 required vascular resection, 14 had microscopically negative margins, 5 had less than 5% residual cancer cells, and 2 had pathologically complete response. The median OS was 21.7 months. Although the aim of the study was designed to meet feasibility and not survival, the median OS is remarkable in the setting of borderline resectable pancreatic cancer.

To improve outcomes of locally advanced pancreatic cancer, a multicenter, international phase II trial (LAPACT) was conducted recently that examined the safety and efficacy of nab-P/G.[51] Sixty-two patients completed induction treatment after which the majority received chemoradiation and 17 underwent surgery (7 achieved R0 resection status, whereas 9 had R1). The treatment was deemed tolerable with a median OS of 18.8 months and median time to treatment failure of 9 months. With the rising incidence of pancreatic cancer, the need to strategize methods in which patients can achieve surgical resection through multimodality approach becomes crucial.

Neoadjuvant Chemoradiation

Preoperative modified FOLFIRINOX or modified FOLFIRINOX plus hypofractionated RT for borderline resectable pancreatic adenocarcinoma was evaluated in a phase II trial (ALLIANCE A021501) was investigated recently and showed favorable OS with neoadjuvant modified FOLFIRINOX relative to historical data, whereas modified FOLFIRINOX with hypofractionated RT did not improve OS.[52] Twenty-eight patients (42%) achieved R0 pancreatectomy in the modified FOLFIRINOX cohort compared with fourteen patients (25%) in the modified FOLFIRNOX plus RT cohort.

ESPAC-5F phase II trial evaluating immediate surgery compared with neoadjuvant gemcitabine plus capecitabine or FOLFIRINOX or chemoradiotherapy in 90 patients with borderline resectable pancreatic cancer was recently conducted.[53] R0 resection rate was 15% for immediate surgery and 23% with neoadjuvant therapy. The overall resection rates did not vary between the various arms of the study, and there was a significant survival advantage with neoadjuvant therapy compared with immediate surgery.

More recently, the updated long-term results of the PREOPANC trial, a multicenter phase III trial that randomized 246 patients with resectable and borderline resectable pancreatic cancer to receive either neoadjuvant chemoradiotherapy with 3 cycles of gemcitabine combined with radiation during the second cycle versus upfront surgery with both arms receiving adjuvant gemcitabine, showed superior OS of the gemcitabine-based chemoradiotherapy followed by surgery and adjuvant gemcitabine versus upfront surgery and adjuvant gemcitabine. ADDIN EN.CITE [54] The difference in survival was 1.4 months between the two arms. However, the 5-year OS was 20.5% with neoadjuvant chemoradiotherapy versus 6.5% with upfront surgery in both patients with resectable and borderline resectable pancreatic cancer.

Preclinical data has evaluated the role of the renin-angiotensin system (RAS) in exerting antitumor activity in pancreatic cancer. Activation of RAS pathway has been implicated in mediation of cell proliferation, metabolism and growth.[55] Angiotensin-receptor blockers have demonstrated manipulation of the tumor microenvironment and activation of immunity to enhance deliver of chemotherapy.[56,57] A single-arm phase II trial evaluated 49 patients with untreated locally advanced unresectable pancreatic cancer that received either FOLFIRINOX and losartan for 8 cycles followed by short-course radiotherapy and capecitabine if radiographic evidence of resectable disease was noted versus long-course of chemoradiotherapy with fluorouracil or capecitabine if persistent vascular involvement was evident radiographically.[58] R0 resection was achieved in 34 of the 42 patients who underwent attempted surgery with a median PFS of 21.3 months and median OS of 33 months among those that underwent surgical resection. Lack of randomization in this study limit clinical implications of and derived benefit of losartan. However, the study highlighted the importance of achieving local control with either long or short course of chemoradiation in improving odds of R0 resection.

Although the notion of neoadjuvant systemic therapy for localized resectable pancreatic cancer remains uncertain, further prospective studies are required to elucidate patient- and disease-related factors that highlight the ideal candidate for neoadjuvant therapy in cases of resectable disease without high-risk features. Based on the current data, the preferred initial approach for patients with borderline resectable disease incorporates neoadjuvant therapy in place of immediate surgery.

Clinical trials

Beyond combination chemotherapy, over the past two decades, there has been little shift in the treatment paradigm for pancreatic cancer which is in stark contrast to novel targeted therapies and immunotherapy noted in various solid and hematological malignancies.[54] Given the aggressive nature of pancreatic cancer, there remains a dire unmet need for the development of novel and effective therapeutic advances. As of 2019, there were 430 registered interventional trials for pancreatic cancer of which 134 were phase I, 94 in phase I/II testing, 165 in phase II testing, and 32 in phase II testing.[55] Of the 430 clinical trials, 135 focused on patients with localized pancreatic adenocarcinoma.

Emerging novel combination therapies, novel immune checkpoint inhibitor combinations, therapeutic vaccines and small drug compounds with current clinical trials are summarized in **Table 1**.

Novel combination therapies

Perioperative chemotherapy with FOLFIRINOX (administered before and after surgery) versus adjuvant chemotherapy for the treatment of resectable pancreatic cancer is currently under investigation in a phase III ALLIANCE trial (NCT04340141) with the primary outcome measure of OS. Another phase II trial is currently evaluating the additional efficacy of adding chemotherapy with FOLFIRINOX before resection of a pancreatic head malignancy to avoid early mortality in those ultimately resected (NCT02919787). Metabolic treatment including atorvastatin, metformin,

Table 1
Clinical trials evaluating novel therapeutic approaches in pancreatic cancer

Treatment	Indication	Clinical Trial ID
Novel combination therapies		
Perioperative FOLFIRINOX vs adjuvant chemotherapy	Resectable pancreatic ca	NCT04340141
Neoadjuvant FOLFIRINOX	Resectable pancreatic head ca	NCT02919787
Atorvastatin, metformin, doxycycline and mebendazole	Any malignancy	NCT02201381
Gemcitabine with or without erlotinib followed by same chemo regimen with or without radiation therapy and capecitabine or 5-FU	Resectable pancreatic ca	NCT01013649
Chemoradiation with gemcitabine or FOLFIRNOX	Locally advanced unresectable pancreatic ca	NCT01827553
Early switching from modified FOLFIRINOX to combination gemcitabine and nab-paclitaxel prior to surgery	Resectable, borderline resectable, or locally advanced pancreatic ca	NCT04539808
Hyperthermic therapies		
Gemcitabine/cisplatin/regional hyperthermia vs gemcitabine/capecitabine	Resectable pancreatic ca	NCT01077427
Adjuvant hyperthermic intra-abdominal chemotherapy with gemcitabine	Resectable pancreatic ca	NCT03251365
Immunotherapy		
Pembrolizumab and paricalcitol with or without chemotherapy	Resectable pancreatic ca	NCT02930902
BMS-813160 with nivolumab and gemcitabine and nab-paclitaxel	Borderline resectable and locally advanced pancreatic adenocarcinoma	NCT03496662
Nivolumab/ipilumab/chemoradiation with gemcitabine/nab-paclitaxel	Locally advanced pancreatic ca	NCT04247165
Neoadjuvant nivolumab with FOLFIRINOX	Borderline resectable pancreatic ca	NCT03970252
Durvalumab/CSF-1R TKI (pexidartinib)	Metastatic/advanced pancreatic or colorectal ca	NCT02777710
Tumor treating field		
Tumor treating fields with gemcitabine/nab-paclitaxel	Locally advanced pancreatic ca	NCT03377491
Small drug compounds		
EndoTAG-1 in combination with gemcitabine vs gemcitabine alone	Locally advanced/metastatic pancreatic adenocarcinoma failed on FOLFIRINOX	NCT03126435
Neoadjuvant nab-paclitaxel and S-1	Borderline resectable pancreatic ca	NCT03850769
CDX-301 and CDX-1140	Resectable pancreatic ca	NCT04536077
GC4711 in Combination With SBRT	Nonmetastatic pancreatic ca	NCT04698915
CPI-613/mFOLFIRINOX vs FOLFIRINOX	Metastatic pancreatic ca	NCT03504423

(continued on next page)

		Clinical Trial
Treatment	**Indication**	**ID**
Olaparib vs placebo	Resected pancreatic ca with BRCA1, BRCA2 or PALB2 mutation	NCT04858334
Cobimetinib/olaparib/onvansertinib/ temuterkib	Pancreatic ca	NCT04005690
Pyrvinium Pamoate	unresectable pancreatic ca	NCT05055323
Vaccines		
Adjuvant RO7198457/atezolizumab/ mFOLFIRINOX	Resectable pancreatic ca	NCT04161755
Adjuvant YE-NEO-001	Previously treated solid tumors	NCT03552718
KRAS peptide vaccine/nivolumab/ ipilumab	Resected MMR-p colorectal and pancreatic ca	NCT04117087
Personalized neoantigen cancer vaccine	Resectable pancreatic ca	NCT04810910
Th-1 dendritic autologous DC vaccine	Pancreatic adenocarcinoma	NCT04157127
mDC3/8-KRAS Vaccine	Pancreatic ductal adenocarcinoma	NCT03592888
MRx0518 with preoperative hypofractionated radiation	Resectable pancreatic ca	NCT04193904

Abbreviations: 5-FU, fluorouracil; FOLFIRINOX, folic acid, fluorouracil, irinotecan, oxaliplatin; mFOLFIRINOX, modified FOLIRINOX; TKI, tyrosine kinase inhibitor.

doxycycline, and mebendazole every 3 months is also under investigation for patients diagnosed with any malignancy and will be receiving the standard of care therapy shortly (NCT02201381). There is an ongoing phase II trial evaluating gemcitabine with or without erlotinib followed by the same chemotherapy regimen with or without RT and capecitabine or 5-FU in patients with pancreatic cancer that has been surgically resected (NCT01013649). In locally advanced, unresectable pancreatic cancer, CONKO-007 phase III trial is evaluating the significance of chemoradiation compared with chemotherapy alone after induction chemotherapy with three cycles of gemcitabine or six cycles of FOLFIRINOX (NCT01827553). NeoOPTIMIZE, a phase II trial, is studying the clinical effectiveness of early switching from modified FOLFIRINOX to combination gemcitabine and nab-paclitaxel before surgery for patients with resectable or borderline resectable pancreatic cancer (NCT04539808).

Hyperthermic therapies
Owing to the hypoxic pancreatic tumor microenvironment which contributes to the survival and proliferation of more aggressive tumor cells, hyperthermia has been considered to enhance the effects of chemoradiotherapy and improve clinical outcomes.[56,57] Hyperthermia has been shown to achieves cytotoxicity and radio- and chemosensitization with enhancement of the sensitization effects of gemcitabine at 43°C.[63,64] The HEATPAC Phase II trial evaluated 7 patients with locally advanced inoperable pancreatic cancer who received 4 cycles of FOLFIRINOX chemotherapy followed by gemcitabine-based chemoradiation combined with weekly deep hyperthermia and then an additional 8 cycles of FOLFIRINOX.[65] Deep hyperthermia was defined as BSD 2000 unit with Sigma-60 or Sigma-Eye phased array applicator. The study noted that following treatment, 2 tumors became unresectable and the median OS was 24 months. Intensified adjuvant regional deep hyperthermia and

gemcitabine and cisplatin compared with standard chemotherapy is under investigation in patients with R0/R1 resected pancreatic carcinoma (NCT01077427). Another phase II/III randomized, multidisciplinary study is examining the use of hyperthermic intra-abdominal chemotherapy with gemcitabine after surgical resection with curative intent in patients with resectable pancreatic cancer to decrease future tumor progression by reducing neoplastic volume and a subpopulation of pancreatic cancer stem cells (NCT03251365). The study will essentially randomize patients to two treatment arms following curative intent surgical resection of pancreatic adenocarcinoma; one arm will receive adjuvant gemcitabine for 4 cycles while the other arm will receive hyperthermic intraperitoneal chemotherapy with gemcitabine and adjuvant gemcitabine for at least 4 cycles.

Immunotherapy

Immunotherapy has thus far proven disappointing reflecting the complex tumor microenvironment and non-immunogenic nature of pancreatic cancer.[58,59] Pancreatic cancer is characterized by low tumor mutational burden compared with those found other solid malignancies which limits the expression of neoantigens by pancreatic tumors leading to poor immunogenic surveillance. The tumor microenvironment of pancreatic tumors is immunosuppressive with reduced cytotoxic and helper T cells, creating an environment resistant to immune recognition and elimination.[57] Pembrolizumab has shown a clinical benefit in mismatch-repair (MMR) deficiency noted in 1% to 3% of pancreatic cancers leading to the first FDA approval of a checkpoint inhibitor for tumor agnostic indication in MMR-deficient malignancies.[60,61] BL-8040, a CXCR antagonist, was recently evaluated in combination with pembrolizumab and chemotherapy for metastatic pancreatic cancer in a phase II trial (COMBAT trial) and showed that the novel combination may expand the therapeutic benefits of chemotherapy.[62] The combination of stereotactic body RT with pembrolizumab and trametinib has shown promising survival benefit in a phase II study for patients with local recurrence after surgical resection.[63]

A number of trials are currently exploring the role of immunotherapy in localized pancreatic cancer including a phase Ib study examining pembrolizumab and paricalcitol, a synthetic vitamin D analog, with or without chemotherapy in patients with pancreatic cancer that can be surgically resected (NCT02930902). BMS-813160 with nivolumab and gemcitabine and nab-paclitaxel is also being evaluated in a phase I/II study in borderline resectable and locally advanced pancreatic ductal adenocarcinoma (NCT03496662). Nivolumab, ipilimumab in combination with gemcitabine and nab-paclitaxel followed by immune-chemoradiation for patients with locally advanced pancreatic cancer is under investigation in a phase I/II study (NCT04247165). A pilot study is currently evaluating nivolumab in combination with chemotherapy (FOLFIRINOX) in the neoadjuvant setting for patients with borderline resectable pancreatic cancer (NCT03970252).

Durvalumab in combination with pexidartinib, a CSF-1R TKI, is undergoing evaluation for safety and efficacy in advanced and metastatic pancreatic cancer (NCT02777710).

Tumor treating field

Noninvasive, regional antimitotic treatment modality which has been approved for glioblastoma is increasingly becoming examined in the setting of pancreatic cancer.[64] Tumor treating fields (TTFs) deliver a specific frequency (150 to 200 kHz) via transducer arrays placed on the skin in close proximity to the tumor site. The phase III P-ANOVA trial (NCT03377491) evaluating the efficacy and safety of combination TTF with nab-paclitaxel and gemcitabine in unresectable locally advanced pancreatic cancer is ongoing after the phase II study demonstrated safety and preliminary efficacy.[65,66]

Immunomodulatory drugs
Lenalidomide with its antiangiogenic properties and enhanced immunomodulatory activity has shown to decrease the expression of phosphorylated ERK in three pancreatic cell lines was investigated in combination with gemcitabine in a phase II study to evaluate the antitumor activity and safety in the treatment of advanced pancreatic cancer. The study did not demonstrate any improvement in survival compared with historical results with this novel combination with additional dose-limited toxicity.[67,68]

Small drug compounds
EndoTAG-1 is a formulation of novel cationic liposomes embedded in paclitaxel to achieve antivascular and antiangiogenic properties.[69] The cytostatic activity of paclitaxel will be targeted to the activated tumor endothelial cell once it has been bound and internalized at the tumor endothelial cells after intravenous administration. EndoTAG-1 plus gemcitabine versus gemcitabine alone in patients with locally advanced pancreatic cancer who have failed prior FOLFIRINOX treatment is under investigation in a phase III trial (NCT03126435).

S-1, an oral fluoropyrimidine derivative, in combination with nab-paclitaxel is under investigation for borderline resectable pancreatic cancer (NCT03850769).[70] CDX-301 is a soluble recombinant human protein form of the Fms-related tyrosine kinase 3 ligand, a hematopoietic cytokine.[71] CDX-1140 is a fully human antibody that targets CD40, an activator in the immune response.[72] The immunological effects of CDX-301 in combination with CDX-1140 are under investigation in individuals with resectable pancreatic cancer (NCT04536077).

GC4711, a selective superoxide dismutase mimetic that converts superoxide to hydrogen peroxide, has been shown to tumor control in combination with RT.[73] A phase IIb study is currently investigating the combination GC4711 with stereotactic body RT for nonmetastatic pancreatic cancer (NCT04698915).

Masitinib is a small molecule agent that targets innate immune cells including mast cell and macrophage activity critical in the tumor microenvironment.[74] In a randomized phase III trial, masitinib plus gemcitabine was evaluated in the treatment of advanced pancreatic adenocarcinoma found no difference in median OS but noted a survival benefit among patients that overexpressed ACOX1 or baseline pain (visual analog scale of pain intensity >20 mm).[75] Results from the study concluded this novel combination as serving a therapeutic benefit in patients with unresectable locally advanced pancreatic cancer with associated pain.[74]

A phase III, multicenter, randomized trial (AVENGER 500) evaluating the safety and efficacy of FOLFIRINOX versus devimistat (CPI-613) in combination with FOLFIRINOX is under evaluation for individuals with metastatic pancreatic adenocarcinoma (NCT03504423). Olaparib is also under investigation as in a randomized study in patients harboring a BRCA1, BRCA2, or PALB2 mutation who have undergone surgical resection of the pancreatic cancer in the APOLLO trial (NCT04858334). Targeted PARP or MEK/ERK inhibition with olaparib or cobimetinib is also being evaluated for resectable and borderline resectable pancreatic cancer in an early phase I trial (NCT04005690).

Antihelminthic pyrvinium pamoate has been shown to target the mitochondrial pathway and is effective in low glucose settings. It has demonstrated preclinical efficacy in the nutrient-depleted pancreatic cancer tumor microenvironment.[76] A phase I trial is ongoing to determine the safety and tolerability of pyrvinium pamoate in unresectable early-stage pancreatic cancer (NCT05055323).

Vaccines

Another therapeutic strategy used in the immune desert of pancreatic tumor microenvironment is through the utilization of vaccines that serve activate specific T cells that can migrate to pancreatic tumors.[57] Various forms of vaccines including whole-cell vaccine, bacterial-based vaccines, yeast-based vaccines, viral vector-based vaccines, peptide vaccines, dendritic cell-based vaccines, among others are under investigation.

Algenpantucel-L in combination with standard of care chemotherapy and chemoradiation was compared with standard of care chemotherapy and chemoradiation alone in patients with borderline resectable or locally advanced pancreatic ductal adenocarcinoma in a phase III randomized trial. The study found that algenpantucel-L did not improve survival in patients who had received standard of care neoadjuvant chemotherapy and chemoradiation.[77] Cyclophosphamide/GVAX pancreas vaccine followed by Listeria-mesothelin, CRS-207, with or without nivolumab was investigated in patients with pancreatic cancer who had received one prior line of therapy for metastatic cancer with ongoing measurable disease. Objective response was noted but the study did not meet its primary end point in improvement in OS.[78] The role of this vaccine in localized pancreatic cancer has not been investigated.

Personalized tumor vaccine, RO7198457, in combination with atezolizumab and modified FOLFIRINOX in under investigation in a phase I study for patients with surgically resected pancreatic cancer (NCT04161755). QUILT-2.025 NANT neoepitope yeast vaccine, YE-NEO-001, is under study in the adjuvant setting to induce T-cell response in patients with previously treated cancers currently in a period of surveillance for recurrent disease (NCT03552718). Mutant KRAS-targeted long peptide vaccine in combination with nivolumab and ipilimumab for patients with resected MMR-p pancreatic cancer is being evaluated in a phase 1 study (NCT04117087). A new type of pancreatic cancer vaccine, the personalized neoantigen cancer vaccine, following surgical resection and adjuvant chemotherapy is under investigation to provide a potential new therapeutic strategy (NCT04810910). Th-1 dendritic cell vaccine in combination with standard chemotherapy for the adjuvant treatment of surgically resectable pancreatic cancer is in phase I study (NCT04157127). Another dendritic cell vaccine, mDC3/8-KRAS, is in phase I evaluation for patients with resectable pancreatic cancer (NCT03592888). A live biotherapeutic product, MRx0518, with preoperative hypofractionated radiation is under investigation in a phase I study for patients with resectable pancreatic cancer (NCT04193904).

SUMMARY

Although the refinements of surgical skills and approaches, innovation in radiographical techniques, and identification of biomarkers have demonstrated an incremental increase in clinical outcomes of localized pancreatic cancer, prolonged survival of this population that continues to rise remains dismal. The role of adjuvant and neoadjuvant chemotherapy and chemoradiotherapy has made significant strides and remains an area in need of further prospective studies. Innovative therapeutic strategies including novel combination chemotherapy, immunotherapies, vaccines, small compound drugs, among others that are currently under investigation provide an avenue to shift the perioperative treatment paradigm of localized pancreatic cancer in the future.

CLINICS CARE POINTS

- Clinical trials must be considered in all patients with localized pancreatic cancer.
- The preferred initial approach for patients with borderline resectable disease incorporates neoadjuvant therapy in place of immediate surgery.
- Given the current data, further prospective studies are required to define the role of adjuvant chemoradiation in resectable, non-high-risk local pancreatic cancer.

AUTHOR CONTRIBUTIONS

Conceptualization, R.T.S. and M.S.; writing—original draft preparation, M.S.; writing—review and editing, R.T.S. and M.S.; supervision, R.T.S. All authors have read and agreed to the published version of the article.

FUNDING

This research received no external funding.
    Institutional Review Board Statement: Not applicable.
    Informed Consent Statement: Not applicable.

DISCLOSURE

The authors have nothing to disclose.

REFERENCES

1. Siegel RL, Miller KD, Fuchs HE, et al. Cancer statistics, 2021. CA Cancer J Clin 2021;71(1):7–33.
2. Ruhl JL, C. C., Hurlbut, A, Ries LAG, Adamo P, Dickie L, Schussler N (eds), Summary stage 2018: codes and coding instructions. 2018.
3. Cancer Facts & Figures 2021. 2021.
4. Rahib L, Wehner MR, Matrisian LM, et al. Estimated projection of US cancer incidence and death to 2040. JAMA Netw Open 2021;4(4):e214708.
5. Burris HA 3rd, Moore MJ, Andersen J, et al. Improvements in survival and clinical benefit with gemcitabine as first-line therapy for patients with advanced pancreas cancer: a randomized trial. J Clin Oncol 1997;15(6):2403–13.
6. Conroy T, Desseigne F, Ychou M, et al. FOLFIRINOX versus gemcitabine for metastatic pancreatic cancer. N Engl J Med 2011;364(19):1817–25.
7. Von Hoff DD, Ervin T, Arena FP, et al. Increased survival in pancreatic cancer with nab-paclitaxel plus gemcitabine. N Engl J Med 2013;369(18):1691–703.
8. Chen L-T, Hoff DDV, Li C-P, et al. Expanded analyses of napoli-1: Phase 3 study of MM-398 (nal-IRI), with or without 5-fluorouracil and leucovorin, versus 5-fluorouracil and leucovorin, in metastatic pancreatic cancer (mPAC) previously treated with gemcitabine-based therapy. J Clin Oncol 2015; 33(3_suppl):234.
9. Golan T, Hammel P, Reni M, et al. Maintenance Olaparib for Germline BRCA-Mutated Metastatic Pancreatic Cancer. N Engl J Med 2019;381(4):317–27.
10. Tempero MA, Malafa MP, Al-Hawary M, et al. Pancreatic adenocarcinoma, version 2.2021, NCCN clinical practice guidelines in oncology. J Natl Compr Canc Netw 2021;19(4):439–57.

11. Kommalapati A, Tella SH, Goyal G, et al. Contemporary management of localized resectable pancreatic cancer. Cancers (Basel) 2018;10(1).

12. Ho WJ, Jaffee EM, Zheng L. The tumour microenvironment in pancreatic cancer - clinical challenges and opportunities. Nat Rev Clin Oncol 2020;17(9):527–40.

13. Qian Y, Gong Y, Fan Z, et al. Molecular alterations and targeted therapy in pancreatic ductal adenocarcinoma. J Hematol Oncol 2020;13(1):130.

14. Hung YH, Hsu MC, Chen LT, et al. Alteration of epigenetic modifiers in pancreatic cancer and its clinical implication. J Clin Med 2019;8(6).

15. Kleeff J, Korc M, Apte M, et al. Pancreatic cancer. Nat Rev Dis Primers 2016;2: 16022.

16. Neoptolemos JP, Stocken DD, Friess H, et al. European study group for pancreatic, C., a randomized trial of chemoradiotherapy and chemotherapy after resection of pancreatic cancer. N Engl J Med 2004;350(12):1200–10.

17. Oettle H, Neuhaus P, Hochhaus A, et al. Adjuvant chemotherapy with gemcitabine and long-term outcomes among patients with resected pancreatic cancer: the CONKO-001 randomized trial. JAMA 2013;310(14):1473–81.

18. Neoptolemos JP, Palmer DH, Ghaneh P, et al. European study group for pancreatic, C., Comparison of adjuvant gemcitabine and capecitabine with gemcitabine monotherapy in patients with resected pancreatic cancer (ESPAC-4): a multicentre, open-label, randomised, phase 3 trial. Lancet 2017;389(10073):1011–24.

19. Conroy T, Hammel P, Hebbar M, et al. FOLFIRINOX or gemcitabine as adjuvant therapy for pancreatic cancer. N Engl J Med 2018;379(25):2395–406.

20. Buanes TA. Role of surgery in pancreatic cancer. World J Gastroenterol 2017; 23(21):3765–70.

21. Varadhachary GR, Tamm EP, Abbruzzese JL, et al. Borderline resectable pancreatic cancer: definitions, management, and role of preoperative therapy. Ann Surg Oncol 2006;13(8):1035–46.

22. Tempero MA, Malafa MP, Al-Hawary M, et al. Pancreatic adenocarcinoma, version 2.2017, NCCN clinical practice guidelines in oncology. J Natl Compr Canc Netw 2017;15(8):1028–61.

23. Vauthey JN, Dixon E. AHPBA/SSO/SSAt consensus conference on resectable and borderline resectable pancreatic cancer: rationale and overview of the conference. Ann Surg Oncol 2009;16(7):1725–6.

24. Hong SB, Lee SS, Kim JH, et al. Pancreatic cancer CT: prediction of resectability according to NCCN criteria. Radiology 2018;289(3):710–8.

25. Callery MP, Chang KJ, Fishman EK, et al. Pretreatment assessment of resectable and borderline resectable pancreatic cancer: expert consensus statement. Ann Surg Oncol 2009;16(7):1727–33.

26. Klauss M, Schobinger M, Wolf I, et al. Value of three-dimensional reconstructions in pancreatic carcinoma using multidetector CT: initial results. World J Gastroenterol 2009;15(46):5827–32.

27. House MG, Yeo CJ, Cameron JL, et al. Predicting resectability of periampullary cancer with three-dimensional computed tomography. J Gastrointest Surg 2004;8(3):280–8.

28. Horton KM, Fishman EK. Adenocarcinoma of the pancreas: CT imaging. Radiol Clin North Am 2002;40(6):1263–72.

29. Al-Hawary MM, Francis IR, Chari ST, et al. Pancreatic ductal adenocarcinoma radiology reporting template: consensus statement of the society of abdominal radiology and the american pancreatic association. Radiology 2014;270(1): 248–60.

30. Kamarajah SK, Burns WR, Frankel TL, et al. Validation of the american joint commission on cancer (AJCC) 8th edition staging system for patients with pancreatic adenocarcinoma: a surveillance, epidemiology and end results (SEER) analysis. Ann Surg Oncol 2017;24(7):2023–30.
31. Sohal DPS. Adjuvant and neoadjuvant therapy for resectable pancreatic adenocarcinoma. Chin Clin Oncol 2017;6(3):26.
32. Bilimoria KY, Bentrem DJ, Ko CY, et al. National failure to operate on early stage pancreatic cancer. Ann Surg 2007;246(2):173–80.
33. Huang L, Jansen L, Balavarca Y, et al. Resection of pancreatic cancer in Europe and USA: an international large-scale study highlighting large variations. Gut 2019;68(1):130–9.
34. Hartwig W, Strobel O, Hinz U, et al. CA19-9 in potentially resectable pancreatic cancer: perspective to adjust surgical and perioperative therapy. Ann Surg Oncol 2013;20(7):2188–96.
35. Ghaneh P, Hanson R, Titman A, et al. PET-PANC: multicentre prospective diagnostic accuracy and health economic analysis study of the impact of combined modality 18fluorine-2-fluoro-2-deoxy-d-glucose positron emission tomography with computed tomography scanning in the diagnosis and management of pancreatic cancer. Health Technol Assess 2018;22(7):1–114.
36. Tsurusaki M, Sofue K, Murakami T. Current evidence for the diagnostic value of gadoxetic acid-enhanced magnetic resonance imaging for liver metastasis. Hepatol Res 2016;46(9):853–61.
37. Shah A, Chao KS, Ostbye T, et al. Trends in racial disparities in pancreatic cancer surgery. J Gastrointest Surg 2013;17(11):1897–906.
38. Strobel O, Neoptolemos J, Jager D, et al. Optimizing the outcomes of pancreatic cancer surgery. Nat Rev Clin Oncol 2019;16(1):11–26.
39. Kalser MH, Ellenberg SS. Pancreatic cancer. Adjuvant combined radiation and chemotherapy following curative resection. Arch Surg 1985;120(8):899–903.
40. Klinkenbijl JH, Jeekel J, Sahmoud T, et al. Adjuvant radiotherapy and 5-fluorouracil after curative resection of cancer of the pancreas and periampullary region: phase III trial of the EORTC gastrointestinal tract cancer cooperative group. Ann Surg 1999;230(6):776–82 [discussion: 782-4].
41. Winer LK, Cortez AR, Ahmad SA, et al. Evaluating the impact of ESPAC-1 on shifting the paradigm of pancreatic cancer treatment. J Surg Res 2021;259:442–50.
42. Regine WF, Winter KA, Abrams RA, et al. Fluorouracil vs gemcitabine chemotherapy before and after fluorouracil-based chemoradiation following resection of pancreatic adenocarcinoma: a randomized controlled trial. JAMA 2008; 299(9):1019–26.
43. Hammel P, Huguet F, van Laethem JL, et al. Effect of chemoradiotherapy vs chemotherapy on survival in patients with locally advanced pancreatic cancer controlled after 4 months of gemcitabine with or without erlotinib: the LAP07 randomized clinical trial. JAMA 2016;315(17):1844–53.
44. Sinn M, Sinn BV, Treue D, et al. TP53 mutations predict sensitivity to adjuvant gemcitabine in patients with pancreatic ductal adenocarcinoma: next-generation sequencing results from the CONKO-001 trial. Clin Cancer Res 2020;26(14):3732–9.
45. Neoptolemos JP, Stocken DD, Bassi C, et al. European Study Group for Pancreatic, C., Adjuvant chemotherapy with fluorouracil plus folinic acid vs gemcitabine following pancreatic cancer resection: a randomized controlled trial. JAMA 2010; 304(10):1073–81.

46. Xu JZ, Wang WQ, Zhang SR, et al. Neoadjuvant therapy is essential for resectable pancreatic cancer. Curr Med Chem 2019;26(40):7196–211.

47. Antonios A, Gharios J, Tohme C. Resectable pancreatic adenocarcinomas: will neoadjuvant FOLFIRINOX replace upfront surgery in the standard of care? Future Oncol 2017;13(11):951–3.

48. Sohal DPS, Duong M, Ahmad SA, et al. Efficacy of Perioperative Chemotherapy for Resectable Pancreatic Adenocarcinoma: A Phase 2 Randomized Clinical Trial. JAMA Oncol 2021;7(3):421–7.

49. Katz MH, Shi Q, Ahmad SA, et al. Preoperative modified FOLFIRINOX Treatment followed by capecitabine-based chemoradiation for borderline resectable pancreatic cancer: alliance for clinical trials in oncology trial A021101. JAMA Surg 2016;151(8):e161137.

50. Al-Batran S-E, Reichart A, Bankstahl US, et al. Randomized multicenter phase II/III study with adjuvant gemcitabine versus neoadjuvant/adjuvant FOLFIRINOX in resectable pancreatic cancer: The NEPAFOX trial. J Clin Oncol 2021;39(3_suppl):406.

51. Philip PA, Lacy J, Portales F, et al. Nab-paclitaxel plus gemcitabine in patients with locally advanced pancreatic cancer (LAPACT): a multicentre, open-label phase 2 study. Lancet Gastroenterol Hepatol 2020;5(3):285–94.

52. Katz MHG, Shi Q, Meyers JP, et al. Alliance A021501: Preoperative mFOLFIRINOX or mFOLFIRINOX plus hypofractionated radiation therapy (RT) for borderline resectable (BR) adenocarcinoma of the pancreas. J Clin Oncol 2021;39(3_suppl):377.

53. Ghaneh P, Palmer DH, Cicconi S, et al. ESPAC-5F: Four-arm, prospective, multicenter, international randomized phase II trial of immediate surgery compared with neoadjuvant gemcitabine plus capecitabine (GEMCAP) or FOLFIRINOX or chemoradiotherapy (CRT) in patients with borderline resectable pancreatic cancer. J Clin Oncol 2020;38(15_suppl):4505.

54. Gotwals P, Cameron S, Cipolletta D, et al. Prospects for combining targeted and conventional cancer therapy with immunotherapy. Nat Rev Cancer 2017;17(5):286–301.

55. Katayama ES, Hue JJ, Bajor DL, et al. A comprehensive analysis of clinical trials in pancreatic cancer: what is coming down the pike? Oncotarget 2020;11(38):3489–501.

56. van der Horst A, Versteijne E, Besselink MGH, et al. The clinical benefit of hyperthermia in pancreatic cancer: a systematic review. Int J Hyperthermia 2018;34(7):969–79.

57. Chi J PR, Rehman H, Goyal S, et al. Recent advances in immunotherapy for pancreatic cancer. Cancer Metastasis Treat 2020;6:43.

58. Kamath SD, Kalyan A, Kircher S, et al. Ipilimumab and Gemcitabine for Advanced Pancreatic Cancer: A Phase Ib Study. Oncologist 2020;25(5):e808–15.

59. O'Reilly EM, Oh DY, Dhani N, et al. Durvalumab with or without tremelimumab for patients with metastatic pancreatic ductal adenocarcinoma: a phase 2 randomized clinical trial. JAMA Oncol 2019;5(10):1431–8.

60. Le DT, Uram JN, Wang H, et al. PD-1 blockade in tumors with mismatch-repair deficiency. N Engl J Med 2015;372(26):2509–20.

61. Hu ZI, Shia J, Stadler ZK, et al. Evaluating mismatch repair deficiency in pancreatic adenocarcinoma: challenges and recommendations. Clin Cancer Res 2018;24(6):1326–36.

62. Bockorny B, Semenisty V, Macarulla T, et al. 8040, a CXCR4 antagonist, in combination with pembrolizumab and chemotherapy for pancreatic cancer: the COMBAT trial. Nat Med 2020;26(6):878–85.
63. Zhu X, Cao Y, Liu W, et al. Stereotactic body radiotherapy plus pembrolizumab and trametinib versus stereotactic body radiotherapy plus gemcitabine for locally recurrent pancreatic cancer after surgical resection: an open-label, randomised, controlled, phase 2 trial. Lancet Oncol 2021;22(8):1093–102.
64. Stupp R, Taillibert S, Kanner A, et al. Effect of tumor-treating fields plus maintenance temozolomide vs maintenance temozolomide alone on survival in patients with glioblastoma: a randomized clinical trial. JAMA 2017;318(23):2306–16.
65. Picozzi VJ, Macarulla T, Philip PA, et al. A phase III trial of tumor-treating fields with nab-paclitaxel and gemcitabine for front-line treatment of locally-advanced pancreatic adenocarcinoma (LAPC): PANOVA-3. J Clin Oncol 2021; 39(3_suppl):TPS448.
66. Rivera F, Benavides M, Gallego J, et al. Tumor treating fields in combination with gemcitabine or gemcitabine plus nab-paclitaxel in pancreatic cancer: Results of the PANOVA phase 2 study. Pancreatology 2019;19(1):64–72.
67. Infante JR, Arkenau HT, Bendell JC, et al. Lenalidomide in combination with gemcitabine as first-line treatment for patients with metastatic carcinoma of the pancreas: a Sarah Cannon Research Institute phase II trial. Cancer Biol Ther 2013;14(4):340–6.
68. Ullenhag GJ, Mozaffari F, Broberg M, et al. Clinical and immune effects of lenalidomide in combination with gemcitabine in patients with advanced pancreatic cancer. PLoS One 2017;12(1):e0169736.
69. Chen L-T, Su M-H. EndoTAG-1 plus gemcitabine versus gemcitabine alone in patients with measurable locally advanced and/or metastatic adenocarcinoma of the pancreas failed on FOLFIRINOX treatment (NCT03126435). J Clin Oncol 2020;38(15_suppl):TPS4669.
70. Zong Y, Yuan J, Peng Z, et al. Nab-paclitaxel plus S-1 versus nab-paclitaxel plus gemcitabine as first-line chemotherapy in patients with advanced pancreatic ductal adenocarcinoma: a randomized study. J Cancer Res Clin Oncol 2021; 147(5):1529–36.
71. Satyamitra M, Cary L, Dunn D, et al. CDX-301: a novel medical countermeasure for hematopoietic acute radiation syndrome in mice. Sci Rep 2020;10(1):1757.
72. Sanborn R, Hauke R, Gabrail N, et al. 405 CDX1140–01, a phase 1 dose-escalation/expansion study of CDX-1140 alone (Part 1) and in combination with CDX-301 (Part 2) or pembrolizumab (Part 3). J ImmunoTherapy Cancer 2020; 8(Suppl 3):A246.
73. Hoffe SE, Kim DW, Costello J, et al. GRECO-2: A randomized, phase 2 study of stereotactic body radiation therapy (SBRT) in combination with GC4711 in the treatment of unresectable or borderline resectable nonmetastatic pancreatic cancer (PC). J Clin Oncol 2021;39(15_suppl):TPS4175.
74. Ezenfis J, Hermine O, Group AS. Masitinib plus gemcitabine as first-line treatment of pancreatic cancer with pain: Results from phase 3 study AB12005. J Clin Oncol 2021;39(15_suppl):4018.
75. Deplanque G, Demarchi M, Hebbar M, et al. A randomized, placebo-controlled phase III trial of masitinib plus gemcitabine in the treatment of advanced pancreatic cancer. Ann Oncol 2015;26(6):1194–200.
76. Schultz CW, McCarthy GA, Nerwal T, et al. The FDA-approved anthelmintic pyrvinium pamoate inhibits pancreatic cancer cells in nutrient-depleted conditions by targeting the mitochondria. Mol Cancer Ther 2021;20(11):2166–76.

77. Hewitt DB, Nissen N, Hatoum H, et al. A phase 3 randomized clinical trial of chemotherapy with or without algenpantucel-L (HyperAcute-Pancreas) immuno-therapy in subjects with borderline resectable or locally advanced unresectable pancreatic cancer. Ann Surg 2022;275(1):45–53.
78. Tsujikawa T, Crocenzi T, Durham JN, et al. Evaluation of cyclophosphamide/GVAX pancreas followed by listeria-mesothelin (CRS-207) with or without nivolumab in patients with pancreatic cancer. Clin Cancer Res 2020;26(14):3578–88.

Novel Considerations in Surgical Management of Individuals with Pancreatic Adenocarcinoma

Chad A. Barnes, MD[a], Susan Tsai, MD, MHS[a,b],*

KEYWORDS

- Pancreatic cancer • Surgery • Neoadjuvant therapy • Survival • Pancreas Cancer
- Borderline Resectable • Chemotherapy • Radiation

KEY POINTS

- Clinical staging with a pancreas protocol CT scan, prior to any endoscopic interventions, is fundamental to assessing operability and facilitates stage-specific treatment planning.
- Multimodality therapy is recommended for all patients with operable disease and may be most reliably delivered in the neoadjuvant setting.
- Surgical resection provides a significant benefit to patients who demonstrate a clinical, radiographic, and tumor marker response to neoadjuvant therapy.
- CA19-9 is a useful prognostic marker. Patients who normalize their CA19-9 after completing all neoadjuvant therapy and surgery experience an improved survival.
- Improvements in chemotherapeutic regimens has resulted in an increased number of patients with locally advanced pancreatic cancer who are offered surgery. These patients are best treated at high-volume centers.

INTRODUCTION

The management of localized pancreatic cancer (PC) has evolved significantly in the last decade, moving away from prioritizing surgery as the primary treatment modality and embracing the need for preoperative (neoadjuvant) multimodality therapy to achieve durable disease-free control.[1] The use of neoadjuvant therapy was initially proposed as a means to identify patients with aggressive disease biology who are at risk for developing early postoperative disease progression. Among the early trials using neoadjuvant therapy, approximately 30% of patients who initiated neoadjuvant

[a] Department of Surgery, Medical College of Wisconsin, 8701 Watertown Plank Road, Milwaukee, WI 53226, USA; [b] LaBahn Pancreatic Cancer Program, Medical College of Wisconsin, 8701 W Watertown Plank Road, Milwaukee, WI 53226, USA
* Corresponding author. Department of Surgery, 8701 Watertown Plank Road, Milwaukee, WI 53226.
E-mail address: stsai@mcw.edu

Hematol Oncol Clin N Am 36 (2022) 979–994
https://doi.org/10.1016/j.hoc.2022.07.004
0889-8588/22/Published by Elsevier Inc.
hemonc.theclinics.com

therapy did not undergo surgical resection, primarily due to metastatic disease progression.[2] These patients were spared the morbidity of a surgical procedure with little oncologic value. However, the broader acceptance of neoadjuvant therapy for patients with localized PC was modest until multiple small series reported unexpected gains in the overall survival experienced by patients who were able to complete all intended neoadjuvant therapy and surgery, with median overall survivals ranging from 33 to 44 months.[2–4] Currently, neoadjuvant therapy is recommended for all patients with borderline and locally advanced PC, and at many centers, it is being used for patients with resectable disease, as well.[1] This article focuses on the diagnostic approach, staging, and treatment of operable PC and highlights 5 guiding principles for the use of neoadjuvant therapy in patients with localized PC.

CLINICAL PRESENTATION AND DIAGNOSTIC WORKUP
Clinical Presentation

The most common symptoms experienced by patients with PC are jaundice, upper abdominal or back pain, and weight loss. A history of significant unintentional weight loss is not uncommon and may be related to exocrine insufficiency, subclinical gastric outlet obstruction, or cancer-related cachexia. In addition, approximately 40% of patients with PC present with new-onset (within 2 years of diagnosis) diabetes in the setting of weight loss, which is consistent with pancreatogenic (type 3c) diabetes mellitus related to the PC. Although physical examination is often unrevealing, the presence of palpable periumbilical or left supraclavicular lymph nodes may indicate metastatic disease. Metastases in these locations may be subtle findings on computed tomography (CT) and may warrant further workup with a PET or biopsy.

Careful questioning regarding family history of cancer may reveal a history of PC, breast, ovarian, colon cancer, or melanoma. As detailed in Mohindroo and colleagues' article, "Genetics of Pancreatic Neuroendocrine Tumors," in this issue, approximately 10% to 15% of PC are thought to be related to a heritable pathogenic variant, and the most common alterations occur in the BRCA2 gene.[5] National Comprehensive Cancer Network guidelines now recommend routine genetic counseling and genetic testing for all patients diagnosed with PC. If an alteration is identified, cascade testing (and high-risk cancer screening) may be offered to additional family members. In addition, identification of germline pathogenic variants may have therapeutic implications for the patient, as some genetic variants may predict responsiveness to specific chemotherapeutics.[6]

Principle #1: Accurate Determination of Clinical Stage

Accurate clinical staging is fundamental to an assessment of operability and helps to facilitate not only stage-specific treatment planning but also shared decision-making with patients and their families. Because most patients with PC present with jaundice, there is an impulse to perform an endoscopic retrograde cholangiopancreatography (ERCP) as the first diagnostic study, as it may be both diagnostic and therapeutic. In contrast to benign biliary obstruction (such as choledocholithiasis), which can occur acutely and is often associated with significant pain and cholangitis, PCs usually present with gradual painless jaundice that is rarely associated with cholangitis. For this reason, although patients may present with jaundice, emergent therapeutic endoscopic interventions are rarely needed. An emphasis should be placed instead on obtaining high-quality CT imaging before any invasive intervention, such as an ERCP. Rarely does the clinical presentation mandate an invasive procedure before obtaining a diagnostic CT scan. The incidence of ERCP-associated pancreatitis is

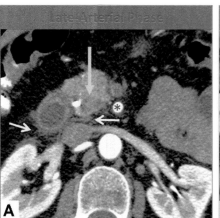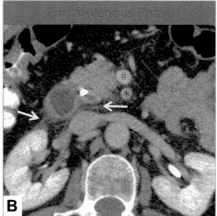

Fig. 1. Resectable pancreatic adenocarcinoma (*orange arrow*). CT in the late-arterial (*A*) and portal-venous (*B*) phases demonstrates a low-attenuation mass completely confined to the pancreas with no tumor contact of the superior mesenteric artery (*red**) and vein (*blue#*) with primary tumor seen best on the arterial phase. Note that a plastic endobiliary stent was placed before this staging CT, with subtle peripancreatic and periduodenal fat stranding likely representing postplacement pancreatitis/inflammation (*yellow arrows*). Sometimes inflammation can be confused with extrapancreatic tumor extension and confound interpretation for accurate staging. Typically, the staging CT should be performed before stent placement to avoid this pitfall.

approximately 4%, and procedure-related complications can result in significant peripancreatic inflammation, which obfuscates the relationship of the primary tumor and adjacent vasculature, resulting in inaccurate assessment of the clinical stage (**Fig. 1**). Prioritizing a high-quality CT scan before any invasive intervention ensures accurate initial staging of the cancer.

Imaging for PC will be explored in greater detail in Chittenden and colleagues' article, "12. Germline Testing for Individuals with Pancreatic Adenocarcinoma and Novel Genetic Risk Factors," in this issue. Herein, we will detail the anatomic features that define the clinical stage of PC. From a surgical perspective, CT scans are the preferred diagnostic study to assess the location of the primary tumor in relation to adjacent vascular structures and to evaluate for distant metastases. The CT scan should include the chest as well as a pancreatic protocol CT scan. The latter includes thin (1 mm slice thickness) image acquisition of the pancreas through both late arterial and venous phases. The late-arterial phase is usually the best phase to identify PC, as the timing provides the maximum contrast difference between normally enhancing pancreatic parenchyma and the PCs that are generally hypoenhancing. In addition, this is the best phase for analyzing the tumor-artery relationships and to note the presence of any aberrant arterial anatomy. The portal venous phase is valuable for assessing variant venous anatomy and tumor-vessel abutment or encasement. In addition, metastatic lesions in the liver are often best appreciated in the venous phase. Additional diagnostic studies, such as a MRI study or PET scan, may be helpful if indeterminate liver lesions or suspicious nodal involvement are detected on CT imaging.

Accurate clinical staging provides the framework for multidisciplinary management, and although consensus among clinicians may not exist (**Tables 1**), all published guidelines generally agree on 2 overarching clinical stages of PC: potentially operable (resectable and borderline resectable disease) and likely inoperable (locally advanced

Table 1
Comparison of radiographic differences in definitions for resectable, borderline resectable, and locally advanced pancreatic cancer

	Commonality	NCCN[1]	AHPBA/SSO/SSAT[2]	MDA[3]/MCW[4]
Resectable				
SMA, celiac artery, CHA	No abutment	No abutment	No abutment, with clear fat planes	No abutment
SMV/PV	No abutment	No abutment, or ≤180° contact without contour irregularity	No abutment, distortion, thrombus, or encasement	No abutment, or <50% narrowing
Borderline Resectable				
SMV/PV	Abutment	Abutment, ≤180° with contour irregularity, or thrombosis	Abutment, impingement, encasement, or short-segment occlusion	Abutment, short-segment occlusion, or >50% narrowing with reconstruction
SMA	Abutment	Abutment	Abutment	Abutment
Celiac artery	Abutment	Abutment	Abutment	Abutment
CHA	Abutment or short-segment encasement	Abutment or short-segment encasement	Abutment or short-segment encasement	Abutment or short-segment encasement
Locally Advanced				
SMV/PV	Involvement or occlusion without reconstruction options	Unreconstructable SMV/PV	Major extensive thrombosis	Occlusion without reconstruction options
SMA	Encasement	Encasement	Circumferential encasement	Encasement
Celiac artery	Encasement	Encasement	Circumferential encasement	Encasement without reconstruction options
CHA	Encasement	Encasement	Circumferential encasement	Encasement without reconstruction options

Abutment = tumor involves ≤ 180° vessel circumference. Encasement = tumor involves > 180° vessel circumference.

Abbreviations: AHPBA/SSO/SSAT, Americas Hepatopancreaticobiliary Association/Society of Surgical Oncology/Society for Surgery of the Alimentary Tract; CHA, common hepatic artery; MDA/MCW, MD Anderson/Medical College of Wisconsin; NCCN, National Comprehensive Cancer Network; SMA, superior mesenteric artery; SMV/PV, superior mesenteric vein/portal vein.

Table 2		
Locally advanced pancreatic cancer subclassification		
	Type	
	A	**B**
Tumor-Artery Anatomy		
SMA	>180° encasement but ≤ 270°	≥270°
Celiac axis	>180° encasement but does not extend to aorta	>180° and abutment/encasement of aorta
CHA	>180° encasement with extension to celiac artery	>180° encasement with extension beyond bifurcation of proper hepatic arteries
Tumor-Vein Anatomy (SMV/PV)		Occlusion without option for reconstruction

Abbreviations: CHA, common hepatic artery; SMA, superior mesenteric artery; SMV/PV, superior mesenteric vein/portal vein.

and metastatic disease). Resectable disease (**Fig. 2**) is defined by an absence of tumor extension to the superior mesenteric artery (SMA), celiac axis, or hepatic artery with a patent superior mesenteric vein (SMV)/portal vein (PV) confluence. Lack of arterial abutment is characterized by the presence of normal soft tissue planes between the tumor and the arteries. Associated SMV/PV abutment/encasement may be acceptable, provided that adequate inflow and outflow targets are identified for potential reconstruction. The distinction between borderline resectable (**Fig. 3**) and locally advanced disease (**Fig. 4**) is determined by the degree of tumor-artery interface (abutment is defined as ≤180° and encasement >180°). Borderline resectable disease is defined as tumor abutment less than or equal to 180° of the SMA or celiac axis. Because of the extent of disease, tumors that are borderline resectable are considered at high risk for having a positive margin, and indeed, the rate of margin positive (R1) resections with a surgery-first approach is consistently around 40%.[7,8] Neoadjuvant therapy (particularly neoadjuvant radiotherapy) has been advocated as a means to sterilize at least the periphery of the tumor, thereby facilitating a margin negative (R0) resection. As the tumor-artery interface increases from abutment to encasement, a complete gross resection of all disease is likely not possible without arterial resection. The borderline resectable category also includes tumor abutment/encasement of a short segment of the hepatic artery, usually at the origin of the gastroduodenal artery, or an occluded SMV/PV, amenable to reconstruction. Locally advanced tumors historically were considered inoperable, but with recent contemporary multimodality therapy, an increasing number of patients with locally advanced tumors are being considered for resection. Although locally advanced tumors are defined by arterial encasement (≥180° of contact) of the celiac artery or SMA, or SMV/PV occlusion with no technical option for reconstruction, at our institution we have found it helpful to subclassify locally advanced tumors into potentially operable (type A) and likely inoperable (type B) (**Table 2**).[9] The dichotomy between A and B largely arises from whether an oncologic resection, R0 resection, could be performed without violation of the tumor. For example, with 360° of arterial encasement, oncologic resection would mandate en bloc resection of the artery. If the tumor involves the celiac axis, resection (with or without reconstruction) may be possible if adequate collateral blood supply to the liver can be preserved—and a growing number of institutions have

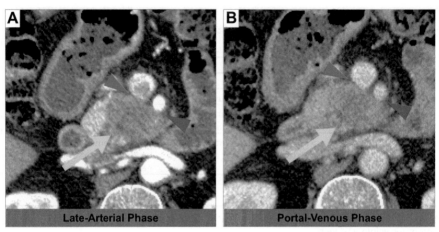

Fig. 2. Borderline resectable pancreatic adenocarcinoma. Late-arterial (*A*) and portal-venous (*B*) phases demonstrate a large low-attenuation mass compatible with pancreatic adenocarcinoma (*orange arrow*). The anterior margin of the tumor abuts (less than 180°) the posterior walls of the superior mesenteric artery (*red arrowhead*) and vein (*blue arrowhead*).

experience with these procedures.[10] For these reasons, select tumors with encasement of the celiac axis may be potentially operable (type A). However, en bloc resection and reconstruction of the superior mesenteric artery is associated with high significant morbidity and mortality and are generally not performed at most institutions. Therefore, 360° encasement of the superior mesenteric artery would generally be considered inoperable (type B). Given the anatomic complexities of patients with locally advanced PC, a multidisciplinary review of the imaging by dedicated abdominal radiologists and surgeons at the time of diagnosis and each restaging interval is critical for staging consensus and to facilitate treatment planning.

Endoscopic Procedures

Following CT imaging, the next procedure usually is an endoscopic ultrasound (EUS) with fine-needle aspiration or fine-needle biopsy for tissue diagnosis. EUS is preferred over percutaneous CT-guided biopsy, which has been associated with up to a 16% rate of peritoneal carcinomatosis presumably related to dissemination of malignant cells along the biopsy tract. For tissue diagnosis, rapid on-site cytopathologic evaluation increases the diagnostic success of EUS/FNA biopsies. Rapid on-site evaluation allows for repeated endoscopic sampling until an adequate cytologic specimen can be obtained and facilitates the simultaneous placement of a decompressive metal stent in patients with obstructive jaundice. Thus rapid on-site cytopathologic evaluation allows for a "one-stop shop" approach, such that a diagnosis can be made and durable biliary drainage can be achieved during one anesthetic procedure. In general, uncovered metal endobiliary stents are preferred over plastic stents for higher patency rates (104 days vs 83 days) and lower rates of complications (12 vs 35%).[11] Covered metal stents have higher rates of stent migration and higher rates of stent-related cholecystitis, as the stents can cover and occlude the cystic duct orifice. In the uncommon circumstance in which an endobiliary stent cannot be placed, a percutaneous transhepatic catheter may be placed with potential for converting this to an endobiliary stent in the future.

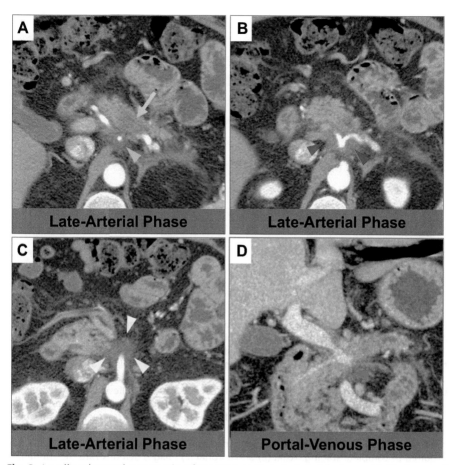

Fig. 3. Locally advanced pancreatic adenocarcinoma. Late-arterial phases (*A–C*) at several levels demonstrate a low-attenuation mass in the pancreatic body (*orange arrow*) with advanced locoregional extrapancreatic tumor extension with soft tissue encasing (greater than 180°) the left-gastric artery (*green arrowhead*), celiac bifurcation (*red arrowheads*), and superior mesenteric artery (*yellow arrowheads*). Portal-venous phase coronal image (*D*) demonstrates the mass causing severe narrowing of the cephalad superior mesenteric vein with a "gap" below the portal-splenic-SMV venous confluence (*blue arrowhead*).

Management of the Symptomatic Patient

If the plan is for neoadjuvant therapy, this can be particularly challenging in the setting of a gastric outlet obstruction or biliary stent–related complication. Management of a gastric outlet obstruction with endoscopic duodenal stenting has been well established in the palliative setting. For palliation, duodenal stenting has been associated with oral intake within 24 hours after placement, and the rates of reintervention for recurrent symptoms occurred in 18% of patients at a median of 125 days. In the preoperative setting, the benefits of duodenal stenting must be weighed against additional considerations. Once an endoluminal stent is placed in the duodenum, access to the biliary system becomes much more complicated, if not impossible. Coordinated planning with the advanced gastrointestinal endoscopist team is helpful to

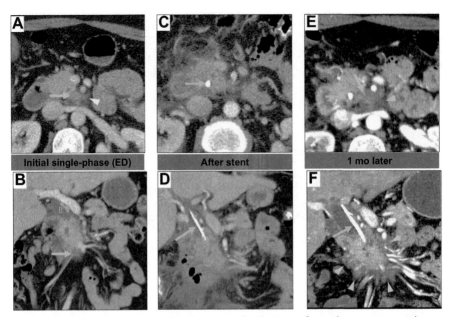

Fig. 4. Postintervention pancreatitis. Initial single-phase CT from the emergency department (ED) in the axial (*A*) and coronal (*B*) planes demonstrate a subtle uncinate process low-attenuation mass (*orange arrow*) with subtle extrapancreatic fat stranding (inflammation and/or tumor) abutting the superior mesenteric artery (*yellow arrowhead*). Note obstruction with dilation of the extrahepatic bile duct (*green B*). Before obtaining a dual-phase CT, the patient was emergently taken to endoscopy to relieve biliary obstruction with a plastic stent (*green arrows*). CT after biliary stenting in the axial (*C*) and coronal (*D*) planes demonstrated the subtle tumor in the uncinate process is not well seen and there is extensive peripancreatic, periduodenal, and transverse mesocolonic inflammation (*red arrowheads*) compatible with postprocedure pancreatitis. One month later, dual-phase CT was acquired to complete staging. Axial (*E*) and coronal (*F*) images demonstrate the subtle uncinate process mass can be visible again, and there is now extensive peripancreatic soft-tissue entrapping/encasing several superior mesenteric artery and vein branches (*orange arrowheads*). The soft tissue is likely post-pancreatitis inflammation; however, these findings are indeterminate by CT and confound accurate staging.

coordinate the placement of durable biliary and luminal stents, as to ensure that the placement of one does not complicate or preclude the placement of the other. In addition, duodenal stents placed in the second and third portions of the duodenum can inadvertently make the surgical resection more challenging. Tumors of the pancreas that generally involve this area usually also involve distal branches of the superior mesenteric artery and vein. Exposure to the root of mesentery in this area can sometimes be made more challenging with the placement of the metal endoluminal stent that may limit the ability of the surgeon to rotate the surgical specimen to allow for optimal exposure.

Biliary stent–related complications occur in approximately 15% of patients during neoadjuvant therapy and occur with more frequency with longer therapy, as the patency rates of the stents decline over time. In general, monitoring of liver function tests may be a harbinger of impending stent occlusion. Also, on CT imaging, the presence of pneumobilia both within the liver and within the stent is usually a good indicator of stent patency. When a stent becomes occluded, often this can be managed with the placement of a covered stent inside the existing uncovered stent. Occasionally, because of placement of a covered stent or from tumor ingrowth, patients can develop cholecystitis during neoadjuvant therapy. In our experience, in patients with potentially operable PC, acute cholecystitis is best managed with the placement of a cholecystostomy tube rather than a cholecystectomy[12]; this prevents a significant interruption of neoadjuvant therapy and does not compromise rates of completion of neoadjuvant therapy and surgery. In the absence of disease progression, the gallbladder can then be addressed at the time of pancreatectomy.

MANAGEMENT OF OPERABLE PANCREATIC CANCER
Principle #2: Prioritize Treatment Sequencing to Address Disease Biology

The rationale for neoadjuvant therapy is based on the observation that most of the patients with localized PC succumb to metastatic disease after curative-intent surgery; this has led to an evolving understanding of PC as a systemic disease with universal agreement that all patients with PC should receive chemotherapy, independent of stage of disease. For several decades, adjuvant therapy has been the standard of care based on the results of several large randomized controlled trials.[13,14] Although a recent randomized controlled trial comparing adjuvant gemcitabine versus 5-fluorouracil/irinotecan/oxaliplatin (PRODIGE-24) demonstrated historic improvements in median overall survival (54 months) with the experimental arm, it is important to remember that the design of adjuvant clinical trials have an inherent selection bias.[14] Patients who are enrolled in adjuvant trials must have recovered from a pancreatectomy with minimal complication, have preserved performance status, and no evidence of disease progression. Unfortunately, retrospective data from large cancer registries have demonstrated that the delivery of adjuvant therapy is unpredictable, with up to 50% of patients who underwent surgical resection never receiving adjuvant therapy.[15,16] This finding was recapitulated in a recent randomized controlled trial that compared perioperative (neoadjuvant and adjuvant) therapy to surgery followed by adjuvant therapy (PREOPANC trial) in patients with localized PC.[3] Only 65 (51%) of the 128 patients in the surgery-first arm received any adjuvant therapy. Even within this subset of patients, not all patients were able to complete the full course of adjuvant chemotherapy. In addition, in the adjuvant setting the primary tumor has been removed, so the ability to assess treatment response to the chemotherapy is limited. Because response to chemotherapeutic regimens is not uniform across all patients, it is reasonable to assume that some patients may be subjected to ineffective systemic therapy and incur unnecessary toxicity.

In contrast to a surgery-first approach, neoadjuvant therapy has several advantages: (1) early delivery of systemic therapy for presumed micrometastases, (2) the ability to identify aggressive tumor biology that may be resistant to available systemic therapies, (3) assessment of treatment response in the primary tumor, and (4) improved selection of patients for surgery by stage of disease and response to therapy. Several institutions have reported initial outcomes with neoadjuvant therapy, and among patients who are able to complete neoadjuvant therapy and surgery the median overall survival exceeds 40 months at most centers.[17,18] Neoadjuvant therapy with contemporary multidrug regimens have been studied in the recent Southwestern Oncology Group S1505 trial. Approximately 70% to 80% of patients with operable PC who initiated neoadjuvant therapy completed neoadjuvant therapy and surgical resection.[19] The long-term results of the PREOPANC trial that randomized patients to receive perioperative (neoadjuvant and adjuvant therapy) therapy or surgery followed by adjuvant therapy demonstrated improved overall survival among the patients with operable PC who received perioperative therapy (hazard ratio: 0.73; $P = .025$).[3] The ongoing clinical trial (Alliance A021806) that will further evaluate neoadjuvant versus surgery-first treatment approaches using contemporary chemotherapeutic regimens. Many centers have already adopted neoadjuvant therapy for patients with localized PC. Currently, all consensus guidelines recommend neoadjuvant therapy for borderline resectable disease, and an increasing number of centers advocate neoadjuvant therapy for resectable disease as well. Likely, future investigations will move away from comparing neoadjuvant versus adjuvant treatment sequencing and focus instead on defining the optimal neoadjuvant therapy for patients, including the best chemotherapeutic regimen, duration of treatment, and whether to include chemoradiation. At the Medical College of Wisconsin, patients with PC are currently being treated with total neoadjuvant therapy approach; this consists of 4 months of neoadjuvant chemotherapy (with interval restaging at 2 months to assess for treatment response and change in chemotherapy in the absence of response) followed by neoadjuvant chemoradiation with a 4-week break before surgery.

Principle #3: Minimize risk for Local-Only Failures

Although PC is increasingly being recognized as a systemic disease, local control remains a significant clinical problem. Previous studies have characterized the patterns of disease recurrence for patients with operable PC treated with a surgery-first approach and demonstrated that local-only recurrences occurred in 20% of patients and are primarily a late event (occurring > 2 years from surgery).[20–22] The high rate of local-only recurrences for patients with PC is not unexpected, as the disease is associated with high rates of R1 resection (40% +) and node positive disease (>70%)[7]; this may be attributed to both the infiltrative nature of PC, which has high rates of perineural and vascular invasion, as well as the close proximity of these tumors to critical vascular structures, such as the SMA, which places them at the highest risk for an R1 resection. The timing of local recurrences as predominantly a late pattern is also not unexpected, as patients must have survived the gauntlet of metastatic disease recurrence to be alive to have a local-only recurrence. Indeed, this pattern of recurrence also explains why clinical trials using neoadjuvant radiation that are designed for primary endpoint of overall survival may only demonstrate a difference in survival with more mature follow-up, as was observed in the PREOPANC study, which was initially reported as a negative study, but then demonstrated a survival benefit with longer follow-up.[3]

Unfortunately, patients with local-only disease recurrence represent a cohort of patients who may have been potentially curable—either with improved surgical technique or as with other solid tumors, the addition of radiotherapy. Novel dose and fractionation approaches for radiotherapy will be discussed in further detail in Rosenthal and colleagues' article, "What Can We Learn About Pancreatic Adenocarcinoma from Imaging?," in this issue. Not surprisingly, the addition of neoadjuvant radiotherapy has been demonstrated reproducibly to halve the rates of node positive disease and R1 resections in PC.[3,23–25] These pathologic changes also translate into decreased rates of local recurrence with the addition of neoadjuvant radiotherapy, from 20% to less than 10%.[26] Furthermore, the addition of radiotherapy is also associated with pancreatic gland fibrosis. From a surgical perspective, this is an advantage, as a fibrotic gland is more likely to hold suture and less likely to result in a postoperative pancreatic fistula. Indeed, surgical complications overall are reduced following neoadjuvant radiotherapy as compared with upfront surgical resection.[27]

Principle #4: Define Clinically Important Treatment Responses

Although there is a growing acceptance of neoadjuvant therapy for patients with localized PC, the optimal neoadjuvant treatment remains controversial and undefined. There is variability in the duration of systemic therapy, utilization of radiotherapy, and the use of adjuvant therapy. The heterogeneity of treatment is somewhat rooted in a lack of consensus as to what the endpoint of neoadjuvant therapy should be: whether surgical resection of the primary tumor is an adequate endpoint independent of treatment response? Currently, the threshold for proceeding with surgery after neoadjuvant therapy is the absence of disease progression, rather than the presence of a treatment response. In patients with localized PC, defining treatment response to therapy can be particularly challenging as, by definition, measurable extrapancreatic disease does not exist and the primary tumors are often enriched with stroma and therefore may not demonstrate marked radiographic responses.[28] The inability to accurately assess response to neoadjuvant therapy may account for the subset of patients with the early postoperative recurrences following neoadjuvant therapy. Therefore, there is an urgent need to better define treatment response in the neoadjuvant setting.

At the Medical College of Wisconsin, we assess treatment response based on 3 criteria: the presence or absence of clinical benefit (eg, the resolution of pain), CT findings to suggest stable or responding disease versus disease progression (change in cross-sectional diameter of the tumor), and the decrease or increase in serum level of carbohydrate antigen (CA) 19-9. Clinical benefit and CA19-9 response are used as surrogate markers of response under the assumption that extrapancreatic micro-metastatic disease has likely responded to therapy if the condition of the patient improves and the level of CA19-9 declines. Although modern chemotherapy regimens have been associated with 30% to 40% response rates among patients with more advanced disease, most of the patients with localized PC are likely to have minimal to modest changes in tumor size.[28–31] Moreover, although tumors may demonstrate a decrease in overall size, the relationship of the tumor to adjacent vessels generally does not change. A change in clinical stage, reflecting a change in local tumor-vessel anatomy, in response to neoadjuvant therapy has been reported to occur in less than 1% of cases.[28] Therefore, restaging imaging should primarily be performed to (1) identify disease progression, whether it be local or distant, which would alter clinical management and (2) facilitate operative planning. Importantly, careful attention to radiographic findings allows for a detailed preoperative plan, especially when vascular reconstruction is anticipated. It is especially important that vascular resections occur as planned events rather than an emergent response to vascular injury, as unexpected vascular injuries can ultimately compromise the completeness of the resection, resulting in a positive margin as well as the durability of the surgical reconstruction.[32,33]

CA19-9 has been demonstrated to be a useful prognostic marker in patients with PC.[34] Among patients with localized PC, a decrease in CA19-9 in response to neoadjuvant therapy has previously been reported to correlate with overall survival.[35] A greater than 50% reduction in CA19-9 levels in response to neoadjuvant therapy has been associated with an improved overall survival.[36,37] For patients with an elevated CA19-9 level at the time of diagnosis, changes in CA19-9 levels have been demonstrated to correspond to treatment response and be prognostic of overall survival.[35,36] Among patients who receive neoadjuvant therapy, approximately one-third of patients will normalize their CA19-9 levels before surgery, one-third of patients will normalize their CA19-9 levels after surgery, and one-third of patients will never normalize their CA19-9 levels even after neoadjuvant therapy and surgery.

Importantly, among patients who undergo neoadjuvant therapy and pancreatic resection, the normalization of CA19-9 in response to therapy has been a highly favorable prognostic factor and has been associated with a median survival of 46 months.[35] Equally important is the recognition that an increase in CA19-9 level after therapy correlates with disease progression. Although most of the patients will experience a decline in CA19-9 in response to neoadjuvant therapy, approximately 20% of patients will have an increase in CA19-9, and among these patients, metastatic disease was detected in 50% of cases.[38] Therefore, clinicians should have a low threshold for expanding the diagnostic workup (MRI of liver or PET) before surgery in patients who have an increasing CA19-9 after neoadjuvant therapy.

EXPANDING SURGICAL SELECTION
Pushing the Boundaries—Surgery for Locally Advanced Pancreatic Cancer

Locally advanced PC has historically been treated with chemotherapy alone or in combination with chemoradiation with median overall survival rates ranging from 13 to 18 months.[39,40] Patients with locally advanced PC who received chemoradiation following chemotherapy represent a select cohort of patients did not progress on prior systemic therapy. With improvements in systemic therapy, the number of patients with locally advanced PC who demonstrate responding or stable disease to systemic therapy is expanding. After 4 to 6 months of systemic therapy, in the absence of metastatic disease, the options for management of the primary tumor include best supportive care, maintenance chemotherapy, chemoradiation, noncurative therapies (such as irreversible electroporation), or surgery. For many patients, surgery is the most attractive option, as it is a potentially curative treatment and signals an end of treatment. However, owing to the complexity of the tumor-vessel relationships, surgery for locally advanced PC is inherently more complicated than a standard pancreatectomy and carries a higher risk of morbidity and mortality. The vascular reconstruction requires resection and reconstruction of critical vascular structures as well as additional vascular procedures (mesocaval shunts, distal splenorenal shunt) that may be performed to facilitate safe exposure for resection.[41,42] Nevertheless, in a subset of highly selected patients who have undergone an extensive course of neoadjuvant therapy (including chemotherapy and chemoradiation), surgical resection may be of value. In our institutional experience of 108 consecutive patients with locally advanced PC, 40 (42%) were able to complete neoadjuvant therapy and surgery (28 [62%] were type A and 12 [24%] were type B). R0 resection was achieved in 32 (80%) of the patients, and there were no postoperative mortalities. The patients who completed neoadjuvant therapy and surgery had a median overall survival of 38.9 months. Increasing complex vascular resections are being performed for locally advanced PC. Not only is it important that such cases be directed to high-volume centers with appropriate technical expertise, but a coordinated multidisciplinary approach is necessary to ensure that such patients benefit from neoadjuvant therapy while minimizing the toxicity of prolonged multimodality therapy.

Principle #5: Avoid High-Risk Operations in High-Risk Patients

Although eligibility for surgery continues to expand, it is important that the decision for surgery be aligned with the overall goals of the patient, realizing that the long-term goal of a potentially curative resection must be weighed against potential loss of independence and quality of life. A careful assessment of the patient's performance status and medical comorbidities should be reevaluated repeatedly before surgery. Several studies have demonstrated that patients with poor performance status or uncontrolled comorbidities are likely to experience postoperative morbidity and mortality.[43–45] The physiologic stress associated with preoperative therapy has the potential to identify/expose patients with poor physiologic reserve who may not tolerate a large operation or the prolonged postoperative recovery. If a given patient cannot tolerate induction therapy, they are unlikely to recover to their prediagnosis level of independence with self-care. Identification of such patients at the time of diagnosis without the "stress test" of induction therapy may be difficult—a surgery-first treatment approach may incur a higher morbidity and mortality in the absence of the selection advantage afforded by neoadjuvant treatment sequencing. During and after induction therapy, physicians can more accurately assess the physiologic tolerance of an individual patient to undergo major surgery. Perhaps even more importantly, after neoadjuvant therapy, the patient and their family have an improved understanding of the disease, are in a better position to evaluate the impact of therapy on their physical health and support systems, and evolve a much more educated opinion regarding their physicians' recommendation for or against an operation.

In our experience, among older patients who completed neoadjuvant therapy but did not undergo surgery (due to either disease progression seen on restaging or a decline in performance status due to the combination of treatment toxicity and underlying comorbidities), the median overall survival was the same regardless of why surgery was not performed.[46] A decline in performance status due to evolving medical comorbidities or the failure to recover from treatment-related toxicity was just as powerful a predictor of poor outcome as was the development of metastatic disease; this confirms previous reports of the powerful impact of performance status on response to anticancer therapy and overall survival in patients with solid tumors.

SUMMARY

Surgery is necessary but not sufficient for long-term survival for patients with PC. Multimodality therapy is recommended for all patients with operable disease and may be most reliably delivered in the neoadjuvant setting. From a surgical perspective, operability depends on 3 factors: clinical stage of disease, response to neoadjuvant therapy, and patient performance status. Increasingly, the complexity of delivering multidisciplinary care will require close coordination of care between surgeons, medical oncologists, and radiation oncologists, to best optimize and individualize treatments to each patient. During neoadjuvant therapy, treatment response may help to further guide surgical selection. In patients who demonstrate a clinical, radiographic, and tumor marker response, surgical resection may be of significant benefit, even in select patients with locally advanced PC.

CLINICS CARE POINTS

Pearls.

- Clinical staging with a pancreatic protocol CT scan at diagnosis, prior to endoscopic biliary interventions, is critical to the assessment of operability.

- Multimodality therapy is recommended for all patients with operable disease and may be most reliably delivered in the neoadjuvant setting.

- The delivery of neoadjuvant chemoradiation reduces local-only recurrences.

- Assessment of treatment response should be based on 3 criteria: the presence or absence of clinical benefit, CT findings to suggest stable or responding disease versus disease progression, and the decrease or increase in CA 19-9 levels.Pitfalls.

Pitfalls

- Patients may experience biliary complications, such as cholecystitis or biliary stent occlusion, during neoadjuvant therapy. When possible, these complications should be temporized with medical management without immediate surgery to avoid significant interruption of neoadjuvant therapy.
- Approximately 20% of patients will have an increase in CA19-9 during neoadjuvant therapy and this is often a harbinger of metastatic disease progression.
- A decline in performance status due to evolving medical comorbidities or from treatment-related toxicity is associated with poor oncologic and surgical outcomes.

REFERENCES

1. Pancreatic Adenocarcinoma. NCCN Clinical Practice Guidlines in Oncology (NCCN Guidelines) 2021; 2.2021. 2021. Available at: http://www.nccn.org/professionals/physician_gls/pdf/pancreatic.pdf. Accessed April 1, 2022.
2. Evans DB, Varadhachary GR, Crane CH, et al. Preoperative gemcitabine-based chemoradiation for patients with resectable adenocarcinoma of the pancreatic head. J Clin Oncol 2008;26(21):3496–502.
3. Versteijne E, Suker M, Groothuis K, et al. Preoperative Chemoradiotherapy Versus Immediate Surgery for Resectable and Borderline Resectable Pancreatic Cancer: Results of the Dutch Randomized Phase III PREOPANC Trial. J Clin Oncol 2020;38(16):1763–73.
4. Tsai S, Christians KK, George B, et al. A Phase II Clinical Trial of Molecular Profiled Neoadjuvant Therapy for Localized Pancreatic Ductal Adenocarcinoma. Ann Surg 2018;268(4):610–9.
5. Canto MI, Harinck F, Hruban RH, et al. International Cancer of the Pancreas Screening (CAPS) Consortium summit on the management of patients with increased risk for familial pancreatic cancer. Gut 2013;62(3):339–47.
6. Golan T, Hammel P, Reni M, et al. Maintenance Olaparib for Germline BRCA-Mutated Metastatic Pancreatic Cancer. N Engl J Med 2019;381(4):317–27.
7. Winter JM, Cameron JL, Campbell KA, et al. 1423 pancreaticoduodenectomies for pancreatic cancer: A single-institution experience. J Gastrointest Surg 2006;10(9):1199–210.
8. Winter JM, Brennan MF, Tang LH, et al. Survival after resection of pancreatic adenocarcinoma: results from a single institution over three decades. Ann Surg Oncol 2012;19(1):169–75.
9. Evans DB, Kamgar M, Tsai S. Goals of Treatment Sequencing for Localized Pancreatic Cancer. Ann Surg Oncol 2019;26(12):3815–9.
10. Christians KK, Pilgrim CH, Tsai S, et al. Arterial resection at the time of pancreatectomy for cancer. Surgery 2014;155(5):919–26.
11. Aadam AA, Evans DB, Khan A, et al. Efficacy and safety of self-expandable metal stents for biliary decompression in patients receiving neoadjuvant therapy for pancreatic cancer: a prospective study. Gastrointest Endosc 2012;76(1):67–75.
12. Jariwalla NR, Khan AH, Dua K, et al. Management of Acute Cholecystitis during Neoadjuvant Therapy in Patients with Pancreatic Adenocarcinoma. Ann Surg Oncol 2019;26(13):4515–21.
13. Sohal DP, Walsh RM, Ramanathan RK, et al. Pancreatic adenocarcinoma: treating a systemic disease with systemic therapy. J Natl Cancer Inst 2014;106(3):dju011.
14. Conroy T, Hammal P, Hebbar M, et al. Unicancer GI PRODIGE 24/CCTG PA.6 trial: A multicenter international randomized phase III trial of adjuvant

mFOLFIRIONX versus gemcitabine in patients wtih resected pancreatic ductal adenocarcinomas. JCO 2018;36(Suppl). abstr LABA4001).

15. Mayo SC, Gilson MM, Herman JM, et al. Management of patients with pancreatic adenocarcinoma: national trends in patient selection, operative management, and use of adjuvant therapy. J Am Coll Surg 2012;214(1):33–45.

16. Merkow RP, Bilimoria KY, Tomlinson JS, et al. Postoperative complications reduce adjuvant chemotherapy use in resectable pancreatic cancer. Ann Surg 2014; 260(2):372–7.

17. Katz MH, Wang H, Fleming JB, et al. Long-term survival after multidisciplinary management of resected pancreatic adenocarcinoma. Ann Surg Oncol 2009; 16(4):836–47.

18. Ward EP, Evans DB, Tsai S. Ten-year experience in optimizing neoadjuvant therapy for localized pancreatic cancer-Medical college of Wisconsin perspective. J Surg Oncol 2021;123(6):1405–13.

19. Sohal DPS, Duong M, Ahmad SA, et al. Efficacy of Perioperative Chemotherapy for Resectable Pancreatic Adenocarcinoma: A Phase 2 Randomized Clinical Trial. JAMA Oncol 2021;7(3):421–7.

20. Barnes CA, Aldakkak M, Christians KK, et al. Radiographic patterns of first disease recurrence after neoadjuvant therapy and surgery for patients with resectable and borderline resectable pancreatic cancer. Surgery 2020;168(3):440–7.

21. Groot VP, Gemenetzis G, Blair AB, et al. Defining and Predicting Early Recurrence in 957 Patients With Resected Pancreatic Ductal Adenocarcinoma. Ann Surg 2019;269(6):1154–62.

22. Groot VP, Rezaee N, Wu W, et al. Patterns, Timing, and Predictors of Recurrence Following Pancreatectomy for Pancreatic Ductal Adenocarcinoma. Ann Surg 2018;267(5):936–45.

23. Cloyd JM, Heh V, Pawlik TM, et al. Neoadjuvant Therapy for Resectable and Borderline Resectable Pancreatic Cancer: A Meta-Analysis of Randomized Controlled Trials. J Clin Med 2020;9(4).

24. Bradley A, Van Der Meer R. Upfront Surgery versus Neoadjuvant Therapy for Resectable Pancreatic Cancer: Systematic Review and Bayesian Network Meta-analysis. Sci Rep 2019;9(1):4354.

25. Versteijne E, Vogel JA, Besselink MG, et al. Meta-analysis comparing upfront surgery with neoadjuvant treatment in patients with resectable or borderline resectable pancreatic cancer. Br J Surg 2018;105(8):946–58.

26. Wittmann D, Hall WA, Christians KK, et al. Impact of Neoadjuvant Chemoradiation on Pathologic Response in Patients With Localized Pancreatic Cancer. Front Oncol 2020;10:460.

27. Cooper AB, Parmar AD, Riall TS, et al. Does the use of neoadjuvant therapy for pancreatic adenocarcinoma increase postoperative morbidity and mortality rates? J Gastrointest Surg 2015;19(1):80–6 [discussion: 86–7].

28. Katz MH, Fleming JB, Bhosale P, et al. Response of borderline resectable pancreatic cancer to neoadjuvant therapy is not reflected by radiographic indicators. Cancer 2012;118(23):5749–56.

29. Tran Cao HS, Balachandran A, Wang H, et al. Radiographic tumor-vein interface as a predictor of intraoperative, pathologic, and oncologic outcomes in resectable and borderline resectable pancreatic cancer. J Gastrointest Surg 2014; 18(2):269–78 [discussion: 278].

30. Von Hoff DD, Goldstein D, Renschler MF. Albumin-bound paclitaxel plus gemcitabine in pancreatic cancer. The New Engl J Med 2014;370(5):479–80.

31. Conroy T, Desseigne F, Ychou M, et al. FOLFIRINOX versus gemcitabine for metastatic pancreatic cancer. The New Engl J Med 2011;364(19):1817–25.

32. Ravikumar R, Sabin C, Abu Hilal M, et al. Portal vein resection in borderline resectable pancreatic cancer: a United kingdom multicenter study. J Am Coll Surgeons 2014;218(3):401–11.

33. Smoot RL, Christein JD, Farnell MB. Durability of portal venous reconstruction following resection during pancreaticoduodenectomy. J Gastrointest Surg 2006;10(10):1371–5.

34. Humphris JL, Chang DK, Johns AL, et al. The prognostic and predictive value of serum CA19.9 in pancreatic cancer. Ann Oncol 2012;23(7):1713–22.

35. Tsai S, George B, Wittmann D, et al. Importance of Normalization of CA19-9 Levels Following Neoadjuvant Therapy in Patients With Localized Pancreatic Cancer. Ann Surg 2018;271(4):740–7.

36. Boone BA, Steve J, Zenati MS, et al. Serum CA 19-9 response to neoadjuvant therapy is associated with outcome in pancreatic adenocarcinoma. Ann Surg Oncol 2014;21(13):4351–8.

37. Katz MH, Varadhachary GR, Fleming JB, et al. Serum CA 19-9 as a marker of resectability and survival in patients with potentially resectable pancreatic cancer treated with neoadjuvant chemoradiation. Ann Surg Oncol 2010;17(7):1794–801.

38. Aldakkak M, Christians KK, Krepline AN, et al. Pre-treatment carbohydrate antigen 19-9 does not predict the response to neoadjuvant therapy in patients with localized pancreatic cancer. HPB (Oxford) 2015;17(10):942–52.

39. Hammel P, Huguet F, van Laethem JL, et al. Effect of Chemoradiotherapy vs Chemotherapy on Survival in Patients With Locally Advanced Pancreatic Cancer Controlled After 4 Months of Gemcitabine With or Without Erlotinib: The LAP07 Randomized Clinical Trial. JAMA 2016;315(17):1844–53.

40. Krishnan S, Chadha AS, Suh Y, et al. Focal Radiation Therapy Dose Escalation Improves Overall Survival in Locally Advanced Pancreatic Cancer Patients Receiving Induction Chemotherapy and Consolidative Chemoradiation. Int J Radiat Oncol Biol Phys 2016;94(4):755–65.

41. Pilgrim CH, Tsai S, Tolat P, et al. Optimal management of the splenic vein at the time of venous resection for pancreatic cancer: importance of the inferior mesenteric vein. J Gastrointest Surg 2014;18(5):917–21.

42. Pilgrim CH, Tsai S, Evans DB, et al. Mesocaval shunting: a novel technique to facilitate venous resection and reconstruction and enhance exposure of the superior mesenteric and celiac arteries during pancreaticoduodenectomy. J Am Coll Surg 2013;217(3):e17–20.

43. Cohen ME, Bilimoria KY, Ko CY, et al. Effect of subjective preoperative variables on risk-adjusted assessment of hospital morbidity and mortality. Ann Surg 2009; 249(4):682–9.

44. Scarborough JE, Bennett KM, Englum BR, et al. The impact of functional dependency on outcomes after complex general and vascular surgery. Ann Surg 2015; 261(3):432–7.

45. Robinson TN, Eiseman B, Wallace JI, et al. Redefining geriatric preoperative assessment using frailty, disability and co-morbidity. Ann Surg 2009;250(3): 449–55.

46. Miura JT, Krepline AN, George B, et al. Use of neoadjuvant therapy in patients 75 years of age and older with pancreatic cancer. Surgery 2015;158(6):1545–55.

Radiotherapy for Pancreatic Adenocarcinoma

Recent Developments and Advances on the Horizon

Samer Salamekh, MD, Sujana Gottumukkala, MD,
Chunjoo Park, PhD, Mu-han Lin, PhD, Nina N. Sanford, MD*

KEYWORDS

- Pancreatic ductal adenocarcinoma • Neoadjuvant therapy • Radiation therapy
- Stereotactic ablative radiation therapy

KEY POINTS

- Indications for radiotherapy in pancreatic cancer vary by surgical resectability status of the tumor: resectable, borderline resectable, and locally advanced unresectable.
- For tumors deemed resectable, radiation is generally not delivered pre-operatively, but may be given adjuvantly particularly in settings of a close or positive surgical margin.
- For borderline resectable tumors, pre-operative radiation has been shown to improve surgical parameters including lowering nodal positivity and positive margin rates.
- For locally advanced unresectable tumors, radiation can improve local control, give patients an interval off of chemotherapy and provide symptomatic relief.
- Multidisciplinary discussion is critical for choosing the best modality and sequencing of care for patients with pancreatic cancer.

INTRODUCTION

Pancreatic ductal adenocarcinoma (PDAC) has one of the lowest survival rates among solid tumors and is currently the fourth leading cause of cancer mortality in men and women.[1] The incidence of PDAC is rising with PDAC expected to become the second most common cause of cancer mortality by 2040.[2,3] Surgery remains the mainstay of curative intent treatment with complete resection being the goal.[4,5] However, approximately 80% of patients are initially either inoperable or borderline operable due to the proximity and involvement of vessels or other critical organs.[6] The most common first

Department of Radiation Oncology, University of Texas Southwestern, 2280 Inwood Road, Dallas, TX 75390, USA
* Corresponding author. Department of Radiation Oncology, University of Texas Southwestern, 2280 Inwood Road, Dallas, TX 75390-9303.
E-mail address: Nina.Sanford@UTSouthwestern.edu

Hematol Oncol Clin N Am 36 (2022) 995–1009
https://doi.org/10.1016/j.hoc.2022.06.002
0889-8588/22/© 2022 Elsevier Inc. All rights reserved.

hemonc.theclinics.com

site of failure after definitive surgery is distant; however, a significant proportion of patients will progress locally with some studies reporting a local failure rate as high as 50% in resected PDAC.[7] Approximately one-third of patients die of locally destructive pancreatic disease, with 15% having only local failure.[3] In this context, the use of radiation therapy (RT) to improve locoregional control in PDAC is highly appealing; however, given conflicting data, the role of RT—when, in whom, and how—remains controversial.

Theoretically, RT can be used in the preoperative setting to improve the rate of R0 resection, in the postoperative setting to sterilize any microscopic residual disease, and in the inoperable setting to maximize local control and slow progression/onset of local symptoms. Historically, the combination of large treatment fields and proximity of the tumor to radiosensitive normal structures such as the duodenum, stomach, and jejunum has limited the delivery of ablative doses of radiation in a safe manner. Randomized trials of RT have shown modest or negative results, which could be related to both low dose and higher toxicity of RT with outdated treatment techniques. In contrast, recent single-arm and single-institution studies have reported favorable outcomes with the use of RT. Recent improvements in systemic therapy for PDAC, as shown in the PRODIGE 24-ACCORD, ESPAC-4, SWOG S1505, and APACT, have demonstrated the need for intensive chemotherapy to provide any chance of long-term disease control for the majority of tumors and also raise further questions regarding the role of RT.[7–10] Furthermore, modern technological developments in radiation delivery, such as stereotactic ablative radiation therapy (SAbR) and MRI-linear accelerators (MR-LINAC) have enabled the safe delivery of higher doses of radiation. The goal of this article is to discuss recent advances and future directions for the role of RT in PDAC.

Resectable Disease

Although resectability status exists on a continuum, PDAC is generally classified as resectable when upfront R0 resection is achievable due to minimal or no contact with critical arterial and venous vessels. The National Comprehensive Cancer Network (NCCN) guidelines recommend adjuvant chemotherapy for resectable PDAC with consideration of neoadjuvant therapy in select patients with high-risk features [very high cancer antigen (CA) 19–9, large tumors, excessive weight loss, and extreme pain].[11] The ongoing Alliance trial, A021806, which randomizes patients to surgery with adjuvant chemotherapy versus perioperative chemotherapy, is anticipated to provide level 1 evidence regarding the optimal chemotherapy sequencing for resectable disease. This trial does not include RT. Generally speaking, adjuvant radiation is recommended in certain situations in which the risk of locoregional recurrence is high, such as positive margins. Neoadjuvant radiation therapy is an emerging treatment paradigm, but additional studies are required to better understand its role in resectable PDAC.

Large retrospective series[6] as well as prospective randomized trials[12] have demonstrated the importance of surgery for patients with resectable PDAC. Despite complete resection, relapses are common, and several studies have attempted to improve survival by adding therapy in the adjuvant setting. One of the earliest such studies is GITSG 91 to 73, a randomized study, that demonstrated a survival benefit with the addition of adjuvant chemoradiation (CRT) with concurrent 5-fluorouracil (5-FU) and 2 years of maintenance 5-FU.[13] It was unclear whether the benefit was from the RT or maintenance chemotherapy. Subsequently, EORTC 40891[14,15] and ESPAC-1[16,17] suggested that the benefit of adjuvant therapy was due to chemotherapy rather than RT but there are several limitations/critiques of these historic trials that is beyond the scope of this review.[18,19] A meta-analysis with patient-level data was published in 2005 of 6 trials and reported that adjuvant chemotherapy provided a 25% reduction in death whereas chemoradiation did not provide a benefit in the overall cohort.[20–22] However, the benefit of chemotherapy was only seen among those with negative resection margins, whereas a trend toward benefit was seen with CRT in patients with positive margins. Based on these and similar studies, adjuvant management has trended toward the use of chemotherapy alone in most patients, except for those with risk factors for local recurrence, for which RT can be considered. Specifically, in current practice, adjuvant RT is generally reserved for resectable disease with surgical pathology demonstrating negative prognostic factors such as positive or close margins, lymphovascular invasion, or high nodal positivity rate.

Modern RT cooperative group studies for resectable pancreatic cancer have also been performed in the adjuvant setting. RTOG 9704 reported on 451 patients with resectable PDAC. After resection, patients were randomized to either 3 weeks of 5-FU followed by CRT (50.4 Gy in 28 fractions with 5-FU) and additional 3 months of standalone 5-FU or 3 weeks of gemcitabine followed by CRT and additional 3 months of gemcitabine. There was no survival difference in the two arms of the trial.[23] Although the radiation protocol was the same in both arms, the trial provided important information regarding predictors of outcomes. Secondary analysis of the trial revealed that patients who received RT per protocol had improved survival compared with those who did not (median survival 20.9 months compared with 17.5 months), without a difference in toxicity.[24] Additional analysis revealed patients without nodal involvement and those with a postoperative CA 19 to 9 <180 U/mL had improved survival (higher CA 19–9 associated with larger tumors).[25] The study was used as a basis for the randomized NRG/RTOG 0848 trial which was designed to answer two questions: whether adding erlotinib to gemcitabine in the postoperative setting improves survival and whether RT improved survival in the adjuvant setting. Patients with PDAC who underwent resection and had postresection serum CA 19 to 9 <180 U/mL were randomized to either 6 months of gemcitabine or 6 months of gemcitabine with erlotinib. After assessing for disease progression and completing systemic therapy, patients underwent a second randomization to receive chemotherapy or CRT (50.4 Gy in 28 fractions with capecitabine or 5-FU). The addition of erlotinib did not improve survival in these patients. The results of the radiotherapy randomization are still pending.

Currently, preoperative RT is generally omitted for resectable disease as, by definition, clear margins are generally felt to be achievable upfront and, as such, the risks of RT are felt to outweigh any potential benefits. One reason for this hesitancy is that delivery of a 6-week course of CRT in the preoperative setting would delay surgery and subsequent adjuvant systemic therapy, which may adversely impact outcomes. Shorter courses of neoadjuvant CRT may provide benefit to patients without the delay of long-course CRT. A phase I/II trial from Massachusetts General Hospital investigated the use of a short course of neoadjuvant chemoradiation with protons (5 fractions of 5Gy-equivalents) and capecitabine followed by early surgery and adjuvant gemcitabine. The study reported favorable rates of toxicity (4.1% grade 3 toxicity and no grade 4/5 toxicity) and no treatment-related delays to surgery.[26] A smaller phase I study from the University of Wisconsin escalated the dose of neoadjuvant chemoradiation to 35 Gy in 5 fractions to the tumor and 25 Gy in 5 to elective nodal volume, with concurrent capecitabine. No acute grade 3 or higher toxicity was seen and all patients who underwent surgery had R0 resection. Although preliminary neoadjuvant CRT studies are encouraging, additional studies are warranted to better understand the role of this paradigm.

Borderline Resectable Disease

PDAC is generally considered borderline resectable if resection is technically feasible but would result in an R1 resection. Historically, management of borderline resectable PDAC has been heterogenous due to the wide range of cancers that fall within this category. This definition has been further complicated after the advent of neoadjuvant therapy that may be able to improve resectability in up to one-third of patients who were initially felt to be unresectable.[27] Per NCCN guidelines, the current treatment paradigm consists of neoadjuvant therapy followed by restaging and consideration of surgery for patients without disease progression.[11] However, there continues to be disagreement between experts on the optimal management of these patients and there is limited evidence to recommend one neoadjuvant regimen over another.

Numerous studies have demonstrated that neoadjuvant therapy improves R0 resection rates for patients with borderline resectable disease but there is still debate over whether neoadjuvant treatment provides a survival benefit. In a retrospective series of 160 patients with borderline resectable PDAC, one of the earliest defining this group, who received neoadjuvant treatment with chemotherapy, CRT (50.4 Gy in 28 fractions or 30 Gy in 10 fractions), or both, Katz and colleagues reported high R0 resection rates and favorable survival for patients able to complete neoadjuvant treatment and subsequent surgery.[28] Of the initial 160 patients, 125 patients (78%) were able to complete neoadjuvant therapy and restaging with 66 patients (41%) ultimately undergoing surgery. Of those patients who underwent surgery, 94% achieved R0 resection with a partial pathologic response noted in 56% of patients. Median survival was significantly higher for patients who were able to undergo resection compared to those who were unable to receive surgery (40 months vs 13 months).

The PREOPANC study randomized 246 patients with resectable or borderline resectable PDAC to immediate surgery followed by adjuvant gemcitabine versus neoadjuvant CRT with gemcitabine followed by surgery and adjuvant chemotherapy. Patients who underwent neoadjuvant CRT had higher R0 resection rates (71% vs 40%) and improved median disease-free survival and locoregional failure-free interval.[29] At median follow-up of 27 months, there was no difference in median overall survival (OS) between arms for the overall cohort. However, a preplanned subgroup analysis of patients with borderline resectable disease demonstrated a median OS benefit with preoperative CRT (17.6 months vs 13.2 months). An update was presented at ASCO 2021 and at median follow-up of 56 months, OS for the overall cohort remained similar between arms; however, 5-yr OS was significantly improved in the neoadjuvant CRT arm (16.5% vs 6.5%).[30] One interpretation of this finding is that neoadjuvant treatment provides a potential long-term survival benefit for those patients who do not develop metastatic disease in the first few years after surgery. A key limitation of the PREOPANC trial is the use of gemcitabine rather than more modern chemotherapy regimens such as FOLFIRINOX or gemcitabine/nab-paclitaxel, which are the current standard of care in the neoadjuvant setting. The ongoing PREOPANC-2 trial seeks to address this limitation by randomizing patients to either 8 cycles of neoadjuvant FOLFIRINOX followed by surgery versus 3 cycles of neoadjuvant gemcitabine with a hypofractionated course of radiation during the second cycle (36 Gy in 15 fractions) followed by surgery and 4 cycles of adjuvant gemcitabine.[31] In a phase II/III Korean study randomizing 58 patients to neoadjuvant gemcitabine-based CRT followed by surgery versus upfront surgery followed by adjuvant CRT, interim analysis demonstrated higher R0 resection rates with neoadjuvant CRT (51.8% vs 26.1%) as well as improved 1-yr OS, 2-yr OS, and median survival.[32]

With the advent of new chemotherapy regimens that improve risk of distant metastasis, there is renewed interest in investigating the role of neoadjuvant RT. The Alliance A021501 trial randomized 126 patients with borderline resectable PDAC to either 8 cycles of neoadjuvant mFOLFIRINOX followed by resection and 4 cycles of adjuvant mFOLFOX or 7 cycles of neoadjuvant mFOLFIRINOX, RT (33–40 Gy in 5 or 25 Gy in 5 fractions), resection, and 4 cycles of adjuvant mFOLFOX.[33] The primary endpoint of the trial was 18-month OS, which was higher with neoadjuvant chemotherapy alone than neoadjuvant chemotherapy with RT (66.4% vs 47.3%) even among patients who underwent pancreatectomy (93.1% vs 78.9%), although the trial was not meant to be a comparison between the two treatment arms. Limitations however of the study were that although randomized, patients in the RT arm had higher baseline CA19 to 9 (median 171 U/mL compared with 248 U/mL), possibly signifying more aggressive disease. Furthermore, fewer patients in the RT arm underwent surgery (51% compared with 58%) and even fewer underwent pancreatectomy (35% compared with 48%). A similar single-institution phase II clinical trial was performed with 48 borderline resectable patients. The patients received 8 cycles of FOLFIRINOX followed by either short-course radiation for those who were resectable based on restaging imaging (25GyE in 5 or 30 Gy in 10 photons) or long-course chemo-radiation for those with persistent vascular involvement (50.4 Gy in 28 with capecitabine or 5-FU).[34] 67% of the patient were able to undergo resection and an R0 resection rate of 97% was achieved. The 2-yr OS was 56% for the overall cohort and 72% for patients who underwent resection. The discordant results between the Alliance phase III trial and the single-institution phase II are likely multifactorial and may include heterogeneity in treatment when enrolled in cooperative setting compared with single institution expertise/bias. In addition, patients in the phase II study received 8 cycles of FOLFOX, which is the same number of cycles patients in the control arm of the Alliance study received, whereas the RT arm in the Alliance study received only 7 cycles. However, the difference in findings is likely too large to be explained by a single cycle of chemotherapy. Final report of the Alliance study is still pending. The ongoing PREOPANC-2 (EudraCT: 2017–002,036–17) is comparing outcomes of neoadjuvant FOLFIRINOX to gemcitabine and CRT (36 Gy in 15 fractions)[31] and PANDAS-PRODIGE 44 (NCT02676349) is investigating the addition of CRT (50.4 Gy in 28 with capecitabine) to FOLFIRINOX. The results of these and other trials will provide additional clarification on the role of neoadjuvant RT.

Locally Advanced Disease

Locally advanced PDAC generally refers to disease which is unresectable due to the involvement of critical vasculature or adjacent organs. Management of patients with locally advanced PDAC typically consists of systemic therapy but subsequent RT may be considered in patients with good performance status and without systemic progression after chemotherapy.[11]

Currently, there is a lack of level 1 data to support the routine use of conventional RT for locally advanced PDAC. In the LAP07 trial, investigators used a two-step randomization process to investigate the effect of gemcitabine versus erlotinib and CRT versus chemotherapy on survival.[35] In the first randomization, patients were randomized to 4 cycles of gemcitabine versus gemcitabine and erlotinib. Patients without disease progression after 4 months underwent a second randomization to long-course CRT with capecitabine versus 2 more months of their initial chemotherapy. There was no difference in survival with the addition of erlotinib. Patients who received CRT had significantly improved local recurrence compared with those who received additional chemotherapy (32% vs 45%); however, there was no difference in survival.

Formal RT quality assurance of the trial suggests that only 32% of patients in the CRT arm were treated per protocol, which may have diminished the impact of CRT.

As hypofractionation has become more common, there has been increasing interest in a potential role for hypofractionated ablative RT for locally advanced PDAC. A prospective cohort study of 119 patients with locally advanced PDAC treated with hypofractionated ablative doses of 75 Gy in 25 fractions, or 67.5 Gy in 15 fractions for tumors within 1 cm from the stomach or intestines, reported favorable survival and locoregional control.[36] In the series, OS was 74% at 1 year and 38% at 2 years. Incidence of local progression was 17.6% at 1 year and 32.8% at 2 years. In the phase II LAPC-1 trial, 50 patients with locally advanced PDAC were treated with 8 cycles of FOLFIRINOX followed by stereotactic ablative radiation therapy (SAbR) with 40 Gy in 5 fractions for those without disease progression.[37] The primary endpoint of 1-yr OS was 64% and following SAbR, 6 patients were able to undergo R0 resection with 2 of these patients demonstrating a complete pathologic response. The ongoing PanCRS study (NCT01926197), a phase III trial randomizing patients to modified FOLFIRINOX versus modified FOLFIRINOX and SAbR may provide further insight into the optimal treatment for locally advanced PDAC, but has halted recruitment at this time.[38]

Stereotactic Ablative Radiation Therapy

Stereotactic ablative radiation therapy (SAbR), also known as stereotactic body radiotherapy (SBRT), provides a method for dose escalation while protecting organs at risk (OARS) and can be used in the neoadjuvant, adjuvant, or definitive setting. Immobilization using SBRT, motion monitoring, and image guided RT provides a process for reducing treatment margins and subsequent dose delivered to organs at risk (OARs). This not only improves the tolerability of treatment but provides an opportunity to escalate the biologically effective dose (BED) with the goal of completely eradicating the tumor and improving local control. Furthermore, an additional advantage of SAbR is that a hypofractionated course of fewer treatments minimizes interruptions in chemotherapy.

Koong and colleagues reported one of the earliest studies of SAbR in PDAC in a phase I dose escalation with 15 patients who were treated from 15 Gy to 25 Gy at a single fraction with no dose limiting toxicity.[39] Metallic fiducial markers were placed and were tracked by orthogonal x-ray during treatment, which was performed with breath hold to minimize target motion during the respiratory cycle. Most centers performing SAbR for PDAC use a similar technique today; however, the radiation is delivered in approximately 5 fractions to provide some averaging/repair of dose received by OARs while still delivering a condensed course of treatment. Pollom and colleagues retrospectively analyzed 167 patients who received a biologically equivalent dose of either 25 Gy in 1 fraction or 33 Gy in 5 fractions using the universal survival curve[40] and found that there was no difference in control rates or survival between the groups. However, there was higher grade $\geq$ 2 GI toxicity in patients who received a single fraction compared with 5 fractions.[41]

Several retrospective[42–45] and prospective single arm studies[41] have been performed demonstrating low toxicity and good LC with SAbR. The results of these studies and multi-institutional analyses have suggested that patients receiving higher BED have improved survival; however, the conclusions are limited by selection bias. The PAULA-1 study analyzed 54 PDAC patients treated with SAbR between 2013 to 2018 and found that both LC and OS was better in patients receiving $\geq$ 48 Gy BED10.[46] Although the majority of studies of SAbR in PDAC are non-randomized, the randomized Alliance A021501 trial did not show a benefit to preoperative hypofractioned radiotherapy in borderline resectable PDAC as described earlier. Ongoing

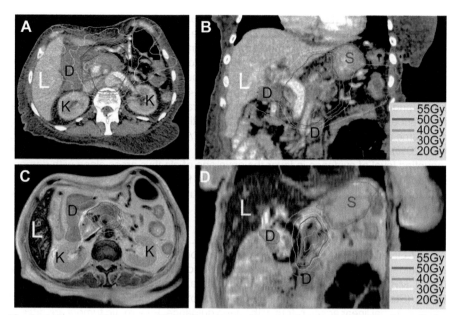

Fig. 1. A 74-year-old woman with locally advanced pancreatic cancer is eligible for radiation treatment with either a conventionally fractionated treatment (CF) of 50.4 Gy in 28 fractions using CT-based planning (*A, B*) or stereotactic ablative radiation treatment (SAbR) of 40 Gy in 5 fractions with MR-based planning (*C, D*). For both plans, the gross tumor volume (GTV) is outlined in orange in all panels while the volume receiving the prescription dose, termed planning target volume (PTV), is outlined in red in all panels. Isodose curves from 20 Gy to 55 Gy are also shown. Note that the dose in CF plan is homogenous with no areas receiving over 50 Gy whereas the SABR plan is more heterogeneous with large portions of GTV receiving over 55 Gy despite nominal prescription dose of 40 Gy. Radiation dose of 50 Gy in 5 fractions is significantly more potent compared with the same dose in 28 fractions. Liver (*L*), duodenum (translucent blue and letter D), kidney (*K*), and stomach (translucent brown and letter S) are adjacent avoidance organs.

randomized studies investigating the role of SAbR in PDAC include AGITG MASTER-PLAN (ACTRN12619000409178)[47] and a Stanford phase III trial (NCT01926197).

Radiation Volume Definition

Historically, conventionally fractionated radiation therapy treatment included the primary tumor as well as the regional lymph nodes (**Fig. 1**). However, initial approaches with hypofractionated treatment/SAbR included only the tumor. This was in part due to concerns of severe GI toxicity, especially with dose-escalated hypofractionated RT. The American Society for Radiation Oncology (ASTRO), European Society for Radiotherapy and Oncology (ESTRO), and the Australasian Gastrointestinal Trials Group/Trans-Tasman Radiation Oncology Group (AGITG/TROG) recommend against treating elective nodal radiation when using SAbR in locally advanced PDAC due to a lack of evidence of benefit.[48–50]

However, a significant proportion of PDAC have perineural and/or lymphovascular involvement, with surgical series suggesting occult metastasis rates as high as 80%.[51] There is increased realization that treating only the tumor with SAbR doses is associated with increased risk of regional recurrence, especially around the celiac and superior mesenteric vasculature.[52,53] These areas are also high risk locations for surgical complications, common sites of positive margins, and are difficult to salvage. Some centers advocate for including the region surrounding the vasculature in an intermediate dose PTV, commonly 25 Gy in 5 fractions. Retrospective studies have demonstrated improved PFS with this approach.[52] A recent retrospective analysis, with propensity score matching, compared outcomes of patients treated at a single institution with either SAbR to the tumor (33–40 Gy in 5 fractions) or SAbR to the tumor and 25 Gy in 5 fractions elective nodal radiation.[54] The 2-year locoregional recurrence was lower with elective nodal radiation (22.6% compared with 44.6%) and came at the expense of higher acute grade 1/grade 2 GI toxicity (60% compared with 20%). Overall survival was similar in the two cohorts. However, given the mounting level of evidence in favor the coverage of elective areas along with demonstrated low toxicity rates, there has been a trend to also treat areas of high risk adjacent to the tumor including vessels and nodal volumes, albeit to a lower dose than the gross tumor.

MRI-Linear Accelerators

An MR-LINAC combines the high energy beam output from a linear accelerator with MRI-guided radiation delivery. There are two commercially available systems: a 0.35 T MRIdian from ViewRay (Oakwood Village, Ohio, USA) and 1.5 T Unity from Elekta (Stockholm, Sweden). These machines offer several advantages compared with traditional linear accelerators with image guidance. Pancreatic tumors are difficult to visualize on CT without using contrast; however, the tumors are readily visualized using MRI. Both commercial systems allow for MR imaging while radiation treatment is being delivered, resulting in true intrafraction motion monitoring. This is particularly important for visualizing stomach, duodenum, and jejunum where radiotherapy hotspots may result in significant toxicity.[55] Imaging during radiation treatment has demonstrated significant variability and unpredictability in the motion of both the tumor as well as the nearby organs at risk (OARs).[56] Furthermore, as MR image is obtained for image alignment at every fraction, MR-LINAC allows for daily adaptation to both the tumor as well as OARS (ie, creation of a new radiotherapy plan with each fraction).

There have been several retrospective reports on using MR-LINAC for the treatment of PDAC. Most of these reports are patients treated with the ViewRay machine because it has been FDA approved longer (initially with a Cobalt-60 radiation source and later with a linear accelerator radiation source). One of the first studies on utilizing MR-LINAC for stereotactic MR-guided adaptive radiation therapy, termed SMART, for the treatment of PDAC was reported by Bohoudi and colleagues, who treated 10 tumors to 40 Gy in 5 fractions.[57] Shortly thereafter, Henke and colleagues reported on a series of 5 PDAC patients treated to 50 Gy in 5 fractions.[58] There have been several larger retrospective studies demonstrating good efficacy with favorable GI toxicity profiles.[59–61] One of these studies divided patients by treatment BED and reported higher OS in patients who received >70 Gy BED10 (49% vs 30%).[59] This is a rapidly evolving area that is driven by continued technological progress and significant opportunities for improvement remain.[62] In a recent multi-institutional review of 148 PDAC patients treated on the MRIdian using SMART (57% locally advanced, 29% borderline resectable, 14% medically inoperable), 23% of patients underwent pancreaticoduodenectomy, and survival (median OS 26 months) was significantly higher than historic controls.[63] Grade 3 acute toxicity was 4.1% and late toxicity 12.8%, with no grade 4 toxicity. Most patients received induction chemotherapy and 50 Gy in 5 fractions. A prospective phase II trial for SMART-based treatment on MRIdian (NCT03621644) and a prospective registry for those treated on Unity (MOMENTUM NCT04075305) are currently underway. An example of an MRI-based treatment plan is shown in **Fig. 1**.

Palliation

Patients with pancreatic cancer may have poor quality of life (QOL) due to tumor progression resulting in jaundice, obstruction, weight loss, and/or pain. Unfortunately, approximately 80% of patients with advanced PDAC will experience severe pain before death, which is most frequently due to the location of the tumor[64] Specifically, the pancreas is near the celiac plexus; compression at this location can result in intense pain that is often difficult to adequately manage. These patients often have poor prognoses, thus, delivering a condensed course of RT to palliate pain while minimizing treatment burden may be a prudent strategy to improve QOL. In one of the largest single institution studies, 61 patients with celiac axis pain related to their PDAC received 8 Gy × 1, 8 Gy × 2, 8 Gy × 3, with at least 66% of patients achieving pain relief.[65] Most other studies utilizing 1 to 6 fractions also demonstrated improvement in pain after RT.[66] However, one study of 22 patients who received 45 Gy in 3 fractions via SAbR demonstrated overall deterioration, increased nausea, and greater pain after RT.[67] Notably, this study used one of the highest doses and was one of the early studies utilizing SAbR, which may have led to poorer outcomes. Importantly however, it demonstrates the need to carefully select patients and design safe treatment plans, particularly when the intent of therapy is palliative. The PAINPANC is a prospective single arm trial currently underway that treats patients with PDAC-related celiac axis pain to 27 Gy in 3 fractions (NL4896, NTR5143).

Oligometastatic Disease

The concept of oligometastasis was first introduced in 1995 as a state of limited systemic metastasis that may be amenable to local treatments that result in cure.[68] This has been shown for several metastatic GI malignancies with liver and lung metastasis such as colorectal cancer.[68] Although PDAC frequently metastasizes to liver and lung, given high rates of early disseminated progression, it is not clear that such a state exists for a meaningful proportion of patients with metastatic PDAC.

There are case reports of long-term survivors of PDAC with metastectomy; however, the clinical course is often of slow progression with recurrences several years after initial resection.[69] Also, most large retrospective series report few long-term survivors after metastectomy.[70] This suggests that some PDAC with limited metastasis may have favorable genomic features that portend a more indolent course that is more amendable to aggressive local therapy rather than identification of a true oligometastatic state. Genomic studies in PDAC suggest that there are metastatic clones in the primary tumor many years before dissemination and that dissemination to distant organs precedes the development of the first clinical site of metastasis by several years.[71] This may explain why an oligometastatic state has been difficult to identify in PDAC.

Advances in biomarkers may better stratify patient's metastatic potential and advances in systemic therapy may slow the growth of metastatic clones such that local therapy may provide a meaningful benefit, whether in overall survival or time off systemic therapy. Several factors have been identified that portend a better prognosis in limited metastatic disease including fewer number of liver metastasis, low CA 19 to 9, and presence of lung metastasis compared to liver metastasis.[70,72] Additional therapy appears to improve survival in those with limited metastatic disease; however, studies are limited by selection bias and there remain limited survivors beyond 5 years.[72]

SAbR provides an appealing treatment option that balances local control and quality of life (QOL) compared with surgical metastectomy. SAbR can be selectively used in patients on chemotherapy to maximize time off systemic therapy, often resulting in improvement in QOL, while minimizing disease progression. The use of SAbR has been shown to improve survival for other disease and may be beneficial for patients with limited metastatic disease. There are at least 2 randomized trials examining the role of SAbR in oligometastatic PDAC (NCT04975516, OligoRARE NCT04498767).

SUMMARY

Improvements in prognosis for patients diagnosed with PDAC have largely attributed to better surgery and advancements in multiagent systemic therapy. Most trials have demonstrated that RT improves locoregional control, but this often has not translated into a survival benefit. However as systemic therapy continues to decrease rates of distant metastasis/recurrence in PDAC, improvements in locoregional control may become more important with greater likelihood of improving survival and quality of life. Although some patients clearly benefit from RT, currently it is difficult to know in whom and when RT should be used. Recent developments in RT delivery with stereotactic body RT (SBRT) as well as MR-LINAC technology can better optimize the therapeutic ratio of RT by providing higher doses of radiation in a more conformal manner that minimizes toxicity. Preliminary studies are highly encouraging but additional randomized studies are necessary to determine the benefit of these new technologies and to optimize the sequencing/timing of RT in relation to systemic therapy and surgery.

CLINICS CARE POINTS

- Multidisciplinary discussion is critical for choosing the best modality and sequencing of care for patients with pancreatic cancer, which may include the use of radiotherapy.
- Careful review of scans is needed to determine surgical resectability status and to design radiation target volumes, the latter which remain an area of controversy. An MRI may help elucidate areas of tumor better than diagnostic CT.
- Our current SAbR dosing is 40 Gy in 5 fractions to the gross tumor with a 25 in 5 Gy elective volume to vascular areas at risk, particularly along the celiac axis and superior mesenteric artery.
- It is important to continue enrolling on prospective randomized trials, so that we can define when and how to most appropriately deliver radiotherapy in patients with pancreatic cancer.

CONFLICTS OF INTEREST

None.

REFERENCES

1. Siegel RL, Miller KD, Jemal A. Cancer statistics, 2020. CA Cancer J Clin 2020; 70(1):7–30.
2. Rahib L, Wehner MR, Matrisian LM, et al. Estimated projection of US cancer incidence and death to 2040. JAMA Netw Open 2021;4(4):e214708.

3. Iacobuzio-Donahue CA, Fu B, Yachida S, et al. DPC4 gene status of the primary carcinoma correlates with patterns of failure in patients with pancreatic cancer. J Clin Oncol 2009;27(11):1806–13.
4. Ducreux M, Cuhna AS, Caramella C, et al. Cancer of the pancreas: ESMO clinical practice guidelines for diagnosis, treatment and follow-up. Ann Oncol 2015; 26(Suppl 5):v56–68.
5. Tempero MA, Malafa MP, Al-Hawary M, et al. Pancreatic adenocarcinoma, version 2.2021, NCCN clinical practice guidelines in oncology. J Natl Compr Canc Netw 2021;19(4):439–57.
6. Geer RJ, Brennan MF. Prognostic indicators for survival after resection of pancreatic adenocarcinoma. Am J Surg 1993;165(1):68–72.
7. Neoptolemos JP, Palmer DH, Ghaneh P, et al. Comparison of adjuvant gemcitabine and capecitabine with gemcitabine monotherapy in patients with resected pancreatic cancer (ESPAC-4): a multicentre, open-label, randomised, phase 3 trial. Lancet 2017;389(10073):1011–24.
8. Von Hoff DD, Ervin T, Arena FP, et al. Increased survival in pancreatic cancer with nab-paclitaxel plus gemcitabine. N Engl J Med 2013;369(18):1691–703.
9. Conroy T, Hammel P, Hebbar M, et al. FOLFIRINOX or gemcitabine as adjuvant therapy for pancreatic cancer. N Engl J Med 2018;379(25):2395–406.
10. Sohal D, Duong MT, Ahmad SA, et al. SWOG S1505: Results of perioperative chemotherapy (peri-op CTx) with mfolfirinox versus gemcitabine/nab-paclitaxel (Gem/nabP) for resectable pancreatic ductal adenocarcinoma (PDA). J Clin Oncol 2020;38(15_suppl):4504.
11. NCCN. Pancreatic Adenocarcinoma (Version 2.2021). 2021. Available at: https://www.nccn.org/professionals/physician_gls/pdf/pancreatic.pdf.
12. Doi R, Imamura M, Hosotani R, et al. Surgery versus radiochemotherapy for resectable locally invasive pancreatic cancer: final results of a randomized multi-institutional trial. Surg Today 2008;38(11):1021–8.
13. Kalser MH, Ellenberg SS. Pancreatic cancer. Adjuvant combined radiation and chemotherapy following curative resection. Arch Surg 1985;120(8):899–903.
14. Klinkenbijl JH, Jeekel J, Sahmoud T, et al. Adjuvant radiotherapy and 5-fluorouracil after curative resection of cancer of the pancreas and periampullary region: phase III trial of the EORTC gastrointestinal tract cancer cooperative group. Ann Surg 1999;230(6):776–82 ; discussion 782-774.
15. Smeenk HG, van Eijck CH, Hop WC, et al. Long-term survival and metastatic pattern of pancreatic and periampullary cancer after adjuvant chemoradiation or observation: long-term results of EORTC trial 40891. Ann Surg 2007;246(5):734–40.
16. Neoptolemos JP, Dunn JA, Stocken DD, et al. Adjuvant chemoradiotherapy and chemotherapy in resectable pancreatic cancer: a randomised controlled trial. Lancet 2001;358(9293):1576–85.
17. Neoptolemos JP, Stocken DD, Friess H, et al. A randomized trial of chemoradiotherapy and chemotherapy after resection of pancreatic cancer. N Engl J Med 2004;350(12):1200–10.
18. Choti MA. Adjuvant therapy for pancreatic cancer–the debate continues. N Engl J Med 2004;350(12):1249–51.
19. Garofalo MC, Nichols EM, Regine WF. Optimal adjuvant therapy for resected pancreatic cancer: chemotherapy or chemoradiotherapy? Gastrointest Cancer Res 2007;1(5):182–7.
20. Stocken DD, Buchler MW, Dervenis C, et al. Meta-analysis of randomised adjuvant therapy trials for pancreatic cancer. Br J Cancer 2005;92(8):1372–81.

21. Tempero M, O'Reilly E, Van Cutsem E, et al. Phase 3 APACT trial of adjuvant nab-paclitaxel plus gemcitabine (nab-P plus Gem) vs gemcitabine (Gem) alone in patients with resected pancreatic cancer (PC): Updated 5-year overall survival. Ann Oncol 2021;32:S226.
22. Jones RP, Psarelli EE, Jackson R, et al. Patterns of recurrence after resection of pancreatic ductal adenocarcinoma: a secondary analysis of the espac-4 randomized adjuvant chemotherapy trial. JAMA Surg 2019;154(11):1038–48.
23. Regine WF, Winter KA, Abrams R, et al. Fluorouracil-based chemoradiation with either gemcitabine or fluorouracil chemotherapy after resection of pancreatic adenocarcinoma: 5-year analysis of the US Intergroup/RTOG 9704 Phase III Trial. Ann Surg Oncol 2011;18(5):1319–26.
24. Abrams RA, Winter KA, Regine WF, et al. Failure to adhere to protocol specified radiation therapy guidelines was associated with decreased survival in RTOG 9704–a phase III trial of adjuvant chemotherapy and chemoradiotherapy for patients with resected adenocarcinoma of the pancreas. Int J Radiat Oncol Biol Phys 2012;82(2):809–16.
25. Berger AC, Garcia M, Hoffman JP, et al. Postresection CA 19-9 predicts overall survival in patients with pancreatic cancer treated with adjuvant chemoradiation: a prospective validation by RTOG 9704. J Clin Oncol 2008;26(36):5918–22.
26. Hong TS, Ryan DP, Borger DR, et al. A phase 1/2 and biomarker study of preoperative short course chemoradiation with proton beam therapy and capecitabine followed by early surgery for resectable pancreatic ductal adenocarcinoma. Int J Radiat Oncol Biol Phys 2014;89(4):830–8.
27. Gillen S, Schuster T, Meyer Z, Buschenfelde C, et al. Preoperative/neoadjuvant therapy in pancreatic cancer: a systematic review and meta-analysis of response and resection percentages. Plos Med 2010;7(4):e1000267.
28. Katz MH, Pisters PW, Evans DB, et al. Borderline resectable pancreatic cancer: the importance of this emerging stage of disease. J Am Coll Surg 2008;206(5): 833–46 ; discussion 846-838.
29. Versteijne E, Suker M, Groothuis K, et al. Preoperative Chemoradiotherapy Versus Immediate Surgery for Resectable and Borderline Resectable Pancreatic Cancer: Results of the Dutch Randomized Phase III PREOPANC Trial. J Clin Oncol 2020;38(16):1763–73.
30. Eijck CHJV, Versteijne E, Suker M, et al. Preoperative chemoradiotherapy to improve overall survival in pancreatic cancer: Long-term results of the multicenter randomized phase III PREOPANC trial. J Clin Oncol 2021;39(15_suppl):4016.
31. Janssen QP, van Dam JL, Bonsing BA, et al. Total neoadjuvant FOLFIRINOX versus neoadjuvant gemcitabine-based chemoradiotherapy and adjuvant gemcitabine for resectable and borderline resectable pancreatic cancer (PREOPANC-2 trial): study protocol for a nationwide multicenter randomized controlled trial. Bmc Cancer 2021;21(1):300.
32. Jang JY, Han Y, Lee H, et al. Oncological Benefits of Neoadjuvant Chemoradiation With Gemcitabine Versus Upfront Surgery in Patients With Borderline Resectable Pancreatic Cancer: A Prospective, Randomized, Open-label, Multicenter Phase 2/3 Trial. Ann Surg 2018;268(2):215–22.
33. Katz MHG, Shi Q, Meyers JP, et al. Alliance A021501: Preoperative mFOLFIRINOX or mFOLFIRINOX plus hypofractionated radiation therapy (RT) for borderline resectable (BR) adenocarcinoma of the pancreas. J Clin Oncol 2021; 39(3_suppl):377.
34. Murphy JE, Wo JY, Ryan DP, et al. Total Neoadjuvant Therapy With FOLFIRINOX Followed by Individualized Chemoradiotherapy for Borderline Resectable

Pancreatic Adenocarcinoma: A Phase 2 Clinical Trial. JAMA Oncol 2018;4(7): 963–9.

35. Hammel P, Huguet F, van Laethem JL, et al. Effect of Chemoradiotherapy vs Chemotherapy on Survival in Patients With Locally Advanced Pancreatic Cancer Controlled After 4 Months of Gemcitabine With or Without Erlotinib: The LAP07 Randomized Clinical Trial. JAMA 2016;315(17):1844–53.

36. Reyngold M, O'Reilly EM, Varghese AM, et al. Association of ablative radiation therapy with survival among patients with inoperable pancreatic cancer. JAMA Oncol 2021;7(5):735–8.

37. Suker M, Nuyttens JJ, Eskens F, et al. Efficacy and feasibility of stereotactic radiotherapy after folfirinox in patients with locally advanced pancreatic cancer (LAPC-1 trial). EClinicalMedicine 2019;17:100200.

38. Gov ClinicalTrials. Phase III FOLFIRINOX (mFFX) +/- SBRT in Locally Advanced Pancreatic Cancer. Available at: https://ClinicalTrials.gov/show/NCT01926197.

39. Koong AC, Le QT, Ho A, et al. Phase I study of stereotactic radiosurgery in patients with locally advanced pancreatic cancer. Int J Radiat Oncol Biol Phys 2004;58(4):1017–21.

40. Park C, Papiez L, Zhang S, et al. Universal survival curve and single fraction equivalent dose: useful tools in understanding potency of ablative radiotherapy. Int J Radiat Oncol Biol Phys 2008;70(3):847–52.

41. Pollom EL, Alagappan M, von Eyben R, et al. Single- versus multifraction stereotactic body radiation therapy for pancreatic adenocarcinoma: outcomes and toxicity. Int J Radiat Oncol Biol Phys 2014;90(4):918–25.

42. Song YC, Yuan ZY, Li FT, et al. Analysis of clinical efficacy of CyberKnife (R) treatment for locally advanced pancreatic cancer. Oncotargets Ther 2015;8.

43. Ryan JF, Rosati LM, Groot VP, et al. Stereotactic body radiation therapy for palliative management of pancreatic adenocarcinoma in elderly and medically inoperable patients. Oncotarget 2018;9(23):16427–36.

44. Mellon EA, Hoffe SE, Springett GM, et al. Long-term outcomes of induction chemotherapy and neoadjuvant stereotactic body radiotherapy for borderline resectable and locally advanced pancreatic adenocarcinoma. Acta Oncol 2015;54(7):979–85.

45. Jung J, Yoon SM, Park JH, et al. Stereotactic body radiation therapy for locally advanced pancreatic cancer. PLoS One 2019;14(4):e0214970.

46. Arcelli A, Guido A, Buwenge M, et al. Higher Biologically Effective Dose Predicts Survival in SBRT of Pancreatic Cancer: A Multicentric Analysis (PAULA-1). Anticancer Res 2020;40(1):465–72.

47. Oar A, Lee M, Le H, et al. AGITG MASTERPLAN: a randomised phase II study of modified FOLFIRINOX alone or in combination with stereotactic body radiotherapy for patients with high-risk and locally advanced pancreatic cancer. Bmc Cancer 2021;21(1).

48. Brunner TB, Haustermans K, Huguet F, et al. ESTRO ACROP guidelines for target volume definition in pancreatic cancer. Radiother Oncol 2021;154:60–9.

49. Oar A, Lee M, Le H, et al. Australasian gastrointestinal trials group (AGITG) and trans-tasman radiation oncology group (TROG) guidelines for pancreatic stereotactic body radiation therapy (SBRT). Pract Radiat Oncol 2020;10(3):e136–46.

50. Palta M, Godfrey D, Goodman KA, et al. Radiation Therapy for Pancreatic Cancer: Executive Summary of an ASTRO Clinical Practice Guideline. Pract Radiat Oncol 2019;9(5):322–32.

51. Brunner TB, Merkel S, Grabenbauer GG, et al. Definition of elective lymphatic target volume in ductal carcinoma of the pancreatic head based on histopathologic analysis. Int J Radiat Oncol Biol Phys 2005;62(4):1021–9.

52. Kharofa J, Mierzwa M, Olowokure O, et al. Pattern of marginal local failure in a phase ii trial of neoadjuvant chemotherapy and stereotactic body radiation therapy for resectable and borderline resectable pancreas cancer. Am J Clin Oncol 2019;42(3):247–52.

53. Zhu X, Ju X, Cao Y, et al. Patterns of local failure after stereotactic body radiation therapy and sequential chemotherapy as initial treatment for pancreatic cancer: implications of target volume design. Int J Radiat Oncol Biol Phys 2019;104(1):101–10.

54. Miller JA, Toesca DAS, Baclay JRM, et al. Pancreatic stereotactic body radiation therapy with or without hypofractionated elective nodal irradiation. Int J Radiat Oncol Biol Phys 2021;112(1):131–42.

55. Elhammali A, Patel M, Weinberg B, et al. Late gastrointestinal tissue effects after hypofractionated radiation therapy of the pancreas. Radiat Oncol 2015;10:186.

56. Heerkens HD, van Vulpen M, van den Berg CA, et al. MRI-based tumor motion characterization and gating schemes for radiation therapy of pancreatic cancer. Radiother Oncol 2014;111(2):252–7.

57. Bohoudi O, Bruynzeel AME, Senan S, et al. Fast and robust online adaptive planning in stereotactic MR-guided adaptive radiation therapy (SMART) for pancreatic cancer. Radiother Oncol 2017;125(3):439–44.

58. Henke L, Kashani R, Robinson C, et al. Phase I trial of stereotactic MR-guided online adaptive radiation therapy (SMART) for the treatment of oligometastatic or unresectable primary malignancies of the abdomen. Radiother Oncol 2018;126(3):519–26.

59. Rudra S, Jiang N, Rosenberg SA, et al. Using adaptive magnetic resonance image-guided radiation therapy for treatment of inoperable pancreatic cancer. Cancer Med 2019;8(5):2123–32.

60. Chuong MD, Bryant J, Mittauer KE, et al. Ablative 5-fraction stereotactic magnetic resonance-guided radiation therapy with on-table adaptive replanning and elective nodal irradiation for inoperable pancreas cancer. Pract Radiat Oncol 2021;11(2):134–47.

61. Hassanzadeh C, Rudra S, Bommireddy A, et al. Ablative five-fraction stereotactic body radiation therapy for inoperable pancreatic cancer using online mr-guided adaptation. Adv Radiat Oncol 2021;6(1):100506.

62. Hall WA, Small C, Paulson E, et al. Magnetic resonance guided radiation therapy for pancreatic adenocarcinoma, advantages, challenges, current approaches, and future directions. Front Oncol 2021;11:628155.

63. Chuong MD, Kirsch C, Herrera R, et al. Long-term multi-institutional outcomes of 5-fraction ablative stereotactic MR-guided adaptive radiation therapy (SMART) for inoperable pancreas cancer with median prescribed biologically effective dose of 100 Gy[10]. Int J Radiat Oncol Biol Phys 2021;111(3):S147–8.

64. Perone JA, Riall TS, Olino K. Palliative Care for Pancreatic and Periampullary Cancer. Surg Clin North Am 2016;96(6):1415–30.

65. Ebrahimi G, Rasch CRN, van Tienhoven G. Pain relief after a short course of palliative radiotherapy in pancreatic cancer, the Academic Medical Center (AMC) experience. Acta Oncol 2018;57(5):697–700.

66. Buwenge M, Macchia G, Arcelli A, et al. Stereotactic radiotherapy of pancreatic cancer: a systematic review on pain relief. J Pain Res 2018;11:2169–78.

67. Hoyer M, Roed H, Sengelov L, et al. Phase-II study on stereotactic radiotherapy of locally advanced pancreatic carcinoma. Radiother Oncol 2005;76(1):48–53.
68. Weichselbaum RR, Hellman S. Oligometastases revisited. Nat Rev Clin Oncol 2011;8(6):378–82.
69. Hagiwara K, Harimoto N, Araki K, et al. Long-term survival of two patients with pancreatic cancer after resection of liver and lung oligometastases: a case report. Surg Case Rep 2020;6(1):309.
70. Saedon M, Maroulis I, Brooks A, et al. Metastasectomy of pancreatic and periampullary adenocarcinoma to solid organ: The current evidence. J BUON 2018; 23(6):1648–54.
71. Yachida S, Jones S, Bozic I, et al. Distant metastasis occurs late during the genetic evolution of pancreatic cancer. Nature 2010;467(7319):1114–7.
72. Yamanaka M, Hayashi M, Yamada S, et al. A Possible Definition of Oligometastasis in Pancreatic Cancer and Associated Survival Outcomes. Anticancer Res 2021;41(8):3933–40.

Cytotoxic Chemotherapy in Advanced Pancreatic Cancer

Muneeb Rehman, MD[a],*, Aakib Khaled[b,1], Marcus Noel, MD[a]

KEYWORDS

- Advanced pancreatic cancer treatment • Chemotherapy for pancreatic cancer
- Metastatic pancreatic cancer

KEY POINTS

- Since the approval of gemcitabine for the treatment of advanced pancreatic cancer in 1997, further advancements in treatments have been slow, with many more negative than positive clinical trials.
- This article examines the specific components of first- and second-line therapies for advanced pancreatic cancer treatment and their effectiveness and concludes with a brief exploration of future directions for targeted therapies.

INTRODUCTION

Pancreatic ductal adenocarcinoma (PDAC) remains of the deadliest malignancies in 2022. Although it was estimated to represent only 3.2% of cancer incidence in 2021, PDAC was expected to account for 7.9% of deaths last year with a 5-year survival rate of 10% combined across all stages of the cancer.[1] Although the 10% overall survival (OS) rate does represent a marked increase in survival over previous years, the reality remains that the disease typically presents in its later stages and in such cases, 5-year survival rates plummet to 3%. At diagnosis, most patients present with advanced, if not metastatic disease, with early diagnosis only accounting for 10% of PDAC incidence.[2] The later-stage diagnosis of PDAC, along with a paucity of symptoms experienced in early stages of the disease, low effectiveness of typical cytotoxic agents, an increased presence of stroma, and overall reduced immunogenicity are among the complex factors contributing to the bleak prognostic outlook for patients diagnosed with PDAC.[3] In addition, large-scale public health crises, that is, the increased prevalence of sedentary lifestyles, dangerous carbohydrate- and fat-

The authors have nothing to disclose.

[a] Georgetown Lombardi Comprehensive Care Center, 3800 Reservoir Road Northwest, Washington, DC 20007, USA; [b] Georgetown University School of Medicine, 3800 Reservoir Road Northwest, Washington, DC 20007, USA

[1] 2001 North Adams St, 631, Arlington, VA 22201, USA

* Corresponding author. 8455 Fenton St Apt 232, Silver Spring, Maryland 20910.

E-mail address: muneeb.s.rehman@medstar.net

heavy diets, and the resulting increased incidence of diabetes and obesity, are strongly implicated as contributing factors to increasing rates of PDAC.[4] This increased incidence is drawn into sharp relief against a backdrop of significant overall decreases in cancer incidence in the past 3 decades.

PDAC is associated with a stromal component that often constitutes a large portion of the mass.[5] The stroma in turn produces a dense extracellular matrix, which, when combined with hyaluronic acid-induced pressure changes, leads to a hypoperfused, effectively isolated microenvironment.[6] This altered microenvironment helps shield the tumor from attempts at therapeutic intervention, including the delivery of cytotoxic chemotherapy. Low immunogenicity is characterized by a relative dearth of effector T cells, and the accumulation of several types of normally functioning immune cells that result in cytotoxic T cell suppression.[7] These unique histologic and immune cell characteristics of PDAC reduce the body's inherent immune surveillance capabilities and are among the typical obstacles to effective treatment.

In recent years, 2 therapies have emerged as the standard of care for the first-line treatment of advanced PDAC: gemcitabine-nab-paclitaxel[8] and FOLFIRINOX,[9] a combination of 5-fluorouracil, leucovorin, irinotecan, and oxaliplatin. These therapies are primarily used to address advanced-stage disease and have limited effectiveness, as is evident in survival rates. Future strategies hoping to reduce PDAC mortality are focused on a variety of factors, including earlier identification of precursor lesions and developing more effective pharmacotherapeutic options. The most common precursor lesion for PDAC is pancreatic intraepithelial neoplasia, the presence of which represents a heavily studied combination of genetic alterations most commonly including point mutations in KRAS and often, inactivation of genes like TP53, SMAD4, and CDKN2A.[10] Continued efforts to understand the genetic profile and specific biomarkers of PDAC will not only support earlier identification of the cancer but also the development of more targeted therapies to help improve patient prognoses, despite the limited success with these strategies to date. The remainder of this review examines the specific components of first- and second-line therapies for PDAC treatment and their effectiveness and concludes with a brief exploration of future directions for targeted therapies.

FIRST-LINE THERAPY

Development of effective treatments for PDAC has been slow and lagged that of other cancers. **Table 1** shows the US Food and Drug Administration (FDA)-approved regimens for the treatment of advanced PDAC. In 1997, Burris and colleagues[11] established first-line standard of care with clinical superiority of first-line gemcitabine monotherapy when compared with 5-fluorouracil (5-FU) (median OS 5.65 vs 4.41 months, $P = .0025$). The survival rate at 12 months was 18% for patients taking gemcitabine and 2% for patients taking 5-FU. In addition, patients in the gemcitabine arm were noted to have improvements in quality-of-life metrics. Pain intensity and/or reduction in analgesic use was reduced in 23.8% of patients in the gemcitabine arm and 4.8% of patients in the 5-FU arm and stable in 39.7% of patients in the gemcitabine arm and 60.3% of patients in the 5-FU arm. Both pain and performance status improved in 4 patients taking gemcitabine, and 11 other patients taking gemcitabine had an improvement in pain with no worsening of performance status. Overall, 15 (23.8%) patients taking gemcitabine were classified as experiencing clinical benefit by primary measures of pain and functional status, whereas 3 (4.8%) patients taking 5-FU experienced clinical benefit.

Over the following 2 decades, several studies investigated adding cytotoxic chemotherapy agents to gemcitabine, but results were mostly disappointing or not

Table 1

Summary of US Food and Drug Administration-approved chemotherapy regimens in advanced pancreatic ductal adenocarcinoma

Composition	FDA Approval	Indication	Survival Rate at 12 months	Median Progression-Free Survival	Median Overall Survival
Gemcitabine[11]	1996	Advanced pancreatic cancer	18% compared with 2% for 5-FU	-	5.65 mo
Nab-paclitaxel and gemcitabine[8]	2013	Metastatic pancreatic cancer	35% compared with 22% for gemcitabine alone	5.5 mo	8.5 mo
5-FU, leucovorin, irinotecan, and oxaliplatin[9]	—	Metastatic pancreatic Cancer	48% compared with 20% for gemcitabine	6.4 mo	11.1 mo
Nanolipossomal irinotecan[18], 5-FU, and leucovorin[22]	2015	Gemcitabine-resistant advanced metastatic pancreatic cancer	26% compared with 16% in 5-FU + folinic acid	3.1 mo	6.1 mo

Abbreviations: 5-FU, 5-fluorouracil; FDA, US Food and Drug Administration.

generalizable. The combination of gemcitabine and capecitabine showed mixed results. A phase 3 trial in 2007 by the Swiss Group for Clinical Cancer Research and the Central European Cooperative Group compared gemcitabine and capecitabine to gemcitabine alone and found no statistical difference in median OS (8.4 months in combination arm vs 7.2 months with capecitabine alone, $P = .234$); however, in the subset of patients with good performance status (Karnofsky Performance Status scale 90–100), there was a significant prolongation in median OS (10.1 vs 7.4 months, $P = .014$).[12] A phase 3 trial in 2009 compared the combination of gemcitabine and capecitabine with gemcitabine in the first-line setting, with results showing a significantly improved progression-free survival (PFS) when compared with gemcitabine (hazard ratio [HR], 0.78; 95% confidence interval [CI], 0.66–0.93; $P = .004$).[13] However, there was a trend but not statistically significant difference in median OS (HR, 0.86; 95% CI, 0.72 to 1.02; $P = .08$).

The combination of gemcitabine with erlotinib, an inhibitor of epidermal growth factor receptor (EGFR) was compared with standard-of-care gemcitabine alone and showed a minimal improvement in median OS (6.24 vs 5.91 months; HR, 0.82; 95% CI, 0.69–0.99; $P = .038$).[14] This combination was approved by the FDA in 2007. However, because of limited clinical benefit, high cost, and increased toxicity (diarrhea, infection, rash, stomatitis), this combination was not widely used, except in a small subgroup of patients with KRAS wild-type PDAC. The combination of gemcitabine and other EGFR and antiangiogenic agents has been tested without a benefit in survival.

Within the last decade, the FDA approved 2 regimens as standard first-line treatments in the metastatic setting. The first regimen—FOLFIRINOX—combined irinotecan, oxaliplatin, and fluorouracil (with leucovorin rescue). The Partenariat de Recherche en Oncologie Digestive (PRODIGE) Group studied this combination versus single agent gemcitabine.[9] A total of 342 patients with Eastern Cooperative Oncology Group (ECOG) performance status of 0 or 1 were randomized to FOLFIRINOX or gemcitabine. Patients were enrolled at 15 centers during phase 2 and expanded to 48 centers during phase 3. Patients were eligible to be included in the study if they were aged 18 years or older and had histologically and cytologically confirmed, measurable metastatic pancreatic adenocarcinoma that had not previously been treated with chemotherapy, ECOG 0 or 1, adequate bone marrow (granulocyte count of at least 1500/mm^3 and platelet count of at least 100,000/mm^3), liver function (bilirubin less than or equal to 1.5 times the upper limit of normal range), and renal function. Exclusion criteria were age 76 years or older, endocrine or acinar pancreatic carcinoma, previous radiotherapy for measurable lesions, cerebral metastases, a history of other major cancer, active infection, chronic diarrhea, a clinically significant history of cardiac disease, and pregnancy or breastfeeding. Outcomes included an overall response rate to FOLFIRINOX of 34.1% and to gemcitabine of 11.3% in the phase 2 trial. In the phase 3 trial, the objective response rate was 31.6% (95% CI, 24.7–39.1) in the FOLFIRINOX group and 9.4% (95% CI, 5.4–14.7) in the gemcitabine group ($P < .001$). There was an improvement in median OS (11.1 vs 6.8 months; HR, 0.57; 95% CI, 0.45–0.74; $P < .001$) and PFS (6.4 vs 3.3 months; HR, 0.47; 95% CI, 0.37–0.59; $P < 0.001$). Although there was statistically significant improvement in outcomes, FOLFIRINOX was noted to have an increased toxicity profile when compared with gemcitabine. The main grade 3 to 4 toxicities were neutropenia (45.7% vs 21%; $P < .001$), febrile neutropenia, thrombocytopenia, neuropathy (9% vs 0%; $P < .001$), vomiting, fatigue, and diarrhea (12.7% vs 1.8%; $P < 0.001$). However, overall-quality-of-life deterioration was less in the FOLFIRINOX arm, likely due to improved disease control.

The second approved regimen is the combination of gemcitabine and nab-paclitaxel, which was compared with gemcitabine in the Metastatic Pancreatic Adenocarcinoma Clinical Trial (MPACT).[8] A total of 861 patients in 151 community and academic centers were enrolled, with 431 patients in the nab-paclitaxel plus gemcitabine arm and 430 in the gemcitabine alone arm. Included patients had an age of at least 18 years, a Karnofsky performance status of 70 (on a scale from 0 to 100, with higher scores indicating better performance status), and histologically or cytologically confirmed metastatic adenocarcinoma of the pancreas that was measurable according to the Response Evaluation Criteria in Solid Tumors (RECIST), version 1.0. Eligible patients could have received treatment with fluorouracil or gemcitabine as a radiation sensitizer in the adjuvant setting if the treatment had been received at least 6 months before randomization. Patients who had received cytotoxic doses of gemcitabine or any other chemotherapy in the adjuvant setting and those with islet cell neoplasms or locally advanced disease were excluded. Included patients had to have adequate hematologic, hepatic, and renal function (absolute neutrophil count of $\geq$1.5 $\times$ 109/L, a hemoglobin level of $\geq$9 g/dL, and a bilirubin level at or below the upper limit of the normal range). Outcomes included an improvement in median OS (8.5 vs 6.7 months; HR, 0.72; 95% CI, 0.62–0.83; $P < .001$) as well as median PFS 5.5 months versus 3.7 months (HR, 0.69; 95% CI, 0.58–0.82; P < .001). Main adverse events of grade 3 or higher in the gemcitabine and nab-paclitaxel arm were neutropenia (38%), fatigue (54%), peripheral neuropathy, and alopecia (50%). There is currently no head-to-head trial comparing FOLFIRINOX versus gemcitabine and nab-paclitaxel in the advanced or metastatic setting. The Southwest Oncology Group (SWOG) compared modified FOLFIRINOX with a dose adjustment (mFOLFIRINOX) versus gemcitabine and nab-paclitaxel in the neoadjuvant setting, with no statistically significant findings. Median OS was 22.4 months in the mFOLFIRINOX arm versus 23.6 months in the gemcitabine and nab-paclitaxel arm, and median disease-free survival (DFS) after resection was 10.9 months in the mFOLFIRINOX arm versus 14.2 months in the gemcitabine and nab-paclitaxel arm (P = .87).[15] The choice of which regimen to use first line in metastatic PDAC is left to physician discretion. Current guidelines suggest first-line use of FOLFIRINOX in patients with an ECOG performance status of 0 or 1, gemcitabine and nab-paclitaxel in patients with ECOG performance status of 0 to 2, and gemcitabine in patients with an ECOG performance status of 2.[1] These 3 regimens are the backbone to which novel agents or cytotoxic drugs are added in clinical trials.

Approaches aimed at intensifying chemotherapy regimens have had promising results, although with associated increased toxicity. A phase 1b/2 pilot trial evaluating cisplatin, gemcitabine, and nab-paclitaxel showed a high response rate, with a complete response rate of 8.3%, partial response 62.5%, stable disease 16.7%, and progressive disease 12.5%. Fatal events occurred for 3 patients (12%); 2 were treatment-related deaths.[16] This combination is currently under study in patients with advanced cholangiocarcinoma and may provide greater insight into the safety and tolerability of this regimen to determine if further investigation of this combination in advanced pancreatic adenocarcinoma is warranted (NCT02392637). Another phase 2 trial evaluated a chemotherapy combination of gemcitabine, nab-paclitaxel, cisplatin, and capecitabine in patients with unresectable or borderline resectable disease with results showing a PFS at 6 months of 100% in the combination arm versus 61% in the control arm.[17] In the metastatic setting, the combination of nab-paclitaxel, gemcitabine, capecitabine, and cisplatin was compared with nab-paclitaxel and

---

[1] Tempero MA, Malafa MP, et al. Pancreatic Adenocarcinoma version 1.2022, NCCN Clinical Practice Guidelines in Oncology. National Comprehensive Cancer Network, Inc. 2022. All rights reserved. Accessed July 11, 2022.

gemcitabine, with the former having a DFS of 74% versus 46% for the latter.[16] Grade 3 adverse events included neutropenia (29% vs 34% in control arm), anemia (21% in both arms), and fatigue (17% in each arm). Grade 4 adverse events included neutropenia (12% vs 5% in the control arm). This combination is promising but needs further study.

SECOND-LINE THERAPY

The FDA-approved regimen for second-line therapy was based on the phase 3 Nanoliposomal Irinotecan-1 (NAPOLI-1) trial, in which patients who progressed after gemcitabine-based therapy in a metastatic, adjuvant, or neoadjuvant setting were randomized to either receive nanoliposomal irinotecan plus 5-FU/leucovorin or 5-FU/leucovorin alone.[18] Patients in the nanoliposomal irinotecan plus 5-FU/leucovorin arm had a median OS of 6.1 months versus 4.2 months (HR, 0.67; 95% CI, 0.49–0.92; $P = .012$). This regimen was approved by the FDA in late 2015. This is the preferred regimen for patients who progressed on gemcitabine-based therapy or who received prior fluoropyrimidine-based therapy if no prior irinotecan was given.

The second-line treatment for patients who received FOLFIRINOX is gemcitabine and nab-paclitaxel. Unfortunately, there are few randomized trials assessing the efficacy of this second-line treatment regimen. A retrospective study reviewed outcomes in patients who had progressed on FOLFIRINOX and received second-line gemcitabine-nab-paclitaxel, which showed a 58% disease control rate and median OS from the first treatment of 18 months.[19]

The Charite-Onkologie-003 (CONKO-003) randomized trial reported a median increase in OS of 2.6 months in patients with gemcitabine-refractory disease who were treated with 5-FU, leucovorin, and oxaliplatin when compared with those patients who only received 5-FU and leucovorin (HR, 0.66; 95% CI, 0.48–0.91; $P = 0.010$) without increased toxicity.[20] The utility of this regimen after FOLFIRINOX has not been established. However, the randomized PANCREOX phase 3 trial investigated the use of biweekly 5-FU, leucovorin, and oxaliplatin (FOLFOX6) versus 5-FU and leucovorin and reached discordant results.[21] Patients in the FOLFOX6 arm had a median OS of 6.1 months versus 9.9 months in patients who received 5-FU and leucovorin (HR, 1.78; 95% CI, 1.08–2.93; $P = .024$). A possible explanation could be that the CONKO-003 trial used a lower dose intensity of oxaliplatin, with the PANCREOX study leading to higher levels of toxicity.

SUMMARY

Despite the progress in our understanding of the molecular tumor biology in PDAC, we have not yet translated these insights into improved treatment options for metastatic pancreatic cancer. Our options are limited to a few key cytotoxic therapies including FOLFIRINOX, gemcitabine-nab-paclitaxel, nanoliposomal irinotecan, and 5-FU, and thus there is still a lot of work to be done in this condition. Better systemic treatment of pancreatic cancer beyond conventional chemotherapy is expected in the near future, thanks to a better understanding of pancreatic cancer tumor biology, the growing availability of noncytotoxic agents, and interest from academia and pharmaceutical companies to meet the challenge. It is unclear whether trials like NCI-MATCH (National Malignancy Institute Molecular Analysis for Therapy Choice) and others that assign drugs based on genetic abnormalities (actionable mutations) would be successful in this cancer because there are not many "hits." However, it is obvious that we can only push the therapeutic envelope in this condition with profound science that includes robust translational applications and vigorous recruitment efforts to research studies. The progress in PDAC has been slow but meaningful.

CLINICS CARE POINTS

- Despite the progress in our understanding of the molecular tumor biology in PDAC, we have not yet translated these insights into improved treatment options for metastatic pancreatic cancer.

- Current guidelines suggest that for patients with metastatic pancreatic cancer and good functional status (ECOG 0-1), first line treatment is the combination of 5-FU, leucovorin, irinotecan, and oxaliplatin (FOLFIRINOX). For patients with borderline functional status, first line therapy is the combination of nab-paclitaxel and gemcitabine. These two regimens have not been compared in the metastatic setting.

- For patients who progress on first line FOLFIRINOX, often gemcitabine and nab-paclitaxel is given as second line treatment, although there are few randomized trials assessing the efficacy of this as a second line regimen.

- For patients who have gemcitabine-resistant metastatic pancreatic cancer, FDA approved treatment is with nanoliposomal irinotecan, 5-FU, and leucovorin.

- Further research is needed to improve outcomes in patients with metastatic or advanced pancreatic cancer.

REFERENCES

1. Facts & figures 2021. Atlanta, GA: American Cancer Society; 2021.
2. Piciucchi M, Capurso G, Valente R, et al. Early onset pancreatic cancer: risk factors, presentation and outcome. Pancreatology 2015;15(2):151–5. https://doi.org/10.1016/j.pan.2015.01.013. Drugs. Author manuscript; available in PMC 2020 September 02. Author Manuscript Author Manuscript Author Manuscript Author Manuscript International Association of Pancreatology (IAP) [et al].
3. Kleeff J, Korc M, Apte M, et al. Pancreatic cancer. Nat Rev Dis Primers 2016;2:16022.
4. Siegel RL, Miller KD, Jemal A. Cancer statistics, 2019. CA: a Cancer J Clinicians 2019;69(1):7–34.
5. Moffitt RA, Marayati R, Flate EL, et al. Virtual microdissection identifies distinct tumor- and stroma-specific subtypes of pancreatic ductal adenocarcinoma. Nat Genet 2015;47(10):1168–78.
6. Stromnes IM, DelGiorno KE, Greenberg PD, et al. Stromal reengineering to treat pancreas cancer. Carcinogenesis 2014;35(7):1451–60.
7. Vonderheide RH, Bayne LJ. Inflammatory networks and immune surveillance of pancreatic carcinoma. Curr Opin Immunol 2013;25(2):200–5.
8. Von Hoff DD, Ervin T, Arena FP, et al. Increased survival in pancreatic cancer with nab-paclitaxel plus gemcitabine. N Engl J Med 2013;369:1691–703.
9. Conroy T, Desseigne F, Ychou M, et al. FOLFIRINOX versus gemcitabine for metastatic pancreatic cancer. N Engl J Med 2011;364:1817–25.
10. Soreide K, Sund M. Epidemiological-molecular evidence of metabolic reprogramming on proliferation, autophagy and cell signaling in pancreas cancer. Cancer Lett 2015;356:281–8.
11. Burris HA, Moore MJ, Andersen J, et al. Improvements in survival and clinical benefit with gemcitabine as first-line therapy for patients with advanced pancreas cancer: a randomized trial. J Clin Oncol 1997;15(6):2403–13.

12. Herrmann R, Bodoky G, Ruhstaller T, et al. Gemcitabine plus capecitabine compared with gemcitabine alone in advanced pancreatic cancer: a randomized, multicenter, phase III trial of the Swiss Group for Clinical Cancer Research and the Central European Cooperative Oncology Group. J Clin Oncol 2007; 25(16):2212–7.

13. Cunningham D, Chau I, Stocken DD, et al. Phase iii randomized comparison of gemcitabine versus gemcitabine plus capecitabine in patients with advanced pancreatic cancer. J Clin Oncol 2009;27(33):5513–8.

14. Moore MJ, Goldstein D, Hamm J, et al. Erlotinib plus gemcitabine compared with gemcitabine alone in patients with advanced pancreatic cancer: a phase III trial of the National Cancer Institute of Canada Clinical Trials Group. J Clin Oncol 2007;25(15):1960–6.

15. Ahmad SA, Duong M, Sohal DPS, et al. Surgical outcome results from swog s1505: a randomized clinical trial of mfolfirinox versus gemcitabine/nab-paclitaxel for perioperative treatment of resectable pancreatic ductal adenocarcinoma. Ann Surg 2020;272(3):481–6.

16. Reni M, Zanon S, Peretti U, et al. Nab-paclitaxel plus gemcitabine with or without capecitabine and cisplatin in metastatic pancreatic adenocarcinoma (PACT-19): a randomised phase 2 trial. Lancet Gastroenterol Hepatol 2018;3(10):691–7.

17. Reni M, Zanon S, Balzano G, et al. A randomised phase 2 trial of nab-paclitaxel plus gemcitabine with or without capecitabine and cisplatin in locally advanced or borderline resectable pancreatic adenocarcinoma. Eur J Cancer 2018;102: 95–102.

18. Wang-Gillam A, Hubner RA, Siveke JT, et al. NAPOLI-1 phase 3 study of liposomal irinotecan in metastatic pancreatic cancer: Final overall survival analysis and characteristics of long-term survivors. Eur J Cancer 2019;108:78–87.

19. Portal A, Pernot S, Tougeron D, et al. Nab-paclitaxel plus gemcitabine for metastatic pancreatic adenocarcinoma after Folfirinox failure: an AGEO prospective multicentre cohort. Br J Cancer 2015;113(7):989–95.

20. Oettle H, Riess H, Stieler JM, et al. Second-line oxaliplatin, folinic acid, and fluorouracil versus folinic acid and fluorouracil alone for gemcitabine-refractory pancreatic cancer: outcomes from the CONKO-003 trial. J Clin Oncol 2014; 32(23):2423–9.

21. Gill S, Ko Y-J, Cripps C, et al. Pancreox: a randomized phase iii study of fluorouracil/leucovorin with or without oxaliplatin for second-line advanced pancreatic cancer in patients who have received gemcitabine-based chemotherapy. J Clin Oncol 2016;34(32):3914–20.

PARPis and Other Novel, Targeted Therapeutics in Pancreatic Adenocarcinoma

William J. Chapin, MD[a,b], Kim A. Reiss, MD[a,b],*

KEYWORDS

- Pancreatic adenocarcinoma • Homologous recombination deficiency • BRCA
- PALB2 • PARP inhibitor • Mismatch repair deficiency • NTRK fusions
- NRG1 fusions

KEY POINTS

- Patients with pancreatic ductal adenocarcinoma (PDAC) and germline pathogenic variants in BRCA1/2 or PALB2 have increased sensitivity to platinum chemotherapy and PARP inhibitors.
- Patients with PDAC and other somatic and germline pathogenic variants in genes involved in DNA damage repair may have a homologous recombination deficiency phenotype. Some may benefit from platinum chemotherapy and/or PARP inhibitors.
- Patients with PDAC with mismatch repair deficiency may benefit from immune checkpoint blockade.
- Patients with advanced PDAC should undergo comprehensive tumor sequencing and fusion analysis due to emerging standard and/or clinical trial options for tumors with NTRK gene fusions, NRG1 gene fusions, and KRAS p.G12C mutations.
- All patients with PDAC should undergo germline sequencing.

INTRODUCTION

Pancreatic ductal adenocarcinoma (PDAC) remains the fourth leading cause of cancer death in the United States, and only 10% of patients survive 5 years from the time of diagnosis.[1] Traditionally, the approach to systemic therapy for PDAC was relatively uniform, with little variation based on patient and tumor characteristics. Recent discoveries have identified biological subsets of patients whom may benefit from novel, targeted therapies.

[a] Department of Medicine, Division of Hematology-Oncology, Perelman School of Medicine, University of Pennsylvania, Philadelphia, PA, USA; [b] Abramson Cancer Center, University of Pennsylvania, 3400 Civic Center Boulevard, 10th Floor South Pavilion, Philadelphia, PA 19104, USA
* Corresponding author. Abramson Cancer Center, University of Pennsylvania, 3400 Civic Center Boulevard, 10th Floor South Pavilion, Philadelphia, PA 19104.
E-mail address: Kim.ReissBinder@pennmedicine.upenn.edu

Hematol Oncol Clin N Am 36 (2022) 1019–1032
https://doi.org/10.1016/j.hoc.2022.07.007
0889-8588/22/© 2022 Elsevier Inc. All rights reserved.

POLY-ADP RIBOSE POLYMERASE INHIBITORS

Germline BRCA1/2 and PALB2 Pathogenic Variants and Homologous Recombination Deficiency

Germline pathogenic variants in *BRCA1* or *BRCA2* (*gBRCA1/2*) predispose to breast, ovarian, prostate, and pancreatic cancer.[2] BRCA1/2 are critical for the repair of double-stranded DNA breaks via the homologous recombination pathway and serve an important role in protecting stalled replication forks from degradation.[3–5] In cells with homologous recombination deficiency (HRD) due to loss of BRCA1 or BRCA2, inhibition of poly ADP-ribose polymerase (PARP) is synthetically lethal due to PARP trapping on DNA lesions leading to collapse of replication forks and an accumulation of double-stranded breaks, and inhibition of PARP activity leading to the accumulation of single strand breaks and stalling of replication forks.[6–8]

The prevalence of *gBRCA1/2* pathogenic variants in unselected populations of patients with PDAC ranges from 4% to 5%, although prevalence is higher in patients with PDAC and Ashkenazi-Jewish heritage.[9] Patients with pathogenic variants in the partner and localizer of the *BRCA2* gene (*PALB2*) are also at increased risk of PDAC, although germline *PALB2* (*gPALB2*) pathogenic variants are identified in less than 1% of unselected patients with PDAC.[9,10]

Platinum Treatment in Patients with Pancreatic Ductal Adenocarcinoma and gBRCA1/2 or gPALB2 Pathogenic Variants

Patients with pathogenic *gBRCA1/2* or *gPALB2* variants benefit preferentially from platinum-based chemotherapy, as has been shown in multiple retrospective studies and in a phase II study in which first-line cisplatin plus gemcitabine in this population had an objective response rate (ORR) exceeding 60%.[11–13]

Maintenance Therapy in Pancreatic Ductal Adenocarcinoma

The depth and durability of responses to platinum-based therapies in the *gBRCA/gPALB2* population can be extraordinary, with responses lasting months or even years. Although this is tremendous in the face of a universally lethal illness, chronic chemotherapy leads to cumulative organ damage and negatively impacts quality of life. Therefore, alternative options for patients with durable responses to treatment, regardless of mutation status, are needed. Maintenance by chemotherapy de-escalation is one strategy, and indeed a recently published trial demonstrated numerically longer median survival without deterioration of quality of life when de-escalation from FOLFIRINOX to 5-fluorouracil and leucovorin (5FU/LV) was used in an all-comer PDAC population.[14]

The POLO trial, published in 2019, was a first-in-kind phase III, randomized, double-blind, placebo-controlled trial examining maintenance therapy with olaparib, a PARP inhibitor (PARPi), in patients with metastatic PDAC and *gBRCA1/2* pathogenic variants whose disease had not progressed during first-line platinum-based chemotherapy.[15] The primary endpoint of progression-free survival (PFS) was significantly longer with olaparib compared with placebo (7.4 vs 3.8 months; hazard ratio (HR) 0.53; 95% confidence interval (CI) 0.35–0.82; $P = .004$), although no difference in overall survival (OS) was observed initially, or in a long-term follow-up (HR 0.83; 95% CI 0.56–1.22; $P = .35$).[15,16] Interestingly, 36 month OS was 33.9% in the olaparib group compared with 17.8% in the placebo group.[16] The trial was underpowered to detect a small but clinically significant benefit in OS for maintenance olaparib compared with placebo. Based on the enrolled sample, the trial had ~22% power to detect a statistically significant benefit in OS for maintenance olaparib with the observed HR of 0.83 (assuming 2-sided alpha of 0.05). An ORR of 20% with median duration of response

(DOR) of 24.9 months was observed in the olaparib group compared with 10% and 3.7 months in the placebo group, respectively.[15] Overall, this indicates that a subgroup of patients has outstanding and durable responses to PARPi maintenance but that identification by genotype alone is insufficient to predict this outcome.

A single-arm phase II study examined maintenance rucaparib in patients with platinum-sensitive advanced PDAC and a pathogenic germline or somatic variant in BRCA1/2 or PALB2.[17] The platinum-sensitivity criteria required that patients had no evidence of platinum resistance, which included steadily rising CA 19-9 and/or increase in lesion size during platinum therapy. PFS at 6 months was 59.5% (95% CI 44.6–74.4) with median OS of 23.5 months (95% CI 20–27). Among patients with measurable disease at baseline, ORR was 41.7% with a disease control rate of 66.7%. The median DOR was 17.3 months (95% CI 8.8–25.8). Objective responses occurred in patients with gBRCA2, gPALB2, and somatic BRCA2 pathogenic variants, although no responses occurred in the 7 patients with gBRCA1 pathogenic variants.[17] In subgroup analyses, those with higher disease burden at study start and those with gBRCA1 variants had inferior outcomes, although the authors point out that the small study sample dictates that these observations be hypothesis generating only. **Table 1** summarizes results of reported trials of PARPi monotherapy in patients with PDAC.

Poly-ADP Ribose Polymerase Inhibitor Toxicity

The POLO trial found that there was no clinically meaningful change from baseline global health-related quality of life score (EORTC QLQ-C30) in either the olaparib or placebo group.[15] A meta-analysis of randomized trials using PARPi compared with placebo found a significantly increased relative risk of myelodysplastic syndrome or acute myeloid leukemia with exposure to PARPi but the absolute incidence remained low (0.73%; 95% CI 0.50–1.07 vs 0.47%; 95% CI 0.26–0.85).[18] These data suggest that the increased risk of myelodysplastic syndrome or acute myeloid leukemia with PARPi treatment is real, although the absolute magnitude of this risk remains small.

PREDICTIVE BIOMARKERS OF POLY-ADP RIBOSE POLYMERASE INHIBITOR IN PANCREATIC DUCTAL ADENOCARCINOMA

Early studies of PARPi were focused on patients with gBRCA1/2 pathogenic variants but genotype alone is an imperfect biomarker because (1) not all tumors with gBRCA pathogenic variants have an HRD and (2) some PDACs without these variants may have an HRD.[19] Other surrogates for HRD may include sensitivity to platinum-based chemotherapy, strong family history of PDAC, other germline and somatic variants involved in DNA damage repair (DDR), and laboratory-based assays for HRD that evaluate DNA scars, mutational patterns, or dynamic homologous recombination function.[19–21]

Platinum Sensitivity as a Predictive Biomarker for Poly-ADP Ribose Polymerase Inhibitor

Platinum sensitivity has emerged as an important requirement for sensitivity to PARPi in PDAC. In a phase II study of rucaparib in patients with advanced PDAC and germline or somatic BRCA1/2 variants, Shroff and her colleagues found that no patients with platinum-resistant PDAC experienced an objective response to rucaparib.[22] In contrast, 28.6% of the platinum-sensitive patients had an objective response and 57.1% had a clinical benefit. Javle and colleagues[21] recently showed that the PFS and OS with olaparib treatment was significantly longer in PDAC patients with platinum-sensitive disease compared with platinum-resistant disease in patients

Table 1
Selected, reported trials evaluating poly-ADP ribose polymerase inhibitors monotherapy in patients with pancreatic ductal adenocarcinoma

Study	Setting	Inclusion	Phase	Treatment	N[a]	Outcome
Golan et al. (POLO)[15]	Maintenance	Advanced PDAC; gBRCA1/2 pathogenic variant; no progression on first-line platinum-based chemotherapy	2	Olaparib 300 mg by mouth twice daily vs placebo	154	PFS: Median 7.4 vs 3.8 mo (HR 0.53; 95% CI 0.35–0.82; P = .004) OS: Median 19.0 vs 19.2 mo (HR 0.83; 95% CI 0.56–1.22; P = .35) ORR: 20% vs 10% DOR: Median 24.9 vs 3.7 mo
Reiss et al. (RUCAPANC2)[17]	Maintenance	Advanced PDAC; germline or somatic pathogenic variants in BRCA1/2 or PALB2; at least 16 wk of platinum-based chemotherapy without platinum resistance	2	Rucaparib 600 mg by mouth twice daily	46	PFS: Median 13.1 mo (95% CI 4.4–21.8) OS: Median 23.5 months (95% CI 20–27) ORR: 41.7% DOR: Median 17.3 mo (95% CI 8.8–25.8)
Javle et al,[21] 2021	Second-line or later therapy	Advanced PDAC; lack of gBRCA1/2 pathogenic variants; personal or family history suggesting HRD, somatic or germline DDR mutations other than gBRCA1/2, or ATM loss by immunohistochemistry	2	Olaparib 300 mg by mouth twice daily	48	PFS: 3.7 mo (95% CI 2.9–5.7) OS: 9.9 mo (95% CI 7.6–16.1) ORR: 2% (one additional unconfirmed response) DOR: 3.9 months (for one responding patient)
Kaufman et al,[57] 2015	Second-line or later therapy	Advanced PDAC; gBRCA1/2 pathogenic variant; prior gemcitabine treatment[b]	2	Olaparib 400mg by mouth twice daily	23	OS: Median 9.8 months ORR: 21.7% DOR: Median 134 days

Shroff et al,[22] 2018	Second-line or third-line therapy	Advanced PDAC; somatic or gBRCA1/2 mutations; 1 or 2 prior therapies	2	Rucaparib 600 mg by mouth twice daily	19	ORR: 15.8%
Lowery et al,[58] 2018	Second-line or third-line therapy	Advanced PDAC; gBRCA1/2 or gPALB2 pathogenic variant; 1–2 previous lines of treatment[c]	2	Veliparib 300 mg twice daily or veliparib 400 mg twice daily	16	PFS: Median 1.7 mo (95% CI 1.57–1.83); OS: Median 3.1 mo (95% CI 1.9–4.1); ORR: 0%

When multiple groups compared, ordered as experimental vs control.
Abbreviation: NA, not applicable or not reported.
[a] Number of patients with PDAC.
[b] 65% of patients had received previous platinum chemotherapy.
[c] 88% of patients had received previous platinum chemotherapy.

with or without pathogenic germline variants in DDR genes. Although platinum sensitivity is not a sufficient biomarker for PARPi sensitivity, evidence strongly suggest that it is required for PARPi efficacy, likely due to an overlap between the mechanisms of secondary platinum resistance and PARPi resistance.

Somatic and Germline Variants in DNA Damage Repair Genes as Predictive Biomarkers for Poly-ADP Ribose Polymerase Inhibitor Sensitivity in Pancreatic Ductal Adenocarcinoma

Somatic and germline variants in DDR genes other than *BRCA1/2* may result in HRD and, therefore, predict for response to PARPi. There are limited data for PARPi activity in those with somatic *BRCA* pathogenic variants, although of 4 such patients treated on available data, 3 had responses to treatment.[17,22] Similarly, there are limited data for those with *gPALB2* pathogenic variants but available data suggest a high ORR in this population as well.[17] Javle and colleagues recently published 2 parallel phase II single-arm trials testing whether patients with pathogenic variants beyond *BRCA* might benefit from olaparib therapy. The study included patients with non-*BRCA* DDR variants, those with loss of ATM expression (ATM loss) by immunohistochemistry, and patients with a personal and/or family history of *BRCA*-associated cancers but without identified pathogenic germline variants.[21] The primary endpoint of the study was ORR. Out of a total of 46 evaluable patients, 1 patient had a confirmed partial response (2%), whereas 33 patients (72%) experienced stable disease on olaparib.[21] The confirmed partial response occurred in a patient with a *gPALB2* pathogenic variant. PFS was significantly longer among patients with germline genetic alterations in DDR genes compared with patients enrolled based on family history alone.[21] Although the sample was small, there were no responses in patients with ATM loss by immunohistochemistry.[21]

Golan and colleagues[19] identified PDAC tumors from patients harboring germline pathogenic variants in *ATM* and *CHEK2*, including several with specific loss of heterozygosity at these loci, and found that none was associated with genomic features of HRD by multiple classifiers, suggesting a homologous recombination proficient phenotype.

Together, these studies suggest that certain patients with genetic alterations in DDR genes other than *gBRCA1/2* exhibit an HRD phenotype and may derive benefit from PARPi, whereas others do not. Therefore, alternative strategies to refine the identification of HRD phenotypes are required.

Tissue-Based Predictive Biomarkers for Poly-ADP Ribose Polymerase Inhibitor Sensitivity

The myChoice HRD assay (Myriad Genetics, Inc., Salt Lake City, UT) is a genomic instability score (GIS) based on telomeric allelic imbalance, loss of heterozygosity, and large-scale state transitions that is performed in parallel with the identification of tumoral variants in *BRCA1* and *BRCA2*.[23] Tumors are classified as HRD if a pathogenic *BRCA1/2* variant is identified, the composite GIS is 42 or greater, or both.[23] The myChoice HRD assay was predictive of benefit of PARPi maintenance in ovarian cancer and is a Food and Drug Administration (FDA)-approved companion diagnostic for olaparib and niraparib in this setting.[23–26]

Additional laboratory-based biomarkers for HRD have aimed to improve on those that evaluate "DNA scars" by incorporating mutational profiles from whole genome sequencing. Davies and colleagues[27] developed the HRDetect score, which is a weighted score incorporating microhomology-mediated deletions, base substitution signatures, rearrangement signatures, and the GIS, although it requires fresh frozen tissue to implement. In a validation cohort of patients with PDAC, the HRDetect score had a sensitivity of 100% for identifying patients with biallelic inactivation of *BRCA1/2*, and identified additional patients without biallelic *BRCA1/2* inactivation who may have an HRD phenotype.[27]

Golan and colleagues[19] subsequently aimed to evaluate a variety of predictive biomarkers for HRD in PDAC to identify non-*BRCA* mutated patients who may harbor an HRD phenotype and benefit from platinum-based chemotherapy and PARPi. Of 391 samples from patients with PDAC, 43 were from patients with a *gBRCA1/2* or *gPALB2* pathogenic variant and evidence of biallelic inactivation (true HRD). Using the myChoice GIS and HRDetect, 12% of patients with *gBRCA1/2* or *gPALB2* pathogenic variants did not have evidence of biallelic inactivation or any markers of HRD, suggesting a homologous recombination proficient phenotype.[19] The HRDetect score had a sensitivity of 98% and specificity of 100% for detecting biallelic loss of *BRCA1/2* or *PALB2* among all 49 patients with *gBRCA1/2* or *gPALB2* pathogenic variants. When applied to the overall cohort, including patients with sporadic PDAC, an additional 29 patients (7% of the cohort) were identified as HRD by HRDetect. Of these 29 patients, 12 had somatic alterations in homologous recombination repair genes, including somatic biallelic inactivation of *BRCA1/2*, homozygous deletion of *XRCC2*, homozygous deletion of *RAD51C*, and loss of heterozygosity at *RAD51C* and *RAD51D* with low gene expression.[19] Sixteen HRD patients did not have specific DNA alterations or aberrant RNA expression in identifiable homologous recombination genes. There was clear interaction between HRD by HRDetect and myChoice GIS and platinum treatment in multivariable survival analysis ($P = .005$; $P = .02$) with higher response rates for HRD patients (63% vs 23% for HRDetect high/low; 52% vs 22% for myChoice GIS high/low) suggesting that each biomarker was predictive of response to platinum therapy. Given the ability to identify patients with an HRD phenotype—regardless of germline variant status in *BRCA1/2* or *PALB2*—and promising data predicting response to platinum chemotherapy, HRD biomarkers are being incorporated into prospective PARPi clinical trials to further evaluate their potential as predictive biomarkers. Real-time functional assays of HRD, such as evaluating RAD51 foci at sites of DNA damage and RNA-based assays, if successful, may have the ability to dynamically assess HRD as it changes with treatment. These assays remain under investigation as well.[20,28,29]

FUTURE DIRECTIONS FOR POLY-ADP RIBOSE POLYMERASE INHIBITOR IN PANCREATIC DUCTAL ADENOCARCINOMA

Given the PFS benefit and observed durable responses for subgroups of patients with PDAC and HRD who received maintenance PARPi, there is interest in expanding the use of these agents. The ongoing APOLLO (EA2192; NCT04858334) trial is evaluating a PARPi as adjuvant therapy following surgical resection and chemotherapy for patients with PDAC and *gBRCA1/2* or *gPALB2* pathogenic variants.

Additionally, PARPi therapy is being examined in combination with other agents to enhance efficacy. In a 2-arm, randomized phase II trial of patients with gBRCA/gPALB2 variants with untreated, advanced PDAC, the combination of PARPi (veliparib) with chemotherapy (gemcitabine plus cisplatin) did not improve ORR, PFS, or OS beyond chemotherapy alone.[13] Veliparib is less effective at PARP trapping on DNA compared with other PARPi, which may partially explain its lower potency and improved toxicity profile.[30] This result does not rule out benefit to chemotherapy combinations with PARPi in other settings or with PARPis that more effectively trap PARP on DNA.[30] Preclinical mouse models of breast and ovarian cancers have demonstrated that PARPis trigger T-cell dependent antitumor immunity and that treatment with concurrent programmed cell deth protein 1 (PD-1) blockade may enhance antitumor response.[31] This finding has led to multiple ongoing trials that aim to combine PARPi with PD-1 or cytotoxic T-lymphocyte-associated protein 4 (CTLA-4) blockade in patients with PDAC (NCT04666740; NCT03404960; NCT04548752). These studies also aim to expand the population that might benefit from PARPi. The PARPVAX and POLAR studies examine immunotherapy plus PARPi as maintenance therapy and include cohorts for patients who have not progressed on platinum-based chemotherapy regardless of mutational status (NCT03404960; NCT04666740). Additional combination therapies with PARPi that target resistance mechanisms and aim to induce HRD—including with ataxia telangiectasia and Rad3-related protein (ATR) inhibitors, WEE1 G2 Checkpoint Kinase (WEE1) inhibitors, and vascular endothelial growth factor (VEGF) inhibitors—remain under development and have been reviewed elsewhere.[20,32]

NTRK FUSIONS

NTRK1, *NTRK2*, and *NTRK3* encode the neurotrophin receptors TRKA, TRKB, and TRKC, respectively.[33] *NTRK* gene fusions leading to TRK fusion proteins have been shown to be oncogenic drivers across multiple tumor types.[33] Across cancers, *NTRK* fusions are uncommon, occurring in ~0.3% of analyzed tumors.[34] In the largest unselected cohort of patients with PDAC evaluated to date, 0.8% were noted to have *NTRK* fusions, although 6.25% of *KRAS* wild-type tumors were found to have *NTRK* fusions.[35] Larotrectinib and entrectinib have been evaluated across cancer types in patients with *NTRK* fusions (**Table 2**), including in patients with PDAC.[36,37] Pooled analyses of early phase trials for larotrectinib and entrectinib in patients with refractory, advanced solid tumors observed ORRs of 79% and 57% and median durations of response of 35.2 and 10 months, respectively.[36,37] One of 2 patients with PDAC (ORR 50%) experienced a partial response to larotrectinib with duration of 3.5 months, and 2 of 3 patients with PDAC experienced a response to entrectinib (ORR 67%), with the other experiencing stable disease. Larotrectinib and entrectinib were approved by the FDA for any solid tumor with *NTRK* fusion and no alternative standard therapy.[38,39]

NEUREGULIN 1 FUSIONS

Fusions involving neuregulin 1 (*NRG1*) are recurrent across cancer types.[40,41] NRG1 activates the ERBB3 (HER3) and ERBB4 (HER4) receptors, which then form heterodimers with other human epidermal growth factor receptor (HER)-family receptors leading to stimulation of downstream signaling pathways.[40,41] Several case-series identified 6 patients with PDAC and *KRAS* wild-type tumors that harbored *NRG1* fusions and observed promising rates of clinical responses on therapies that targeted HER-family receptors.[40,41] These promising data prompted the development and evaluation of a bispecific antibody, zenocutuzumab, which blocks heterodimerization of ERBB2 and ERBB3 in *NRG1* fusion-positive cancers (see **Table 2**).[42] In a phase II trial, 53 patients with refractory solid tumors with *NRG1* fusions were treated with zenocutuzumab. Of the 10 patients with PDAC that were evaluable, ORR was 40% (95% CI 15%–70%) and disease control rate was 90% (95% CI 15%–70%), with a CA19-9 decline of more than 50% observed in all patients with elevated CA19-9 at baseline.[42] No patients required dose reduction for toxicity. Targeting *NRG1* fusions in patients with PDAC and wild-type *KRAS* has shown significant promise and results from the ongoing research in this patient population are eagerly anticipated (NCT02912949).

Table 2
Prospective trials of biomarker-directed therapies including patients with pancreatic ductal adenocarcinoma

Study	Biomarker	Inclusion	Treatment	N[a]	Outcome
Hong et al,[36] 2020	NTRK fusion	Advanced NTRK fusion-positive solid tumor; had received standard therapy previously, if available	Larotrectinib 100 mg by mouth twice daily	2	ORR: 50% DOR: 3.5 mo (in 1 patient)
Doebele et al,[37] 2020	NTRK fusion	Advanced NTRK fusion-positive solid tumor; may have received prior anticancer therapies	Entrectinib 600 mg by mouth once daily	3	ORR: 66%
Le et al,[49] 2017	MMRd/MSI-H	Advanced solid tumor; MMRd or MSI-H; progression on at least 1 prior therapy	Pembrolizumab 10 mg/kg IV every 14 d	8	ORR: 62%
Marabelle et al. (KEYNOTE-158)[47]	MMRd/MSI-H	Advanced noncolorectal cancer; MMRd or MSI-H; progression on prior standard therapies	Pembrolizumab 200 mg IV every 3 wk	22	ORR: 18.2% (5.2%–40.3%) DOR: Median 13.4 mo (range 8.1–16.0[b], mo)
Schram et al,[42] 2021,[c]	NRG1 fusion	Advanced NRG1 fusion-positive solid tumors; previously treated with standard therapies	Zenocutuzumab 750 mg IV every 2 wk	13	ORR: 40% (95% CI 15%–70%)
Hong et al,[56] 2020	KRAS p.G12C	Advanced solid tumor; KRAS p.G12C mutation on tumor tissue; at least one previous line of systemic therapy	Sotorasib 960 mg by mouth daily (dose in the expansion cohort)	12	ORR: 9%

Abbreviations: MMRd, mismatch repair deficient; MSI-H, microsatellite instability–high.
[a] Number of patients with PDAC.
[b] Longest response was ongoing at the time of data cutoff.
[c] Trial is ongoing.

MISMATCH REPAIR DEFICIENCY IN PANCREATIC DUCTAL ADENOCARCINOMA

Mismatch repair deficiency (MMRd) results from the biallelic loss of expression of genes involved in DNA mismatch repair, including *MLH1*, *MSH2*, *MSH6*, and *PMS2*.[43] This can occur in the setting of Lynch syndrome or sporadically, in which case biallelic loss of mismatch repair gene expression occurs through somatic mutation and/or epigenetic silencing.[43–46] Although MMRd tumors were initially described in colorectal cancers, they represent 2% to 4% of all cancers and between 0.3% and 1.6% of PDAC.[47,48]

Pembrolizumab was studied in treatment refractory colorectal and noncolorectal MMRd cancers (see **Table 2**).[49] Eighty-six patients with 12 tumor types were treated with pembrolizumab. ORR was 53% (95% CI 42%–46%) with 21% of patients experiencing a complete response.[49] Disease control rate was 77% (95% CI 66%–85%). The trial included 8 patients with PDAC with an observed ORR of 62%.[49] Pembrolizumab was approved by the FDA for the treatment of locally advanced or metastatic MMRd solid tumors with no satisfactory alternative treatment options.[50] KEYNOTE-158 evaluated 233 patients with noncolorectal, locally advanced or metastatic cancers that were MMRd and had no acceptable standard options for treatment.[47] Twenty-two patients with PDAC were enrolled, with 1 patient experiencing a complete response and 2 patients experiencing a partial response (ORR 18.2%; 95% CI 5.2%–40.3%).[47] For patients with PDAC, pembrolizumab therapy should be considered after disease progression on standard therapies, when no subsequent standard options exist or are contraindicated.[47,49]

KRAS G12C MUTATIONS

KRAS is a guanosine triphosphatase that serves as a molecular switch as it cycles between the active guanosine triphosphate bound state and the inactive guanosine diphosphate bound state in response to extracellular signaling.[51,52] The *KRAS* p.G12C mutation favors the active form of KRAS, leading to hyperactivation of downstream oncogenic pathways and uncontrolled cell growth.[53] Small molecule inhibitors, such as sotorasib, covalently bind to a region in KRAS G12C that is present only in the inactive conformation, thereby trapping KRAS G12C in its inactive state and preventing downstream oncogenic signaling.[52] In patients with NSCLC and a *KRAS* p.G12C mutation, sotorasib demonstrated an ORR of 37.1% (95% CI 28.6%–45.2%) and disease control rate of 80.6% (95% CI 72.6%–87.2%), leading to an FDA-accelerated approval in this patient population.[54] *KRAS* mutations are present in more than 90% of PDAC, although *KRAS* p.G12C mutations are present in only 1.6%.[51,55] In the CodeBreak100 trial, which evaluated sotorasib in patients with *KRAS* p.G12C solid tumors, 1/11 patients with PDAC experienced a partial response with a duration of 4.4 months, 8/11 experienced stable disease, and 2/11 experienced progressive disease as best response (see **Table 2**).[56] Ongoing trials for patients with *KRAS* p.G12C mutations that include patients with PDAC aim to evaluate combination therapy approaches with KRAS G12C inhibitors that may address resistance mechanisms to KRAS G12C inhibition (NCT04185883; NCT04330664).

SUMMARY

Although the prognosis for patients with PDAC remains poor, there has been progress in the development of novel, biomarker-directed therapies for subgroups of patients. Patients with HRD derive benefit from platinum-based chemotherapy, and olaparib maintenance treatment is associated with improved PFS among patients with *gBRCA1/2* pathogenic variants. Ongoing trials aim to investigate PARPi in other settings for the treatment of PDAC, to identify patients beyond those with *gBRCA1/2* or *gPALB2* pathogenic variants who may have a HRD phenotype and benefit from PARPi, and to evaluate combinations with PARPi that may improve clinical efficacy. The best way to clinically identify HRD in PDAC patients remains elusive, with substantial effort geared toward answering this question. Biomarker-directed therapies, including pembrolizumab for patients with MMRd and larotrectinib and entrectinib for patients with *NTRK* fusions, have been approved in a disease agnostic fashion. Additional promising biomarker-directed therapies for tumors with *NRG1* fusions and *KRAS* p.G12C mutations remain under development.

CLINICS CARE POINTS

- All patients with a new diagnosis of PDAC should undergo germline genetic testing, as germline mutations in DDR genes have important implications for systemic treatment options and for counseling of family members.

- Patients with advanced PDAC should undergo comprehensive tumor sequencing, fusion analysis, and mismatch repair/microsatellite instability testing due to the availability of effective biomarker-directed therapies for *NTRK* fusions, *NRG1* fusions, and MMRd.

- Patients with advanced PDAC and germline or somatic pathogenic variants in DDR genes, especially *BRCA1/2* and *PALB2*, should receive platinum-containing chemotherapy regimens as first-line treatment whenever possible.

- For patients with advanced PDAC and germline pathogenic variants in *BRCA1/2* without disease progression on platinum chemotherapy after at least 4 months, olaparib can provide a respite from cytotoxic chemotherapy.

DISCLOSURE

Dr K.A. Reiss: Research support from Clovis Oncology, Bristol-Myers Squibb, Tesaro, GlaxoSmithKline; Advisory board for Carisma Therapeutics; Consulting for AstraZeneca. Dr W.J. Chapin has no disclosures to report.

REFERENCES

1. Siegel RL, Miller KD, Fuchs HE, et al. Cancer Statistics, 2021. CA Cancer J Clin 2021;71(1):7–33.
2. Levy-Lahad E, Friedman E. Cancer risks among BRCA1 and BRCA2 mutation carriers. Br J Cancer 2007;96(1):11–5.
3. Chen CC, Feng W, Lim PX, et al. Homology-Directed Repair and the Role of BRCA1, BRCA2, and Related Proteins in Genome Integrity and Cancer. Annu Rev Cancer Biol 2018;2:313–36.
4. Schlacher K, Christ N, Siaud N, et al. Double-strand break repair-independent role for BRCA2 in blocking stalled replication fork degradation by MRE11. Cell 2011;145(4):529–42.
5. Schlacher K, Wu H, Jasin M. A distinct replication fork protection pathway connects Fanconi anemia tumor suppressors to RAD51-BRCA1/2. Cancer Cell 2012;22(1):106–16.
6. Farmer H, McCabe N, Lord CJ, et al. Targeting the DNA repair defect in BRCA mutant cells as a therapeutic strategy. Nature 2005;434(7035):917–21.

7. Bryant HE, Schultz N, Thomas HD, et al. Specific killing of BRCA2-deficient tumours with inhibitors of poly(ADP-ribose) polymerase. Nature 2005;434(7035): 913–7.

8. Dias MP, Moser SC, Ganesan S, et al. Understanding and overcoming resistance to PARP inhibitors in cancer therapy. Nat Rev Clin Oncol 2021;18(12):773–91.

9. Casolino R, Paiella S, Azzolina D, et al. Homologous recombination deficiency in pancreatic cancer: a systematic review and prevalence meta-analysis. J Clin Oncol 2021;39(23):2617–31.

10. Yang X, Leslie G, Doroszuk A, et al. Cancer risks associated with germline PALB2 pathogenic variants: an international study of 524 families. J Clin Oncol 2020; 38(7):674–85.

11. Golan T, Kanji ZS, Epelbaum R, et al. Overall survival and clinical characteristics of pancreatic cancer in BRCA mutation carriers. Br J Cancer 2014;111(6): 1132–8.

12. Wattenberg MM, Asch D, Yu S, et al. Platinum response characteristics of patients with pancreatic ductal adenocarcinoma and a germline BRCA1, BRCA2 or PALB2 mutation. Br J Cancer 2020;122(3):333–9.

13. O'Reilly EM, Lee JW, Zalupski M, et al. Randomized, multicenter, phase II trial of gemcitabine and cisplatin with or without veliparib in patients with pancreas adenocarcinoma and a germline BRCA/PALB2 mutation. J Clin Oncol 2020; 38(13):1378.

14. Dahan L, Williet N, Le Malicot K, et al. Randomized phase II trial evaluating two sequential treatments in first line of metastatic pancreatic cancer: results of the PANOPTIMOX-PRODIGE 35 trial. J Clin Oncol 2021;39(29):3242–50.

15. Golan T, Hammel P, Reni M, et al. Maintenance olaparib for germline BRCA-mutated metastatic pancreatic cancer. N Engl J Med 2019;381(4):317–27.

16. Golan T, Hammel P, Reni M, et al. Overall survival from the phase 3 POLO trial: Maintenance olaparib for germline BRCA-mutated metastatic pancreatic cancer. J Clin Oncol 2021;39(3_suppl):378.

17. Reiss KA, Mick R, O'Hara MH, et al. Phase II study of maintenance rucaparib in patients with platinum-sensitive advanced pancreatic cancer and a pathogenic germline or somatic variant in BRCA1, BRCA2, or PALB2. J Clin Oncol 2021; 39(22):2497–505.

18. Morice PM, Leary A, Dolladille C, et al. Myelodysplastic syndrome and acute myeloid leukaemia in patients treated with PARP inhibitors: a safety meta-analysis of randomised controlled trials and a retrospective study of the WHO pharmacovigilance database. Lancet Haematol 2021;8(2):e122–34.

19. Golan T, O'Kane GM, Denroche RE, et al. Genomic features and classification of homologous recombination deficient pancreatic ductal adenocarcinoma. Gastroenterology 2021;160(6):2119–32.e9.

20. Wattenberg MM, Reiss KA. Determinants of homologous recombination deficiency in pancreatic cancer. Cancers 2021;13(18):4716.

21. Javle M, Shacham-Shmueli E, Xiao L, et al. Olaparib monotherapy for previously treated pancreatic cancer with DNA Damage repair genetic alterations other than germline BRCA variants: findings from 2 phase 2 nonrandomized clinical trials. JAMA Oncol 2021;7(5):693–9.

22. Shroff RT, Hendifar A, McWilliams RR, et al. Rucaparib monotherapy in patients with pancreatic cancer and a known deleterious BRCA mutation. JCO Precis Oncol 2018;2018. https://doi.org/10.1200/PO.17.00316.

23. González-Martín A, Pothuri B, Vergote I, et al. Niraparib in patients with newly diagnosed advanced ovarian cancer. N Engl J Med 2019;381(25):2391–402.

24. Ray-Coquard I, Pautier P, Pignata S, et al. Olaparib plus bevacizumab as first-line maintenance in ovarian cancer. N Engl J Med 2019;381(25):2416–28.
25. FDA approves niraparib for HRD-positive advanced ovarian cancer. FDA. 2019. Available at: https://www.fda.gov/drugs/resources-information-approved-drugs/fda-approves-niraparib-hrd-positive-advanced-ovarian-cancer. Accessed December 29, 2021.
26. FDA approves olaparib plus bevacizumab as maintenance treatment for ovarian, fallopian tube, or primary peritoneal cancers. FDA. 2021. Available at: https://www.fda.gov/drugs/resources-information-approved-drugs/fda-approves-olaparib-plus-bevacizumab-maintenance-treatment-ovarian-fallopian-tube-or-primary. Accessed December 29, 2021.
27. Davies H, Glodzik D, Morganella S, et al. HRDetect is a predictor of BRCA1 and BRCA2 deficiency based on mutational signatures. Nat Med 2017;23(4):517–25.
28. Naipal KAT, Verkaik NS, Ameziane N, et al. Functional ex vivo assay to select homologous recombination-deficient breast tumors for PARP inhibitor treatment. Clin Cancer Res 2014;20(18):4816–26.
29. Leibowitz B, Dougherty BV, Bell JS, et al. Validation of Genomic and Transcriptomic Models of Homologous Recombination Deficiency in a Real-World Pan-Cancer Cohort. BMC Cancer 2021. https://doi.org/10.1101/2021.12.20.21267985. 2021.12.20.21267985.
30. Murai J, Huang S yin N, Das BB, et al. Trapping of PARP1 and PARP2 by clinical PARP inhibitors. Cancer Res 2012;72(21):5588–99.
31. Pantelidou C, Sonzogni O, De Oliveria Taveira M, et al. PARP inhibitor efficacy depends on CD8+ T-cell recruitment via intratumoral STING pathway activation in BRCA-deficient models of triple-negative breast cancer. Cancer Discov 2019;9(6):722–37.
32. Crowley F, Park W, O'Reilly EM. Targeting DNA damage repair pathways in pancreas cancer. Cancer Metastasis Rev 2021;40(3):891–908.
33. Cocco E, Scaltriti M, Drilon A. NTRK fusion-positive cancers and TRK inhibitor therapy. Nat Rev Clin Oncol 2018;15(12):731–47.
34. Solomon JP, Linkov I, Rosado A, et al. NTRK fusion detection across multiple assays and 33,997 cases: diagnostic implications and pitfalls. Mod Pathol 2020;33(1):38–46.
35. Allen MJ, Zhang A, Bavi P, et al. Molecular characterisation of pancreatic ductal adenocarcinoma with NTRK fusions and review of the literature. J Clin Pathol 2021. https://doi.org/10.1136/jclinpath-2021-207781. jclinpath-2021-207781.
36. Hong DS, DuBois SG, Kummar S, et al. Larotrectinib in patients with TRK fusion-positive solid tumours: a pooled analysis of three phase 1/2 clinical trials. Lancet Oncol 2020;21(4):531–40.
37. Doebele RC, Drilon A, Paz-Ares L, et al. Entrectinib in patients with advanced or metastatic NTRK fusion-positive solid tumours: integrated analysis of three phase 1-2 trials. Lancet Oncol 2020;21(2):271–82.
38. FDA approves larotrectinib for solid tumors with NTRK gene fusions. FDA. 2019. Available at: https://www.fda.gov/drugs/fda-approves-larotrectinib-solid-tumors-ntrk-gene-fusions. Accessed December 31, 2021.
39. FDA approves entrectinib for NTRK solid tumors and ROS-1 NSCLC. FDA. 2019. Available at: https://www.fda.gov/drugs/resources-information-approved-drugs/fda-approves-entrectinib-ntrk-solid-tumors-and-ros-1-nsclc. Accessed December 31, 2021.
40. Heining C, Horak P, Uhrig S, et al. NRG1 fusions in KRAS wild-type pancreatic cancer. Cancer Discov 2018;8(9):1087–95.

41. Jones MR, Williamson LM, Topham JT, et al. NRG1 gene fusions are recurrent, clinically actionable gene rearrangements in KRAS wild-type pancreatic ductal adenocarcinoma. Clin Cancer Res 2019;25(15):4674–81.

42. Schram AM, O'Reilly EM, O'Kane GM, et al. Efficacy and safety of zenocutuzumab in advanced pancreas cancer and other solid tumors harboring NRG1 fusions. J Clin Oncol 2021;39(15_suppl):3003.

43. Dudley JC, Lin MT, Le DT, et al. Microsatellite instability as a biomarker for PD-1 blockade. Clin Cancer Res Off J Am Assoc Cancer Res 2016;22(4):813–20.

44. Veigl ML, Kasturi L, Olechnowicz J, et al. Biallelic inactivation of hMLH1 by epigenetic gene silencing, a novel mechanism causing human MSI cancers. Proc Natl Acad Sci 1998;95(15):8698–702.

45. Kane MF, Loda M, Gaida GM, et al. Methylation of the hMLH1 promoter correlates with lack of expression of hMLH1 in sporadic colon tumors and mismatch repair-defective human tumor cell lines. Cancer Res 1997;57(5):808–11.

46. Geurts-Giele WR, Leenen CH, Dubbink HJ, et al. Somatic aberrations of mismatch repair genes as a cause of microsatellite-unstable cancers. J Pathol 2014;234(4):548–59.

47. Marabelle A, Le DT, Ascierto PA, et al. Efficacy of pembrolizumab in patients with noncolorectal high microsatellite instability/mismatch repair–deficient cancer: results from the phase II KEYNOTE-158 study. J Clin Oncol 2020;38(1):1–10.

48. Hu ZI, Shia J, Stadler ZK, et al. Evaluating mismatch repair deficiency in pancreatic adenocarcinoma: challenges and recommendations. Clin Cancer Res 2018; 24(6):1326–36.

49. Le DT, Durham JN, Smith KN, et al. Mismatch-repair deficiency predicts response of solid tumors to PD-1 blockade. Science 2017;357(6349):409–13.

50. Marcus L, Lemery SJ, Keegan P, et al. FDA Approval Summary: Pembrolizumab for the Treatment of Microsatellite Instability-High Solid Tumors. Clin Cancer Res 2019;25(13):3753–8.

51. Lee MS, Pant S. Personalizing Medicine With Germline and Somatic Sequencing in Advanced Pancreatic Cancer: Current Treatments and Novel Opportunities. Am Soc Clin Oncol Educ Book Am Soc Clin Oncol Annu Meet 2021;41:1–13.

52. Skoulidis F, Li BT, Dy GK, et al. Sotorasib for lung cancers with KRAS p.G12C mutation. N Engl J Med 2021;384(25):2371–81.

53. Ostrem JM, Peters U, Sos ML, et al. G12C) inhibitors allosterically control GTP affinity and effector interactions. Nature 2013;503(7477):548–51.

54. FDA grants accelerated approval to sotorasib for KRAS G12C mutated NSCLC. FDA. 2021. Available at: https://www.fda.gov/drugs/resources-information-approved-drugs/fda-grants-accelerated-approval-sotorasib-kras-g12c-mutated-nsclc. Accessed January 2, 2022.

55. Bailey P, Chang DK, Nones K, et al. Genomic analyses identify molecular subtypes of pancreatic cancer. Nature 2016;531(7592):47–52.

56. Hong DS, Fakih MG, Strickler JH, et al. KRASG12C Inhibition with sotorasib in advanced solid tumors. N Engl J Med 2020;383(13):1207–17.

57. Kaufman B, Shapira-Frommer R, Schmutzler RK, et al. Olaparib Monotherapy in Patients With Advanced Cancer and a Germline BRCA1/2 Mutation. J Clin Oncol 2015;33(3):244–50.

58. Lowery MA, Kelsen DP, Capanu M, et al. Phase II trial of veliparib in patients with previously treated BRCA-mutated pancreas ductal adenocarcinoma. Eur J Cancer Oxf Engl 1990 2018;89:19–26.

Genetics of Pancreatic Neuroendocrine Tumors

Chirayu Mohindroo, MD[a,b], Florencia McAllister, MD[a,c,d,e],
Ana De Jesus-Acosta, MD[f],*

KEYWORDS

- Pancreatic neuroendocrine tumors • Germline mutations • Somatic mutations
- Precision medicine • Molecular therapies • Targeted therapies

KEY POINTS

- Over the last 20 years, the incidence rates for pNETs have been steadily increasing.
- Most pNETs occur sporadically, with 10% to 17% of the cases associated with germline mutations.
- Sporadically occurring pNETs, are commonly associated with somatic mutations in MEN1, DAXX/ATRX, and genes related to the mTOR pathway.
- Four inherited syndromes associated with mutations in the NF1 gene, VHL gene, MEN1 gene, and TSC genes are commonly implicated in pNET development.

INTRODUCTION

Pancreatic neuroendocrine tumors (pNETs) are characterized as a rare disease with an incidence of less than 1 in 100,000 individuals per year, and accounts for 1% to 2% of all pancreatic tumors.[1–3] That being said, pNETs are the second most common pancreatic neoplasm[4] and relatively indolent in clinical presentation when compared with pancreatic adenocarcinoma (PDAC). During the last 2 decades, the incidence rates for pNETs have been steadily increasing, especially for asymptomatic disease. The increasing incidence can be attributed to advances in imaging and endoscopy

[a] Department of Clinical Cancer Prevention, The University of Texas MD Anderson Cancer Center, 1515 Holcombe, Unit 1360, Houston, TX 77030, USA; [b] Department of Internal Medicine, Sinai Hospital of Baltimore, 2435 W. Belvedere Ave, Ste 56, Baltimore, MD 21215, USA; [c] Department of Gastrointestinal Medical Oncology, The University of Texas MD Anderson Cancer Center, Houston, TX, USA; [d] Department of Immunology, The University of Texas MD Anderson Cancer Center, Houston, TX, USA; [e] Clinical Cancer Genetics Program, The University of Texas MD Anderson Cancer Center, Houston, TX, USA; [f] Department of Oncology, The Sidney Kimmel Comprehensive Cancer Center at Johns Hopkins, Johns Hopkins University School of Medicine, CRB1, 1650 Orleans Street, CRB1 Rm 409, Baltimore, MD 21287
* Corresponding author.
E-mail address: adejesu1@jhmi.edu

Hematol Oncol Clin N Am 36 (2022) 1033–1051
https://doi.org/10.1016/j.hoc.2022.07.005
0889-8588/22/© 2022 Elsevier Inc. All rights reserved.

along with updated staging and grading classifications for NETs, which have allowed better recognition of the disease.[1]

The World Health Organization classifies pNETs, based on proliferative fraction of neoplastic cells, into 3 groups, namely low grade (G1), intermediate grade (G2), and high grade (G3). Ninety percent of the tumors are G1 and G2, and these tend to have an unpredictable clinical course that varies from indolent to highly malignant.[4] G3 tumors, in the range of 20% to 55%, have a relatively well-differentiated histology and better prognosis.[5]

Most pNETs occur sporadically with 10% to 17% of the cases being associated with germline mutations.[6,7] Germline mutations such as multiple endocrine neoplasia type 1 (MEN-1), von Hippel-Lindau syndrome (VHL), neurofibromatosis type 1 (NF1), and occasionally tuberous sclerosis complex (TSC) are the most commonly identified mutations to be associated with pNETs.[4] For sporadically occurring pNETs, MEN1, DAXX/ATRX, and genes related to the mammalian target of rapamycin (mTOR) pathway have been commonly identified as somatic alterations.[7,8] In many cancer types, somatic and germline mutations are of great significance for diagnosis, understanding disease biology and treatment management.

SOMATIC MUTATIONS IN PATIENTS WITH PANCREATIC NEUROENDOCRINE TUMORS

Advances in sequencing have expanded our knowledge in the commonly mutated genes in sporadic pNETs. Jiao and colleagues performed exomic sequencing initially in 10 sporadic pNETs and further expanded the knowledge of commonly mutated genes in 58 additional pNETs. Results revealed that 44% of the tumors had somatic inactivating mutations in MEN1, which encodes for menin, a component of a histone methyltransferase complex, and 43% had mutations in genes encoding either of the 2 subunits of a transcription/chromatin remodeling complex consisting of DAXX (death-domain-associated protein) and ATRX (α thalassemia/mental retardation syndrome X-linked). Around 14% of the tumors also had mutations in the mTOR pathway.[8] Another study, performed by Reit and colleagues[9] in advanced pNETs, showed an enrichment in MEN1 (40%), DAXX (25%), DMD (25%), SETD2 (25%), ATRX (20%), and CREBBP (20%) somatic mutations. A summary of these prominent studies are highlighted in **Table 1**.

Multiple Endocrine Neoplasia Type 1

MEN1 is the most frequently mutated gene in sporadic pNETs, ranging from 25% to 44% of tumors in various studies.[8,10,11] MEN1 is responsible for the production of menin protein, located in the nucleus, due to the presence of 3 nuclear localization signals in the C-terminal region. This is essential to the antitumor functions, namely regulation of DNA replication and repair, histone methylation and acetylation, DNA methylation, positive or negative control of gene expression, cell signaling, control of cell cycle and cell growth, control of apoptosis, and cell mobility.[12] In the context of pNETs, menin is responsible for histone methylation in promoters of specific target genes, which have a role in growth and differentiation of neuroendocrine cells.[13] In sporadic pNETs, 30% of nonfunctioning pancreatic neuroendocrine tumors (NF-pNETs), 7% of insulinomas, 36% of gastrinomas, 67% of glucagonomas, and 44% of vasoactive intestinal peptide tumors (VIPomas) are associated with MEN1 mutations.[14,15] Somatic mutations in MEN1 were associated with prolonged survival compared with tumors that lacked these mutations. The effect was further pronounced in patients with metastatic disease.[8]

Table 1
Prominent studies highlighting the somatic mutations in patients with pancreatic neuroendocrine tumors

Study Group	Number of Patients	WHO Grade Stages	Metastatic Disease	MEN1	DAXX	ATRX	mTOR Pathway	Clinical Findings
Jiao et al,[8] 2011	68	31 (G1), 34 (G2), 3 (G3)	21%	44%	25%	18%	17%	MEN1, DAXX/ATRX, or the combination of both MEN1 and DAXX/ATRX were associated with prolonged survival relative to those patients whose tumors lacked these mutations. More pronounced in patients with metastatic disease and with mutations in both MEN1 and DAXX/ATRX
Scarpa et al[7] 2017	98	36 (G1), 57 (G2), 5 (G3)	54%	36%	22%	11%	15%	DAXX or ATRX or mTOR pathway mutations were associated with a poor prognosis in the G2 subgroups with mutations in mTOR regulators
Raj et al[16] 2018	80	29 (G1), 44 (G2), 23 (G3)	100%	56%	40%	25%	43%	MEN1, DAXX, or ATRX alterations is associated with improved OS in the metastatic setting, BRAF alterations were significantly associated with poor survival, SETD2 alternations with aggressive histopathologic features
Yuan et al,[31] 2014	37	22 (G1), 9 (G2), 6 (G3)	8%	35%	32%	35%	54%	A higher number of gene mutations and the DAXX/ATRX and KRAS gene mutations are correlated with a poor prognosis of patients with pNET

ATRX (alpha-thalassemia/mental retardation syndrome X-linked) and DAXX (death domain associated protein)DAXX/ATRX

More than half of the pNETs are found to have somatic alterations in DAXX ranging from 25% to 40% and in ATRX ranging from 18% to 25%.[8,16] These genes are involved in the production of histone-related proteins that bind to telomeres and pericentric heterochromatin regions of the genome and are involved in genomic stability.[17–19] Loss of these proteins leads to the alternative lengthening of telomeres (ALT) phenotype.[20,21] As expected, the ALT phenotype does correlate with DAXX/ATRX status, whereas pNETs with a DAXX or ATRX mutation were found to have ALT, and pNETs with neither of the 2 mutations did not have the ALT phenotype.[20–22] In the clinical setting, these mutations have been used to correlate with prognosis (see **Table 1**), as discussed below the results have been conflicting.

GENES RELATED TO THE MAMMALIAN TARGET OF RAPAMYCIN

pNETs with somatic mutations in genes encoding for proteins associated with mTOR pathway, ranging from 15% to 54%, with the prominent mutations being identified in PTEN, TSC2, and PIK3CA. Recently, Scarpa and colleagues[7] also identified mutations in DEPDC5, another gene in the mTOR pathway. The phosphatidylinositol 3-kinase (PI3K)-Akt-mTOR pathway is involved in multiple essential functions including modulation of cell growth, proliferation, metabolism, survival, and angiogenesis.[23] A study by Missiaglia and colleagues[24] consisting of 72 pNETs showed that the expression of 2 endogenous inhibitors of the mTOR pathway, PTEN and TSC2, was downregulated in the majority of the tumors, respectively, 35% and 60% of cases. PHLDA3 is another tumor suppressor gene involved in the inhibition of Akt activity in islet cells and found to undergo loss of heterozygosity in 70% of the pNETs tumors.[11] Low prevalence of somatic mutations in mTOR pathway genes does not match the high prevalence of cases with low gene expression. This is suggestive of somatic mutations, which are yet to be discovered. Expression profiling and exome sequencing have highlighted the significance of activated mTOR signaling as potential druggable mechanism in 14% of pNET patients[8,24] but the real-world outcomes are controversial. Studies have shown that the presence of such genetic alterations does not predict response or resistance to therapy but can act as prognostic markers to determine clinical outcomes.[25]

POTENTIAL CLINICAL UTILITY OF SOMATIC TESTING IN PATIENTS WITH NEUROENDOCRINE TUMORS

Somatic mutations may provide guidance for the biology and aggressiveness of the tumor, prognosis, and functionality of pNETs. For example, somatic mutations may vary with the grade and differentiation of tumors and thus explain the difference in disease biology. Pancreatic neuroendocrine carcinomas have been differentiated from well-differentiated pNETs on the presence of TP53 and RB1 recurrent mutations that are found in NECs; however, they are rarely seen in pNETs.[26–30] This may be utilized in cases where the differentiation of the grade cannot be clearly established. Similarly, Raj and colleagues[16] recently highlighted the clinical utility of repeat sequencing at disease progression that revealed increasing tumor grade and genetic evolution, showing that pNETs adopt a more aggressive behavior through time and various therapies.

Ethnicity and racial differences may also contribute. Yuan and colleagues assessed these factors and found higher mutation rates in KRAS, TP53, mTOR pathway genes

(PTEN and TSC2), and VHL genes in Chinese patients compared with Caucasian patients. Furthermore, KRAS and DAXX/ATRX gene mutations were predictive of worse survival in Chinese pNET patients. This could indicate racial differences in somatic mutations among patients with pNETs.[31]

Somatic mutations may also have a role as a prognostic marker in patients with pNETs. In the clinical setting, ATRX/DAXX has often been correlated with prognosis, although studies have been conflicting.[25] Although some study groups such as metastatic group reported an improved overall survival and specific stages,[8,16,32,33] other study groups associated these somatic mutations with a shortened survival time.[31,34–37] A meta-analysis conducted by Wang and colleagues,[25] consisting of 14 studies with 2313 pNET patients, reported that those with ATRX/DAXX gene mutations had poor disease-free survival, whereas altered ATRX/DAXX genes in metastatic patients showed a trend toward improved overall survival, although not statistically significant.

Somatic mutations have also highlighted potentially druggable mechanisms. The mTOR pathway is one of the key targets in this disease. Everolimus, an mTOR inhibitor is Food and Drug Administration (FDA) approved for patients with pancreatic neuroendocrine tumors based on the results of RADIANT study, which showed a significant increase in progression-free survival among patients with advanced pNETs.[38,39] It is still unclear if detecting mutations in the mTOR pathway will lead to alterations in clinical treatment or utilized as a biomarker for treatment selection as discussed above.

Somatic mutations may also differ based on tumor functionality. Functional tumors such as insulinomas lack mutations in MEN1, DAXX/ATRX, and mTOR pathway genes, which are frequently seen in NF-pNETs.[40] Multiple study groups have consistently identified sporadic insulinomas to be associated with YY1 mutation.[40–43]

With the available information, we propose somatic mutations may guide discussions of prognosis for patients with pNET (particularly those with localized and metastatic disease) and assist in cases where the grading of the tumor may not be clear based on histologic assessment.

GERMLINE MUTATIONS IN PATIENTS WITH PANCREAS NEUROENDOCRINE TUMORS

There are 4 inherited syndromes associated with the development of pNETs, which include NF1 gene, VHL gene, MEN1 gene, and TSC (hamartin [TSC1] and tuberin [TSC2] genes).[6] A summary of the commonly associated associated syndromes for familial pNETs have been highlighted in (**Table 2**). In addition, limited literature also exists for germline mutations in MUTYH, CHEK2, BRCA2,[7] CDKN1B,[7,8,24] and PTEN.[44,45]

Multiple Endocrine Neoplasia Type 1

MEN1 is one of the most common inherited pNET syndromes causing up to 10% of pNETs. MEN1 is an autosomal dominant disorder characterized by an increased risk of neuroendocrine tumors of the parathyroid, pituitary, and pancreas. MEN1 gene is located on chromosome 11q13.[46,47] Most MEN1-associated pNETs are nonfunctional but approximately 10% to 25% can develop functional insulinomas.[48] A study conducted by Kfir and colleagues, comparing MEN1-related pNETs to sporadic pNETs, showed that age at diagnosis with MEN1-related pNET was significantly younger than with sporadic pNETs (mean age 49.2 ± 16.7 vs 61.6 ± 12.7 years). A survival analysis showed a trend for better outcomes in patients with MEN1-related pNETs and lower all-causes mortality.[49]

Table 2
Commonly associated syndromes along with clinical features for familial pancreatic neuroendocrine tumors

Associated Syndromes	Clinical Features	Causative Genes	Prevalence of pNET Associated with the Disease
MEN1	Primary hyperparathyroidism, functional and NF-pNETs, and functional/ nonfunctional pituitary tumors	MEN1 gene on 11q13	30%–80%[121–124]
MEN4	Parathyroid tumors, neuroendocrine tumors including pituitary, adrenal, enteropancreatic tumors, lipomas, and meningiomas	CDKN1B gene on 12p13.1-p12	25%[55]
VHL	Renal cell carcinoma, pheochromocytoma, serous cystadenoma and neuroendocrine tumors of the pancreas, endolymphatic sac tumors, epididymal and broad ligament cysts and hemangioblastomas of the retina and central nervous system	VHL gene 3p25.3	9%–17%[59–61]
NF1	Pigmentary lesions (café-au-lait macules, skinfold freckling, and Lisch nodules), dermal neurofibromas, brain tumors (optic pathway gliomas and glioblastoma), peripheral nerve tumors (spinal neurofibromas, plexiform neurofibromas, and malignant peripheral nerve sheath tumors)	NF1 gene 17q11.2	10%[72–74]
TSC	Disabling neurologic disorders, facial angiofibromas, renal angiomyolipomas, and pulmonary lymphangiomyomatosis	9q34 TSC1 gene, 16p13 TSC2 gene	1%[125]

Multiple Endocrine Neoplasia Type 4

More recently, familial cases of MEN1 syndrome with similar clinical features but no identified causative gene variant were found to have cyclin-dependent kinase inhibitor 1b gene (CDKN1B) and led to the discovery of MEN4 syndrome. CDKN1B encodes for p27, and mutations in CDKN1B lead to increased cell cycle progression and proliferation. The most common phenotype associated with MEN4 is primary hyperparathyroidism due to parathyroid tumors, followed by pituitary tumors and gastroenteropancreatic neuroendocrine tumors.[50] Given its recent discovery, the prevalence and natural history of pNETs in this genetic syndrome is not well known.[51,52] The prevalence of gastrinomas and NF-pNETs in MEN4 is regarded to be around 25%.[53] However, few case reports exist for pNETs in context of MEN4 syndrome.[7,54–56]

Von Hippel Lindau Syndrome

VHL is an autosomal dominant disease, related with mutations of the VHL gene on chromosome 3. The gene encodes a protein involved in the ubiquitination and degradation of hypoxia-inducible-factor (HIF). The lack of HIF degradation drives overexpression of vascular endothelial growth factor F (VEGF).[57] It is related to retinal and central nervous system hemangioblastomas and less likely associated with renal cell carcinomas, pheochromocytomas, paragangliomas, and pNETs.[58] Prevalence of pNETs in VHL disease ranges from 9% to 17%, and most commonly, the tumors are multiple and nonfunctional.[59–61] De mestier and colleagues[59] reported that patients with VHL-associated pNETs had better prognosis VHL-related pNETs compared with sporadic pNETs. Risk factors for pNET metastasis in VHL syndrome include greatest tumor diameter greater than 3 cm, blood type O, tumor doubling time less than 500 days, pathogenic missense variants, or any pathogenic variant in exon 3 of the VHL gene.[61–63]

In patients with VHL who develop pNET, around 40% of these patients have no tumor growth or a decrease in tumor size, and around 20% of the tumors will be malignant (defined based on locoregional invasion, and/or regional or distant metastasis).[64–66] Limited data exists on the optimal indication for surgical resection in VHL-associated, localized pancreatic solid lesions that could possibly progress to malignancy.[60]

Neurofibromatosis Type 1

NF1 is an autosomal dominant tumor predisposition syndrome with a frequency of 1 in 3000 births, with approximately half of cases occurring due to de novo mutation.[67] It is caused by a mutation in the tumor suppressor gene NF1, located at the long arm of chromosome 17. Generally, it functions as a negative regulator of the ras oncogene signaling pathway.[68–70] NF is largely characterized by nervous system involvement including neurofibromas and cutaneous findings. It is a less frequent cause of pNETs,[71] with gastroenteropancreatic-NET tumors reported in up to 10% of patients with NF1 syndrome, most frequently nonfunctioning somatostatinomas originating from the duodenum.[72–74] These tumors can increase morbidity but rarely contribute to the mortality of NF-1 patients.[46]

Tuberous Sclerosis Complex

TSC is an autosomal dominant genetic disorder, characterized by the formation of benign hamartomas and malignant tumors in various organs including the brain, heart, eyes, kidney, skin, and lungs. TSC is caused by mutations of 2 tumor suppressor genes, encoding for TSC1 and TSC2, regulating cell growth and proliferation pathways, including the mTOR pathway and PI3K. pNETs are a rare manifestation for this syndrome occurring in 1.8% to 9% of these patients.[48,75,76] In a study conducted by Larson and colleagues, which included 219 patients with TSC, 6 patients were diagnosed with pNET. Compared with the general population developing pNETs, the lesions in the TSC cohort occurred at a younger age and were more frequently cystic.[76] Targeted therapy using mTOR inhibitors such as everolimus has been successfully tried in pNET patients.[77]

OTHERS

Besides the above-mentioned germline mutations, few others have also been described in the literature. Scarpa and colleagues performed whole genome sequencing of 102 primary pNETs and reported a prevalence of germline mutations in 17% of these cases. Besides VHL, MEN1, and CDKN1B, the authors also identified for the first time germline mutations in MUTYH, CHEK2, and BRCA2.[7] Moreover, the study discovered a larger-than-anticipated germline contribution to clinically sporadic pNETs, which potentially affects surveillance, diagnosis, and treatment of pNETs.

Case reports have identified germline PTEN mutation in pNETs.[44,45] Patients with Cowden syndrome have a germline PTEN mutation, and have a 6-fold increased risk for the development of neuroendocrine tumors.[44] Petignot and colleagues[78] described the first case of pNET associated with germline mutation in MAXX. Germline mutations in MAX are typically associated with sporadic and familial pheochromocytoma-paragangliomas. Li-Fraumeni syndrome, associated with germline TP53 has been extensively described with breast, brain, adrenal, hematological, and colorectal cancers, along with bone and soft tissue sarcomas. Aversa and colleagues[79] described the first case associated with pNET.

POTENTIAL CLINICAL UTILITY OF GERMLINE TESTING IN PATIENTS WITH NEUROENDOCRINE TUMORS

National Cancer Comprehensive Network (NCCN) guidelines have recently been updated and recommend genetic counseling and testing for inherited genetic syndromes in patients with pancreatic and duodenal NETs.[80] The first step is a detailed history, which should include family history, personal history of cancers followed by a clinical examination, paying particular attention to the syndromic associations to MEN, VHL, NF, and TSC, which are more frequently described. Another important consideration would be age, and patients aged younger than 40 years presenting with pNET should be considered for genetic testing. Other important factors to consider would be tumor type, tumor size, and number.[69]

Until recently, germline testing for PDAC was indicated only for individuals with a personal or family history of cancer. However, it was shown that approximately 42% of individuals with a germline alteration in PDAC would be missed by a testing strategy focusing on specific factors such as family history, personal history, age, and ethnicity.[81] This led to a change in the NCCN guidelines to recommending universal germline testing for patients being diagnosed with PDAC.

Studies by Scarpa and colleagues[7] and Raj and colleagues[16] reported a larger-than anticipated germline mutation contribution to pNET development in clinically sporadic appearing patients without any of the traditional risk factors such as family history. These findings do suggest having a lower threshold to germline testing in patients with pNETs may be further investigated. A summary of multigene panel studies representing germline mutations in patients with pNETs have been shown in (**Table 3**).

Germline testing would also be relevant for therapy in pNET patients. Although data is limited, case reports have shown targeted directed treatment of germline-mutated pNETs. Nuñez and colleagues[82] showed a numerical benefit in disease control rate with everolimus in patients with germline mutations versus those with sporadic ones.

From a therapeutic standpoint, in patients with suspected VHL syndrome, testing may provide further treatment options.,86 The recent FDA approval of belzutifan can be considered in patients with VHL germline mutations.[83,84] Patients with pNET

Table 3
Multigene panel studies representing germline mutations in patients with pancreatic neuroendocrine tumors

Study Groups	Number of Genes Analyzed	Number of Genes Detected	Prevalence	Detected Gene Mutations
Scarpa et al[7] 2017	683	6	16/102 (15.6%)	BRCA2 (1), CDKN1B (1), CHEK2 (4), MEN1 (5), MUTYH (5), and VHL1 (1)
Raj et al[16] 2018	76	6	14/88 (16%)	MEN1 (1), VHL (1), TSC2 (1),CHEK2 (4), MUTYH (4), and APC (3)
Whitman et al[126] 2018	1 to 130	3	11 (N/A)[a]	MEN1(8), MUTYH (2), and APC (1)

[a] 31/107, (Total number of pNETs not specified).

and underlying germline mutation may be incredibly responsive to this therapy.[85] Ongoing trials (NCT04924075) are currently evaluating the use of HIF-1 inhibitors in patients with pNET irrespective of germline status.[86]

The presence of germline mutations has also important consequences for patient's family members. Larger studies in the context to germline mutations would be beneficial for diagnosis, treatment, and screening.

Importance/Future Perspective: Surveillance Strategy for High-Risk Cases

Surveillance for pNETs is complex and depends on a variety of factors including, size, functionality, pathological features, and treatment.[87] We will discuss surveillance in the context of high-risk cases based on inherited syndromes specifically MEN1 and VHL. In patients with MEN1 subjects with pNETs less than 2 cm in size are not recommended to undergo surgery or receive any medical therapy, unless a functioning endocrine syndrome is detected[88,89]; however, recent studies also indicate potential metastatic spread in this subgroup highlighting the importance of active surveillance.[90,91] In a meta-analysis done by Sallinen and colleagues, consisting of 9 studies including 344 patients with sporadic and 64 patients with MEN1 related to small ($\leq$2 cm), asymptomatic, and NF-pNETs, it was concluded that although it was reasonable to pursue expectant management for sporadic tumors, MEN1-related tumors required a more individualized approach. MEN1-associated NF-pNETs appeared to have higher rates of tumor growth (52%), need for surgical resection (25%), and rate of disseminated disease (9%).[92] In a study by Faggiano and colleagues,[93] consisting of 42 MEN1 patients with pNETs less than 2 cm, **Progression Free Survival (**PFS) was significantly prolonged in the group taking lanreotide (somatostatin analogs) compared with active surveillance group.

Patients with germline mutations in VHL gene follow specific protocols for management.[94,] A study conducted by Tirosh and colleagues has provided unique insights for surveillance in this group. Patients with pNETs less than 1.2 cm had a 100% negative predictive value for developing metastasis and requiring a surgical intervention and were considered appropriate for anatomical imaging every 2 to 3 years, and patients with pNETs greater than 1.2 cm and less than 3 cm, depending on the type of mutation were considered appropriate for surveillance but varying intervals of imaging.[95]

Therapies for Patients Harboring Susceptibility Gene Mutations

Surgical resection of pNETs has been suggested to be the only potentially curative treatment.[96] Depending on the clinical scenario, systemic chemotherapies have gained great importance in the treatment of pNETs. However, unlike PDAC where robust evidence exists fortargeted therapy with agents such as platinum, Poly Adenosine diphosphate-ribose Polymerase(PARP) inhibitors, and checkpoint inhibitor therapy based on genetic alterations,[97] is yet to be established in pNETs. Although, various somatic/germline mutations have been identified in pNETs, only mTOR pathway is common and "potentially" targeted.[98] Everolimus is a first-generation oral mTOR inhibitor approved by FDA for pNETs. The drug acts by inhibiting mTOR kinase binding to 12-kDa FK506-binding protein (FKBP-12) and ultimately reducing the activity of mTOR downstream effectors S6K1 and 4E-BP1.[99,100] RADIANT-3 a phase III study compared everolimus at 10 mg/d as monotherapy (n = 207) versus placebo (n = 203), in pNET patients, showed a prolonged median PFS (11.0 versus 4.6 months; HR = 0.35; 95% CI: 0.27–0.45; $P < .001$) in the arm treated with everolimus.[99] Similarly RADIANT-4, yielded similar results with a prolonged PFS in everolimus arm compared with the placebo arm consisting of advanced GI and Lung NETs.[101] Combinations of mTOR inhibitors have also been tested in multiple studies. Somatostatin receptors (SSR) are overexpressed in 70% of the pNETs,[102] and their efficacy has been shown in the CLARINET study[103] and the PROMID trial,[104] respectively, for lanreotide and octreotide. Numerous trials explored the combination of mTOR inhibitors with SSR,[105,106] with RADIANT-2 being the landmark trial. It compared everolimus, plus octreotide, versus placebo plus octreotide showing a significant benefit in PFS for the everolimus arm[107] but the results did not reach statistical significance for Overall Survival(OS).[108] Italian Trials in Medical Oncology (ITMO) group also showed benefit in the combination of everolimus plus octreotide as a treatment.[109] Pasireotide (second-generation Somatostatin Analog) used in combination with everolimus has shown conflicting results[110,111] but a study combining radioembolization, everolimus, and pasireotide showed survival benefit.[112]

VEGF inhibitors have shown efficacy in the treatment of pNETs.[113] pNETs are considered to be highly vascular tumors, the combination of VEGF inhibitors and mTOR inhibitors have been used in combination to show synergistic activity. mTOR inhibitors have been used in combination with sorafenib,[114] sunitinib,[115] and bevacizumab.[116]

Other drugs used in combination with mTOR inhibitors include temozolomide[117] and lutetium-177-octreotate.[118] However, unlike other malignancies, where precise genetic alterations present in the tumor are used for the choice of therapeutics, this is yet to be established in pNETs.[119] As discussed in the sections above, therapy based on genetic alterations is only limited to a few case reports and small studies.[77,82,120] A currently ongoing open-label phase II clinical trial (NCT02315625) has been designed to determine the role of mutation-targeting therapy with sunitinib or everolimus for patients with advanced low-grade or intermediate-grade NETs. Patients will be either assigned to sunitinib or everolimus based on somatic/germline mutations.[119] Another small retrospective study comparing the use of everolimus in patients with germline mutations (MEN1 and VHL) versus patients with sporadic tumors showed a prolonged PFS and Time to Treatment Failure (TTF), which did not reach statistical significance.[82]

In a phase 2, open-label, single-group trial, evaluating the efficacy and safety of the HIF-2α inhibitor belzutifan, among 22 VHL patients with pNETs, 20 patients (91%) had a confirmed response, including 3 patients [14%] who had a complete response.[85] Belzutifan is now approved for adult patients with VHL disease who require therapy for pNET, not requiring immediate surgery.[83,84] The recent advances in next generation sequencing have greatly increased our understanding of the genetics in context to pNETs. As we enter the era of precision of medicine, deeper understanding of genetics can help guide clinical behaviors, improve disease management, surveillance, and screening for pNETs.

SUMMARY

Genetic testing is becoming increasingly important in the management of pNETs. Although our knowledge in the field is still evolving, advances in genetic sequencing have increased our understanding of the complex genetic mechanisms underlying pNET formation. Clinicians should consider incorporating genomic testing into treatment paradigms and involving genetic counsellors to help patients and family members with decisions regarding genetic testing, interpretation, and follow-up.

CLINICS CARE POINTS

Pearls:

- MEN1 is the most commonly mutated gene in sporadic pNETs, ranging from 25% to 44% of tumors.
- Presence of genetic alterations in the mTOR pathway can act as a prognostic marker to determine clinical outcomes.
- Somatic mutations can help guide the biology and aggressiveness of the tumor, prognosis, and functionality of pNETs.
- NCCN guidelines now recommend genetic counseling and testing for inherited genetic syndromes in all pNET patients.
- Belzutifan (HIF-2α inhibitor) is now FDA-approved for VHL patients with pNETs.

Pitfalls:

- Studies utilizing DAXX or ATRX mutations as prognostic markers have been conflicting.
- Unlike PDAC, where substantial evidence exists for targetted therapy, it is yet to be established for pNETs.

ACKNOWLEDGEMENTS

F. McAllister supported by grants from the NCI (1R37CA237384-01A1), CPRIT (RP200173), V Foundation Translational Award, Andrew Sabin Family Fellowship, SU2C-Lustgarten Foundation Pancreatic Cancer Interception Translational Cancer Research Grant (Grant Number: SU2C- AACR-DT25-17).and philanthropic support from the MD Anderson Moonshot Programs.

COI: F. McAllister is an SAB Member at Neologics Bio.

REFERENCES

1. Dasari A, Shen C, Halperin D, et al. Trends in the incidence, prevalence, and survival outcomes in patients with neuroendocrine tumors in the United States. JAMA Oncol 2017;3(10):1335–42.

2. Hallet J, Law CHL, Cukier M, et al. Exploring the rising incidence of neuroendocrine tumors: a population-based analysis of epidemiology, metastatic presentation, and outcomes. Cancer 2015;121(4):589–97.

3. Klimstra DS. Nonductal neoplasms of the pancreas. Mod Pathol 2007;20(1): S94–112.

4. Bosman FT, Carneiro F, Hruban RH, et al. WHO classification of tumours of the digestive system. Lyon, France: World Health Organization; 2010.

5. Weltgesundheitsorganisation LR, Osamura R, Klöppel G, et al. WHO classification of tumours of endocrine organs. Lyon: International Agency for Research on Cancer; 2017.

6. Marx SJ, Simonds WF. Hereditary hormone excess: genes, molecular pathways, and syndromes. Endocr Rev 2005;26(5):615–61.

7. Scarpa A, Chang DK, Nones K, et al. Whole-genome landscape of pancreatic neuroendocrine tumours. Nature 2017;543(7643):65–71.

8. Jiao Y, Shi C, Edil BH, et al. DAXX/ATRX, MEN1, and mTOR pathway genes are frequently altered in pancreatic neuroendocrine tumors. Science 2011; 331(6021):1199–203.

9. van Riet J, van de Werken HJ, Cuppen E, et al. The genomic landscape of 85 advanced neuroendocrine neoplasms reveals subtype-heterogeneity and potential therapeutic targets. Nat Commun 2021;12(1):1–14.

10. Capelli P, Martignoni G, Pedica F, et al. Endocrine neoplasms of the pancreas: pathologic and genetic features. Arch Pathol Lab Med 2009;133(3):350–64.

11. Corbo V, Dalai I, Scardoni M, et al. MEN1 in pancreatic endocrine tumors: analysis of gene and protein status in 169 sporadic neoplasms reveals alterations in the vast majority of cases. Endocr Relat cancer 2010;17(3):771–83.

12. Marini F, Giusti F, Tonelli F, et al. Pancreatic Neuroendocrine Neoplasms in Multiple Endocrine Neoplasia Type 1. Int J Mol Sci 2021;22(8):4041.

13. Karnik SK, Hughes CM, Gu X, et al. Menin regulates pancreatic islet growth by promoting histone methylation and expression of genes encoding p27Kip1 and p18INK4c. Proc Natl Acad Sci 2005;102(41):14659–64.

14. Kann P, Balakina E, Ivan D, et al. Natural course of small, asymptomatic neuroendocrine pancreatic tumours in multiple endocrine neoplasia type 1: an endoscopic ultrasound imaging study. Endocr Relat cancer 2006;13(4):1195–202.

15. Shen H-CJ, He M, Powell A, et al. Recapitulation of pancreatic neuroendocrine tumors in human multiple endocrine neoplasia type I syndrome via Pdx1-directed inactivation of Men1. Cancer Res 2009;69(5):1858–66.

16. Raj N, Shah R, Stadler Z, et al. Real-time genomic characterization of metastatic pancreatic neuroendocrine tumors has prognostic implications and identifies potential germline actionability. JCO Precision Oncol 2018;2:1–18.

17. Elsaesser S, Allis C. HIRA and Daxx constitute two independent histone H3. 3-containing predeposition complexes. Paper presented at: Cold Spring Harbor symposia on quantitative biology2010.

18. Goldberg AD, Banaszynski LA, Noh K-M, et al. Distinct factors control histone variant H3. 3 localization at specific genomic regions. Cell 2010;140(5):678–91.

19. Lewis PW, Elsaesser SJ, Noh K-M, et al. Daxx is an H3. 3-specific histone chaperone and cooperates with ATRX in replication-independent chromatin assembly at telomeres. Proc Natl Acad Sci 2010;107(32):14075–80.

20. Heaphy CM, De Wilde RF, Jiao Y, et al. Altered telomeres in tumors with ATRX and DAXX mutations. Science 2011;333(6041):425.

21. Marinoni I, Kurrer AS, Vassella E, et al. Loss of DAXX and ATRX are associated with chromosome instability and reduced survival of patients with pancreatic neuroendocrine tumors. Gastroenterology 2014;146(2):453–60. e455.

22. De Wilde RF, Heaphy CM, Maitra A, et al. Loss of ATRX or DAXX expression and concomitant acquisition of the alternative lengthening of telomeres phenotype are late events in a small subset of MEN-1 syndrome pancreatic neuroendocrine tumors. Mod Pathol 2012;25(7):1033–9.

23. Willems L, Tamburini J, Chapuis N, et al. PI3K and mTOR signaling pathways in cancer: new data on targeted therapies. Curr Oncol Rep 2012;14(2):129–38.

24. Missiaglia E, Dalai I, Barbi S, et al. Pancreatic endocrine tumors: expression profiling evidences a role for AKT-mTOR pathway. J Clin Oncol 2010;28(2):245.

25. Wang F, Xu X, Ye Z, et al. Prognostic Significance of Altered ATRX/DAXX Gene in Pancreatic Neuroendocrine Tumors: A Meta-Analysis. Front Endocrinol 2021; 12:719.

26. Basturk O, Tang L, Hruban RH, et al. Poorly differentiated neuroendocrine carcinomas of the pancreas: a clinicopathologic analysis of 44 cases. Am J Surg Pathol 2014;38(4):437.

27. Hijioka S, Hosoda W, Matsuo K, et al. Rb loss and KRAS mutation are predictors of the response to platinum-based chemotherapy in pancreatic neuroendocrine neoplasm with grade 3: a Japanese multicenter pancreatic NEN-G3 study. Clin Cancer Res 2017;23(16):4625–32.

28. Konukiewitz B, Schlitter AM, Jesinghaus M, et al. Somatostatin receptor expression related to TP53 and RB1 alterations in pancreatic and extrapancreatic neuroendocrine neoplasms with a Ki67-index above 20. Mod Pathol 2017; 30(4):587–98.

29. Tang LH, Untch BR, Reidy DL, et al. Well-differentiated neuroendocrine tumors with a morphologically apparent high-grade component: a pathway distinct from poorly differentiated neuroendocrine carcinomas. Clin Cancer Res 2016;22(4): 1011–7.

30. Yachida S, Vakiani E, White CM, et al. Small cell and large cell neuroendocrine carcinomas of the pancreas are genetically similar and distinct from well-differentiated pancreatic neuroendocrine tumors. Am J Surg Pathol 2012; 36(2):173.

31. Yuan F, Shi M, Ji J, et al. KRAS and DAXX/ATRX gene mutations are correlated with the clinicopathological features, advanced diseases, and poor prognosis in Chinese patients with pancreatic neuroendocrine tumors. Int J Biol Sci 2014; 10(9):957.

32. Kim JY, Brosnan-Cashman JA, An S, et al. Alternative lengthening of telomeres in primary pancreatic neuroendocrine tumors is associated with aggressive clinical behavior and poor survival. Clin Cancer Res 2017;23(6):1598–606.

33. Park JK, Paik WH, Lee K, et al. DAXX/ATRX and MEN1 genes are strong prognostic markers in pancreatic neuroendocrine tumors. Oncotarget 2017;8(30): 49796.

34. Chou A, Itchins M, de Reuver PR, et al. ATRX loss is an independent predictor of poor survival in pancreatic neuroendocrine tumors. Hum Pathol 2018;82: 249–57.

35. Cives M, Partelli S, Palmirotta R, et al. DAXX mutations as potential genomic markers of malignant evolution in small nonfunctioning pancreatic neuroendocrine tumors. Scientific Rep 2019;9(1):1–10.

36. Roy S, LaFramboise WA, Liu T-C, et al. Loss of chromatin-remodeling proteins and/or CDKN2A associates with metastasis of pancreatic neuroendocrine

tumors and reduced patient survival times. Gastroenterology 2018;154(8): 2060–3. e2068.

37. Singhi AD, Liu T-C, Roncaioli JL, et al. Alternative lengthening of telomeres and loss of DAXX/ATRX expression predicts metastatic disease and poor survival in patients with pancreatic neuroendocrine tumors. Clin Cancer Res 2017;23(2): 600–9.

38. Yao JC, Shah MH, Ito T, et al. Everolimus for advanced pancreatic neuroendocrine tumors. N Engl J Med 2011;364(6):514–23.

39. Lee L, Ito T, Jensen RT. Everolimus in the treatment of neuroendocrine tumors: Efficacy, side-effects, resistance, and factors affecting its place in the treatment sequence. Expert Opin Pharmacother 2018;19(8):909–28.

40. Wang H, Bender A, Wang P, et al. Insights into beta cell regeneration for diabetes via integration of molecular landscapes in human insulinomas. Nat Commun 2017;8(1):1–15.

41. Cao Y, Gao Z, Li L, et al. Whole exome sequencing of insulinoma reveals recurrent T372R mutations in YY1. Nat Commun 2013;4(1):1–6.

42. Cromer MK, Choi M, Nelson-Williams C, et al. Neomorphic effects of recurrent somatic mutations in Yin Yang 1 in insulin-producing adenomas. Proc Natl Acad Sci 2015;112(13):4062–7.

43. Parekh VI, Modali SD, Welch J, et al. Frequency and consequence of the recurrent YY1 p. T372R mutation in sporadic insulinomas. Endocr Relat Cancer 2018; 25(5):L31–5.

44. Greidinger A, Miller-Samuel S, Giri VN, et al. Neuroendocrine Tumors Are Enriched in Cowden Syndrome. JCO precision Oncol 2020;4. PO. 19.00241.

45. Neychev V, Sadowski S, Zhu J, et al. Neuroendocrine tumor of the pancreas as a manifestation of Cowden syndrome: a case report. J Clin Endocrinol Metab 2016;101(2):353–8.

46. Jensen RT, Berna MJ, Bingham DB, et al. Inherited pancreatic endocrine tumor syndromes: advances in molecular pathogenesis, diagnosis, management, and controversies. Cancer 2008;113(S7):1807–43.

47. Vezzosi D, Cardot-Bauters C, Bouscaren N, et al. Long-term results of the surgical management of insulinoma patients with MEN1: a Groupe d'étude des Tumeurs Endocrines (GTE) retrospective study. Eur J Endocrinol 2015;172(3): 309–19.

48. Anlauf M, Garbrecht N, Bauersfeld J, et al. Hereditary neuroendocrine tumors of the gastroenteropancreatic system. Virchows Archiv 2007;451(1):29–38.

49. Kfir SK, Halperin R, Percik R, et al. Distinct prognostic factors in sporadic and multiple endocrine neoplasia type 1-related pancreatic neuroendocrine tumors. Stuttgart, Germany: Hormone and Metabolic Research; 2021.

50. Ahmed F.W., Majeed M.S., Kirresh O., Multiple Endocrine Neoplasias Type 4. [Updated 2022 Apr 4]. In: StatPearls [Internet]. Treasure Island (FL): StatPearls Publishing; 2022 Jan-. Available from: https://www.ncbi.nlm.nih.gov/books/NBK568728/

51. Pellegata NS. MENX and MEN4. Clinics 2012;67:13–8.

52. Thakker RV. Multiple endocrine neoplasia type 1 (MEN1) and type 4 (MEN4). Mol Cell Endocrinol 2014;386(1–2):2–15.

53. Alrezk R, Hannah-Shmouni F, Stratakis CA. MEN4 and CDKN1B mutations: the latest of the MEN syndromes. Endocr Relat Cancer 2017;24(10):T195–208.

54. Francis JM, Kiezun A, Ramos AH, et al. Somatic mutation of CDKN1B in small intestine neuroendocrine tumors. Nat Genet 2013;45(12):1483–6.

55. Frederiksen A, Rossing M, Hermann P, et al. Clinical features of multiple endocrine neoplasia type 4: novel pathogenic variant and review of published cases. J Clin Endocrinol Metab 2019;104(9):3637–46.

56. Georgitsi M, Raitila A, Karhu A, et al. Germline CDKN1B/p27Kip1 mutation in multiple endocrine neoplasia. J Clin Endocrinol Metab 2007;92(8):3321–5.

57. Kaelin WG. Molecular basis of the VHL hereditary cancer syndrome. Nat Rev Cancer 2002;2(9):673–82.

58. Findeis-Hosey JJ, McMahon KQ, Findeis SK. Hereditary Cancer Syndromes in Children: Von Hippel–Lindau Disease. J Pediatr Genet 2016;5(2):116.

59. de Mestier L, Gaujoux S, Cros J, et al. Long-term prognosis of resected pancreatic neuroendocrine tumors in von Hippel-Lindau disease is favorable and not influenced by small tumors left in place. Ann Surg 2015;262(2):384–8.

60. Keutgen XM, Hammel P, Choyke PL, et al. Evaluation and management of pancreatic lesions in patients with von Hippel–Lindau disease. Nat Rev Clin Oncol 2016;13(9):537.

61. Weisbrod AB, Kitano M, Thomas F, et al. Assessment of tumor growth in pancreatic neuroendocrine tumors in von Hippel Lindau syndrome. J Am Coll Surg 2014;218(2):163–9.

62. Krauss T, Ferrara AM, Links TP, et al. Preventive medicine of von Hippel–Lindau disease-associated pancreatic neuroendocrine tumors. Endocr Relat Cancer 2018;25(9):783–93.

63. Weisbrod AB, Liewehr DJ, Steinberg SM, et al. Association of type O blood with pancreatic neuroendocrine tumors in Von Hippel–Lindau syndrome. Ann Surg Oncol 2012;19(6):2054–9.

64. Blansfield JA, Choyke L, Morita SY, et al. Clinical, genetic and radiographic analysis of 108 patients with von Hippel-Lindau disease (VHL) manifested by pancreatic neuroendocrine tumors (PNETs). Surgery 2007;142(6):814–8. e812.

65. Charlesworth M, Verbeke CS, Falk GA, et al. Pancreatic lesions in von Hippel–Lindau disease? A systematic review and meta-synthesis of the literature. J Gastrointest Surg 2012;16(7):1422–8.

66. Igarashi H, Ito T, Nishimori I, et al. Pancreatic involvement in Japanese patients with von Hippel-Lindau disease: results of a nationwide survey. J Gastroenterol 2014;49(3):511–6.

67. Evans D, Howard E, Giblin C, et al. Birth incidence and prevalence of tumor-prone syndromes: Estimates from a UK family genetic register service. Am J Med Genet A 2010;152(2):327–32.

68. Goldgar D, Green P, Parry D, et al. Multipoint linkage analysis in neurofibromatosis type I: an international collaboration. Am J Hum Genet 1989;44(1):6.

69. O'Shea T, Druce M. When should genetic testing be performed in patients with neuroendocrine tumours? Rev Endocr Metab Disord 2017;18(4):499–515.

70. Viskochil D, Buchberg AM, Xu G, et al. Deletions and a translocation interrupt a cloned gene at the neurofibromatosis type 1 locus. Cell 1990;62(1):187–92.

71. Klöppel G, Rindi G, Anlauf M, et al. Site-specific biology and pathology of gastroenteropancreatic neuroendocrine tumors. Virchows Archiv 2007;451(1):9–27.

72. Caiazzo R, Mariette C, Piessen G, Jany T, Carnaille B, Triboulet J. Type I neurofibromatosis, pheochromocytoma and somatostatinoma of the ampulla. Literature review. Paper presented at: Annales de chirurgie2006.

73. Cantor A, Rigby C, Beck P, et al. Neurofibromatosis, phaeochromocytoma, and somatostatinoma. Br Med J (Clinical Res ed.) 1982;285(6355):1618.

74. Relles D, Baek J, Witkiewicz A, et al. Periampullary and duodenal neoplasms in neurofibromatosis type 1: two cases and an updated 20-year review of the literature yielding 76 cases. J Gastrointest Surg 2010;14(6):1052–61.
75. Koc G, Sugimoto S, Kuperman R, et al. Pancreatic tumors in children and young adults with tuberous sclerosis complex. Pediatr Radiol 2017;47(1):39–45.
76. Larson A, Hedgire S, Deshpande V, et al. Pancreatic neuroendocrine tumors in patients with tuberous sclerosis complex. Clin Genet 2012;82(6):558–63.
77. Schrader J, Henes F, Perez D, et al. Successful mTOR inhibitor therapy for a metastatic neuroendocrine tumour in a patient with a germline TSC2 mutation. Ann Oncol 2017;28(4):904–5.
78. Petignot S, Daly AF, Castermans E, et al. Pancreatic neuroendocrine neoplasm associated with a familial MAX deletion. Horm Metab Res 2020;52(11):784–7.
79. Aversa JG, De Abreu FB, Yano S, et al. The first pancreatic neuroendocrine tumor in Li-Fraumeni syndrome: a case report. BMC cancer 2020;20(1):1–6.
80. Network NCC. NCCN Guidelines Version 4.2021 Neuroendocrine and Adrenal Tumors. 2021. Available at: https://www.nccn.org/professionals/physician_gls/pdf/neuroendocrine.pdf. Accessed 19 Feb, 2022.
81. Lowery MA, Wong W, Jordan EJ, et al. Prospective evaluation of germline alterations in patients with exocrine pancreatic neoplasms. JNCI: J Natl Cancer Inst 2018;110(10):1067–74.
82. Nuñez JE, Donadio M, Rocha Filho D, et al. The efficacy of everolimus and sunitinib in patients with sporadic or germline mutated metastatic pancreatic neuroendocrine tumors. J Gastrointest Oncol 2019;10(4):645.
83. Deeks ED. Belzutifan: First Approval. Drugs 2021;81(16):1921–7.
84. Administration FaD. FDA approves belzutifan for cancers associated with von Hippel-Lindau disease. 2021; https://www.fda.gov/drugs/resources-information-approved-drugs/fda-approves-belzutifan-cancers-associated-von-hippel-lindau-disease. Accessed August 8, 2022.
85. Jonasch E, Donskov F, Iliopoulos O, et al. Belzutifan for renal cell carcinoma in von Hippel–Lindau disease. N Engl J Med 2021;385(22):2036–46.
86. Merck Sharp & Dohme LLC. Belzutifan/MK-6482 for the Treatment of Advanced Pheochromocytoma/Paraganglioma (PPGL), Pancreatic Neuroendocrine Tumor (pNET), or Von Hippel-Lindau (VHL) Disease-Associated Tumors (MK-6482-015) ClinicalTrials.gov identifier: NCT04924075. Updated July 14, 2022. Accessed August 8, 2022 https://clinicaltrials.gov/ct2/show/NCT04924075
87. Halfdanarson TR, Strosberg JR, Tang L, et al. The North American neuroendocrine tumor society consensus guidelines for surveillance and medical management of pancreatic neuroendocrine tumors. Pancreas 2020;49(7):863–81.
88. Thakker RV, Newey PJ, Walls GV, et al. Clinical practice guidelines for multiple endocrine neoplasia type 1 (MEN1). J Clin Endocrinol Metab 2012;97(9):2990–3011.
89. tumors Iaon. AIOM, Linee Guida Neoplasie Neuroendocrine. 2018. Available at: https://www.aiom.it/wp-content/uploads/2018/11/2018_LG_AIOM_Neuroendocrini.pdf. Accessed 9th November, 2021.
90. Donegan D, Singh Ospina N, Rodriguez-Gutierrez R, et al. Long-term outcomes in patients with multiple endocrine neoplasia type 1 and pancreaticoduodenal neuroendocrine tumours. Clin Endocrinol 2017;86(2):199–206.
91. Triponez F, Dosseh D, Goudet P, et al. Epidemiology data on 108 MEN 1 patients from the GTE with isolated nonfunctioning tumors of the pancreas. Ann Surg 2006;243(2):265.

92. Sallinen V, Le Large TY, Galeev S, et al. Surveillance strategy for small asymptomatic non-functional pancreatic neuroendocrine tumors–a systematic review and meta-analysis. HPb 2017;19(4):310–20.

93. Faggiano A, Modica R, Lo Calzo F, et al. Lanreotide therapy vs active surveillance in MEN1-related pancreatic neuroendocrine tumors< 2 centimeters. J Clin Endocrinol Metab 2020;105(1):78–84.

94. Rednam SP, Erez A, Druker H, et al. Von Hippel–Lindau and hereditary pheochromocytoma/paraganglioma syndromes: clinical features, genetics, and surveillance recommendations in childhood. Clin Cancer Res 2017;23(12):e68–75.

95. Tirosh A, Sadowski SM, Linehan WM, et al. Association of VHL genotype with pancreatic neuroendocrine tumor phenotype in patients with von Hippel–Lindau disease. JAMA Oncol 2018;4(1):124–6.

96. Belotto M, do Nascimento Santos Crouzillard B, de Oliveira Araujo K, et al. Pancreatic neuroendocrine tumors: surgical resection. Arq Bras Cir Dig 2019; 32:e1428.

97. Rainone M, Singh I, Salo-Mullen EE, et al. An emerging paradigm for germline testing in pancreatic ductal adenocarcinoma and immediate implications for clinical practice: a review. JAMA Oncol 2020;6(5):764–71.

98. Pipinikas CP, Berner AM, Sposito T, et al. The evolving (epi) genetic landscape of pancreatic neuroendocrine tumours. Endocr Relat Cancer 2019;26(9): R519–44.

99. Capdevila J, Salazar R, Halperín I, et al. Innovations therapy: mammalian target of rapamycin (mTOR) inhibitors for the treatment of neuroendocrine tumors. Cancer Metastasis Rev 2011;30(1):27–34.

100. Capozzi M, Caterina I, De Divitiis C, et al. Everolimus and pancreatic neuroendocrine tumors (PNETs): Activity, resistance and how to overcome it. Int J Surg 2015;21:S89–94.

101. Yao JC, Fazio N, Singh S, et al. Everolimus for the treatment of advanced, non-functional neuroendocrine tumours of the lung or gastrointestinal tract (RADIANT-4): a randomised, placebo-controlled, phase 3 study. The Lancet 2016;387(10022):968–77.

102. Grozinsky-Glasberg S, Shimon I, Korbonits M, et al. Somatostatin analogues in the control of neuroendocrine tumours: efficacy and mechanisms. Endocr Relat cancer 2008;15(3):701–20.

103. Caplin ME, Pavel M, Ćwikła JB, et al. Lanreotide in metastatic enteropancreatic neuroendocrine tumors. N Engl J Med 2014;371(3):224–33.

104. Rinke A, Muller H, Schade-Brittinger C, et al. Placebo-controlled, double-blind, prospective, randomized study on the effect of octreotide LAR in the control of tumor growth in patients with metastatic neuroendocrine midgut tumors: a report from the PROMID Study Group. J Clin Oncol 2009;27(28):4656–63.

105. Yao JC, Lombard-Bohas C, Baudin E, et al. Daily oral everolimus activity in patients with metastatic pancreatic neuroendocrine tumors after failure of cytotoxic chemotherapy: a phase II trial. J Clin Oncol 2010;28(1):69.

106. Yao JC, Phan AT, Chang DZ, et al. Efficacy of RAD001 (everolimus) and octreotide LAR in advanced low-to intermediate-grade neuroendocrine tumors: results of a phase II study. J Clin Oncol 2008;26(26):4311.

107. Pavel ME, Hainsworth JD, Baudin E, et al. Everolimus plus octreotide long-acting repeatable for the treatment of advanced neuroendocrine tumours associated with carcinoid syndrome (RADIANT-2): a randomised, placebo-controlled, phase 3 study. The Lancet 2011;378(9808):2005–12.

108. Pavel M, Baudin E, Öberg K, et al. Efficacy of everolimus plus octreotide LAR in patients with advanced neuroendocrine tumor and carcinoid syndrome: final overall survival from the randomized, placebo-controlled phase 3 RADIANT-2 study. Ann Oncol 2017;28(7):1569–75.

109. Bajetta E, Catena L, Fazio N, et al. Everolimus in combination with octreotide long-acting repeatable in a first-line setting for patients with neuroendocrine tumors: An ITMO group study. Cancer 2014;120(16):2457–63.

110. Chan JA, Ryan DP, Zhu AX, et al. Phase I study of pasireotide (SOM 230) and everolimus (RAD001) in advanced neuroendocrine tumors. Endocr Relat Cancer 2012;19(5):615–23.

111. Kulke MH, Ruszniewski P, Van Cutsem E, et al. A randomized, open-label, phase 2 study of everolimus in combination with pasireotide LAR or everolimus alone in advanced, well-differentiated, progressive pancreatic neuroendocrine tumors: COOPERATE-2 trial. Ann Oncol 2017;28(6):1309–15.

112. Kim HS, Shaib WL, Zhang C, et al. Phase 1b study of pasireotide, everolimus, and selective internal radioembolization therapy for unresectable neuroendocrine tumors with hepatic metastases. Cancer 2018;124(9):1992–2000.

113. Capozzi M, Von Arx C, De Divitiis C, et al. Antiangiogenic therapy in pancreatic neuroendocrine tumors. Anticancer Res 2016;36(10):5025–30.

114. Hobday T, Rubin J, Holen K, et al. MC044h, a phase II trial of sorafenib in patients (pts) with metastatic neuroendocrine tumors (NET): A Phase II Consortium (P2C) study. J Clin Oncol 2007;25(18_suppl):4504.

115. Angelousi A, Kamp K, Kaltsatou M, et al. Sequential everolimus and sunitinib treatment in pancreatic metastatic well-differentiated neuroendocrine tumours resistant to prior treatments. Neuroendocrinology 2017;105(4):394–402.

116. Kulke MH, Niedzwiecki D, Foster NR, et al. Randomized phase II study of everolimus (E) versus everolimus plus bevacizumab (E+ B) in patients (Pts) with locally advanced or metastatic pancreatic neuroendocrine tumors (pNET), CALGB 80701 (Alliance). Am Soc Clin Oncol 2015;33(15).

117. Chan JA, Blaszkowsky L, Stuart K, et al. A prospective, phase 1/2 study of everolimus and temozolomide in patients with advanced pancreatic neuroendocrine tumor. Cancer 2013;119(17):3212–8.

118. Claringbold PG, Turner JH. NeuroEndocrine tumor therapy with lutetium-177-octreotate and everolimus (NETTLE): a phase I study. Cancer Biother Radiopharm 2015;30(6):261–9.

119. Neychev V, Steinberg SM, Cottle-Delisle C, et al. Mutation-targeted therapy with sunitinib or everolimus in patients with advanced low-grade or intermediate-grade neuroendocrine tumours of the gastrointestinal tract and pancreas with or without cytoreductive surgery: protocol for a phase II clinical trial. BMJ open 2015;5(5):e008248.

120. Maia MC, Lourenço DM Jr, Riechelmann R. Efficacy and long-term safety of everolimus in pancreatic neuroendocrine tumor associated with multiple endocrine neoplasia type I: case report. Oncol Res Treat 2016;39(10):643–5.

121. Brandi ML, Gagel RF, Angeli A, et al. Consensus: guidelines for diagnosis and therapy of MEN type 1 and type 2. J Clin Endocrinol Metab 2001;86(12):5658–71.

122. Dralle H, Krohn SL, Karges W, et al. Surgery of resectable nonfunctioning neuroendocrine pancreatic tumors. World J Surg 2004;28(12):1248–60.

123. Goudet P, Bonithon-Kopp C, Murat A, et al. Gender-related differences in MEN1 lesion occurrence and diagnosis: a cohort study of 734 cases from the Groupe d'etude des Tumeurs Endocrines. Eur J Endocrinol 2011;165(1):97–105.

124. Thomas-Marques L, Murat A, Delemer B, et al. Prospective endoscopic ultraso-nographic evaluation of the frequency of nonfunctioning pancreaticoduodenal endocrine tumors in patients with multiple endocrine neoplasia type 1. J Am Gastroenterol 2006;101(2):266–73.
125. Eledrisi MS, Stuart CA, Alshanti M. Insulinoma in a patient with tuberous scle-rosis: is there an association? Endocr Pract 2002;8(2):109–12.
126. Whitman J, Shih B, Blanco A, et al. Emerging value of multigene panels for germline testing in patients with neuroendocrine tumors. Am Soc Clin Oncol 2018;36(4).

Palliative and Supportive Care for Individuals with Pancreatic Adenocarcinoma

Ryan D. Nipp, MD, MPH

KEYWORDS

- Pancreatic cancer • Palliative care • Geriatric oncology • Supportive care
- Quality of life • Symptoms

KEY POINTS

- Individuals with pancreatic adenocarcinoma experience a complex constellation of palliative and supportive care needs. Notably, when caring for patients with pancreatic adenocarcinoma, clinicians must carefully assess and address these individuals' palliative and supportive care needs, as these can have important implications related to their treatment experience and care outcomes.
- Prior research has consistently demonstrated the benefits of palliative and supportive care interventions for patients with cancer to help address symptom burden, illness understanding, coping mechanisms, and informed decision making. However, much of this research did not specifically tailor the interventions to the unique concerns of a pancreatic cancer population.
- Currently, an urgent need exists to design and conduct rigorous research with the goal of enhancing care delivery and outcomes for the highly symptomatic population of individuals with pancreatic adenocarcinoma.

PALLIATIVE AND SUPPORTIVE CARE NEEDS FOR INDIVIDUALS WITH PANCREATIC ADENOCARCINOMA

Individuals with pancreatic adenocarcinoma experience a complex constellation of palliative and supportive care needs. For example, patients with pancreatic cancer frequently endure symptoms from the cancer and the side effects of treatment, including fatigue, pain, nausea, vomiting, diarrhea, neuropathy, and loss of appetite.[1–3] In addition, patients often require urgent care visits and hospital admissions to help address uncontrolled symptoms related to their symptoms and side effects.[2,4,5] Importantly, data suggest that patients' symptoms and quality of life correlate with treatment response, health care use, and survival outcomes.[6] Thus, when

University of Oklahoma Health Sciences Center, Stephenson Cancer Center, 800 Northeast 10th Street, Oklahoma City, OK 73104, USA
E-mail address: ryan-nipp@ouhsc.edu
Twitter: @RyanNipp (R.D.N.)

Hematol Oncol Clin N Am 36 (2022) 1053–1061
https://doi.org/10.1016/j.hoc.2022.07.009
0889-8588/22/© 2022 Elsevier Inc. All rights reserved.

caring for patients with pancreatic adenocarcinoma, clinicians must carefully assess and address these individuals' palliative and supportive care needs, as these can have important implications related to their treatment experience and care outcomes.

Another area related to the palliative and supportive care needs in pancreatic cancer includes the multifaceted topic of patients' illness understanding. Patients' generally report a desire to receive accurate information about their illness and treatment options, yet data suggest that many patients often misunderstand the curability of their cancer.[7-10] For example, patients often cite a more optimistic estimate of their curability than their treating clinicians.[11] Importantly, prior research has shown that patient-clinician communication about illness and prognosis does not take away patients' hope, and rather, these discussions can help patients and their loved ones to make more informed treatment decisions while preparing for their future.[9,12-19] Therefore, patients' understanding of their illness and treatment options represents an important priority for addressing the palliative and supportive care needs of individuals with pancreatic adenocarcinoma.

In addition to challenges with symptom management and the complexities of illness understanding, other examples of the palliative and supportive care needs in pancreatic cancer include patients' quality-of-life concerns, coping mechanisms, care coordination, end-of-life care, caregiver support, as well as physical function, nutrition, comorbid conditions, and polypharmacy.[20-24] Notably, patients frequently report a wide variety of supportive care needs with distinct ranges of severity,[25-27] and therefore, addressing these needs often requires a comprehensive, patient-centered approach to management of each individual's unique palliative and supportive care needs.[28-30]

PALLIATIVE AND SUPPORTIVE CARE SERVICES IN ONCOLOGY

Palliative and supportive care services are often conceptualized as care delivered by a team of specially trained clinicians that provides patient- and family-centered care with the goal of improving quality of life throughout patients' course of illness.[31,32] Based on substantial prior evidence demonstrating the benefits of early integration of palliative care into the care of patients with cancer,[33-37] guidelines recommend early palliative care concurrent with disease-directed treatment of all individuals with advanced cancer.[31,32] Despite these guideline recommendations and the benefits seen in prior work for earlier involvement of palliative care in oncology, many patients still receive palliative and supportive services late in the illness trajectory.[5] Several misperceptions exist that may help explain why these services are forgone or used late, such as the misunderstanding that palliative and supportive care are only appropriate after patients have completed all available life-prolonging therapies.[38] However, a growing literature has sought to demonstrate that the benefits of palliative and supportive care include enhancing patient outcomes without shortening survival.

BENEFITS OF PALLIATIVE AND SUPPORTIVE CARE INTERVENTIONS IN ONCOLOGY

Prior research has consistently demonstrated the benefits of palliative and supportive care interventions for patients with cancer to help address symptom burden, illness understanding, coping mechanisms, and informed decision making.[33-37] Examples of palliative and supportive care interventions include the early integration of palliative care, patient-reported symptom monitoring, and geriatric-assessment interventions, among others.[33-37,39-42]

The early integration of palliative care into routine oncology care represents a potential strategy to ensure appropriate monitoring and management of patients' palliative and supportive care needs. Substantial evidence consistently has shown that earlier involvement of palliative care can improve outcomes for patients with cancer and their loved ones.[33–37,39–42] Specifically, studies demonstrate the benefits of early integration of specialty palliative care for patients with cancer for improving their quality of life, symptom management, illness understanding, coping strategies, and care at the end of life.[33–37,39–41] These data have informed expert guidelines that recommend the incorporation of dedicated palliative care services, early in the disease course, and alongside active treatment for patients with advanced cancer.[31,43] However, limited numbers of palliative care clinicians may hinder the ability for all patients to receive direct care from palliative care specialists. Thus, a growing need exists for additional research to define the role of scalable palliative and supportive care interventions in oncology.

Increasingly, data support the benefits of patient-reported symptom monitoring interventions to help address patients' symptom burden, enhance quality of life, decrease health care utilization, and potentially improve survival.[28–30,44,45] However, symptom monitoring interventions may not always benefit all patient populations equally, and these interventions often require considerable effort from patients and health systems, given the technology and resources required.[46] Notably, with the growing use of telehealth, both palliative care and symptom monitoring interventions have experienced increased utility for helping with remote patient care.[47] Furthermore, the use of symptom monitoring interventions coupled with hospital-at-home care represents a promising opportunity to enhance care delivery and outcomes for patients with cancer.[48] Importantly, as the evidence continues to grow supporting the utility of symptom monitoring and hospital-at-home interventions in oncology, efforts are needed to adapt these interventions to the unique needs of individuals with pancreatic cancer.

As the population ages and the number of older adults with cancer continues to grow exponentially, the proportion of patients with pancreatic cancer increasingly consists of patients from the geriatric oncology population.[49] Older adults with cancer possess a unique set of concerns, including geriatric-specific issues (eg, functional impairment, comorbidity, and polypharmacy) and palliative care-specific concerns (eg, symptom burden, illness understanding, and coping).[20–22] Therefore, older adults with cancer need to have interventions targeting their unique concerns.[22,50–52] Notably, palliative care consultation alone may not always address all the geriatric-specific issues of older individuals with cancer, and geriatric care by itself may not completely address all the palliative care concerns of an oncology population.[53,54] Thus, in order to deliver patient-centered care to an increasingly older population of patients with pancreatic cancer, interventions are needed that address the complex geriatric and palliative care concerns unique to these individuals.

Geriatric assessment-guided care represents a novel strategy with increasing data supporting the benefits of these models of care for targeting older patients' geriatric and palliative care concerns.[51,52,55,56] Geriatric assessment-guided care interventions are designed to address the multifaceted geriatric and palliative care issues unique to older adults with cancer. For example, prior work has demonstrated that the provision of a geriatric assessment-guided intervention could facilitate communication, improve care satisfaction, and increase advance care planning for older adults with advanced cancer.[57] Additional work has shown the feasibility and acceptability of a transdisciplinary geriatric intervention, delivered by geriatricians, which sought to address patients' geriatric and palliative care needs.[58] However, a workforce shortage of geriatricians limits access to these specialists, thus highlighting the importance of additional efforts to find effective ways of delivering geriatric care to older adults with cancer.[59,60] In recent work, an intervention that entailed oncologists receiving a tailored geriatric assessment summary and management recommendations for their older adults receiving cancer treatment demonstrated the ability to reduce the incidence of adverse treatment side effects for these patients.[56] Collectively, these studies add to a growing evidence base espousing the benefits of palliative and supportive care services in oncology, while highlighting the potential for these interventions to address the substantial supportive care needs of individuals with pancreatic cancer.

DATA REGARDING PALLIATIVE AND SUPPORTIVE CARE IN PANCREATIC ADENOCARCINOMA

Data regarding palliative and supportive care interventions specifically for individuals with pancreatic cancer are relatively limited. Several studies of palliative and supportive care interventions enrolled patients with pancreatic adenocarcinoma, which can help to elucidate the potential benefits for this population. For example, multiple practice-changing studies of palliative care interventions enrolled patients with varying cancer types, including individuals with pancreatic cancer.[34–37,61,62] Although these studies demonstrated many benefits for palliative and supportive care interventions, most patients in these studies had cancer types other than pancreatic adenocarcinoma. Notably, data suggest that the benefits of palliative and supportive care interventions may differ based on patients' cancer type.[36] Hence, efforts to understand the benefits of supportive care interventions specifically in a pancreatic cancer population are needed.

Although prospective, randomized trials are regarded as the gold standard of scientific evidence that should be used to inform practice change, many of the efforts to understand the role and benefits of palliative and supportive care interventions for patients with pancreatic cancer originate from retrospective studies.[63–67] The prospective research largely derives from smaller studies and/or descriptions of a single-center experience.[48,68–71] One study with most patients having pancreatic cancer demonstrated that an early palliative care intervention did not meet the primary outcome of reducing pain and depression scores.[69] In a study involving patients with advanced pancreatic cancer, an intervention of early systematic palliative care showed the potential to enhance quality of life, increase hospice use, and foster higher-quality end-of-life care.[70,71] A recent prospective trial sought to determine the feasibility of delivering a Supportive Oncology Care at Home intervention designed to address the needs of patients receiving treatment for pancreatic cancer.[48] The Supportive Oncology Care at Home intervention entailed the following: (1) Remote monitoring of patients' symptoms and vital signs; (2) A hospital-at-home care model for symptom assessment and management; and (3) Structured communication with the oncology team. This trial demonstrated the feasibility and acceptability of the Supportive Oncology Care at Home intervention, and future work will investigate the efficacy of this intervention for improving outcomes in patients with pancreatic cancer. Thus, although the literature in support of palliative care interventions continues to grow, a tremendous need remains for studies focused on understanding the role and benefits of palliative and supportive care interventions for individuals with pancreatic adenocarcinoma.

FUTURE DIRECTIONS FOR PALLIATIVE AND SUPPORTIVE CARE IN PANCREATIC ADENOCARCINOMA

Importantly, ongoing work is critically needed to determine how best to provide optimal supportive care for patients with pancreatic cancer.[36] For patients with pancreatic cancer, whether they are receiving treatment with curative or palliative intent, these individuals and their loved ones would benefit from research investigating how best to address the complex shared decision making for these patients, while also helping to support these patients along their cancer course.[10] As patients with pancreas adenocarcinoma often present with a complex and unique constellation of palliative and supportive care needs, interventions to address these needs will require personalized efforts distinctly designed for this population. Although a growing evidence base continues to support the benefits of palliative care interventions in oncology, much of this research did not specifically tailor the interventions to the unique concerns of a pancreatic cancer population. Therefore, an urgent need exists to design and conduct rigorous research with the goal of enhancing care delivery and outcomes for the highly symptomatic population of individuals with pancreatic adenocarcinoma.

CLINICS CARE POINTS

- Individuals with pancreatic adenocarcinoma experience a complex constellation of palliative and supportive care needs.
- When caring for patients with pancreatic adenocarcinoma, clinicians must carefully assess and address these individuals' palliative and supportive care needs, as these can have important implications related to their treatment experience and care outcomes.
- Prior research has consistently demonstrated the benefits of palliative and supportive care interventions for patients with cancer to help address symptom burden, illness understanding, coping mechanisms, and informed decision making.
- Minimal research has focused on specifically tailoring palliative and supportive care interventions to the unique concerns of a pancreatic cancer population.
- Currently, an urgent need exists to design and conduct rigorous research with the goal of enhancing care delivery and outcomes for the highly symptomatic population of individuals with pancreatic adenocarcinoma.

DISCLOSURE

The authors have nothing to disclose.

REFERENCES

1. Conroy T, Desseigne F, Ychou M, et al. FOLFIRINOX versus gemcitabine for metastatic pancreatic cancer. N Engl J Med 2011;364(19):1817–25.
2. Faris JE, Blaszkowsky LS, McDermott S, et al. FOLFIRINOX in locally advanced pancreatic cancer: the Massachusetts General Hospital Cancer Center experience. The oncologist 2013;18(5):543–8.
3. Von Hoff DD, Ervin T, Arena FP, et al. Increased survival in pancreatic cancer with nab-paclitaxel plus gemcitabine. N Engl J Med 2013;369(18):1691–703.
4. Smyth EN, Bapat B, Ball DE, et al. Metastatic Pancreatic Adenocarcinoma Treatment Patterns, Health Care Resource Use, and Outcomes in France and the United Kingdom Between 2009 and 2012: A Retrospective Study. Clin Ther 2015;37(6):1301–16.
5. Nipp RD, Tramontano AC, Kong CY, et al. Patterns and predictors of end-of-life care in older patients with pancreatic cancer. Cancer Med 2018;7(12):6401–10.

6. van Seventer EE, Fish MG, Fosbenner K, et al. Associations of baseline patient-reported outcomes with treatment outcomes in advanced gastrointestinal cancer. Cancer 2021;127(4):619–27.
7. Greer JA, Pirl WF, Jackson VA, et al. Perceptions of health status and survival in patients with metastatic lung cancer. J Pain Symptom Manag 2014;48(4):548–57.
8. Weeks JC, Catalano PJ, Cronin A, et al. Patients' expectations about effects of chemotherapy for advanced cancer. N Engl J Med 2012;367(17):1616–25.
9. Epstein AS, Prigerson HG, O'Reilly EM, et al. Discussions of Life Expectancy and Changes in Illness Understanding in Patients With Advanced Cancer. J Clin Oncol 2016;34(20):2398–403.
10. Lee HJ Jr, Qian CL, Landay SL, et al. Communicating the Information Needed for Treatment Decision Making Among Patients With Pancreatic Cancer Receiving Preoperative Therapy. JCO Oncol Pract 2021;OP2100388. https://doi.org/10.1200/OP.21.00388.
11. Gramling R, Fiscella K, Xing G, et al. Determinants of Patient-Oncologist Prognostic Discordance in Advanced Cancer. JAMA Oncol 2016. https://doi.org/10.1001/jamaoncol.2016.1861.
12. Steinhauser KE, Christakis NA, Clipp EC, et al. Preparing for the end of life: preferences of patients, families, physicians, and other care providers. J Pain Symptom Manag 2001;22(3):727–37. Available at: http://www.ncbi.nlm.nih.gov/pubmed/11532586.
13. Steinhauser KE, Christakis NA, Clipp EC, et al. Factors considered important at the end of life by patients, family, physicians, and other care providers. JAMA 2000;284(19):2476–82. Available at: http://www.ncbi.nlm.nih.gov/pubmed/11074777.
14. Steinhauser KE, Clipp EC, McNeilly M, et al. In search of a good death: observations of patients, families, and providers. Ann Intern Med 2000;132(10):825–32. Available at: http://www.ncbi.nlm.nih.gov/pubmed/10819707.
15. Lundquist G, Rasmussen BH, Axelsson B. Information of imminent death or not: does it make a difference? J Clin Oncol 2011;29(29):3927–31.
16. Smith TJ, Dow LA, Virago E, et al. Giving honest information to patients with advanced cancer maintains hope. Oncology 2010;24(6):521–5. Available at: http://www.ncbi.nlm.nih.gov/pubmed/20568593.
17. Zhang B, Wright AA, Huskamp HA, et al. Health care costs in the last week of life: associations with end-of-life conversations. Arch Intern Med 2009;169(5):480–8.
18. Cohen MG, Althouse AD, Arnold RM, et al. Is Advance Care Planning Associated With Decreased Hope in Advanced Cancer? JCO Oncol Pract 2020;OP2000039. https://doi.org/10.1200/OP.20.00039.
19. Cohen MG, Althouse AD, Arnold RM, et al. Hope and advance care planning in advanced cancer: Is there a relationship? Cancer 2021. https://doi.org/10.1002/cncr.34034.
20. Mor V, Allen S, Malin M. The psychosocial impact of cancer on older versus younger patients and their families. Cancer 1994;74(7 Suppl):2118–27. Available at: http://www.ncbi.nlm.nih.gov/pubmed/8087779.
21. Nipp RD, Greer JA, El-Jawahri A, et al. Coping and Prognostic Awareness in Patients With Advanced Cancer. J Clin Oncol 2017. https://doi.org/10.1200/JCO.2016.71.3404. JCO2016713404.
22. Cheung WY, Le LW, Gagliese L, et al. Age and gender differences in symptom intensity and symptom clusters among patients with metastatic cancer. Support Care Cancer 2011;19(3):417–23.

23. Ferris FD, Bruera E, Cherny N, et al. Palliative cancer care a decade later: accomplishments, the need, next steps – from the American Society of Clinical Oncology. J Clin Oncol 2009;27(18):3052–8.

24. Nipp RD, Subbiah IM, Loscalzo M. Convergence of Geriatrics and Palliative Care to Deliver Personalized Supportive Care for Older Adults With Cancer. J Clin Oncol 2021;JCO2100158. https://doi.org/10.1200/JCO.21.00158.

25. Mohile SG, Heckler C, Fan L, et al. Age-related Differences in Symptoms and Their Interference with Quality of Life in 903 Cancer Patients Undergoing Radiation Therapy. J Geriatr Oncol 2011;2(4):225–32.

26. Nipp RD, Thompson LL, Temel B, et al. Screening Tool Identifies Older Adults With Cancer at Risk for Poor Outcomes. J Natl Compr Cancer Netw 2020; 18(3):305–13.

27. Nipp RD, El-Jawahri A, Moran SM, et al. The relationship between physical and psychological symptoms and health care utilization in hospitalized patients with advanced cancer. Cancer 2017;123(23):4720–7.

28. Basch E, Deal AM, Kris MG, et al. Symptom Monitoring With Patient-Reported Outcomes During Routine Cancer Treatment: A Randomized Controlled Trial. J Clin Oncol 2016;34(6):557–65.

29. Denis F, Basch E, Septans AL, et al. Two-Year Survival Comparing Web-Based Symptom Monitoring vs Routine Surveillance Following Treatment for Lung Cancer. JAMA 2019;321(3):306–7.

30. Strasser F, Blum D, von Moos R, et al. The effect of real-time electronic monitoring of patient-reported symptoms and clinical syndromes in outpatient workflow of medical oncologists: E-MOSAIC, a multicenter cluster-randomized phase III study (SAKK 95/06). Ann Oncol 2016;27(2):324–32.

31. Ferrell BR, Temel JS, Temin S, et al. Integration of Palliative Care Into Standard Oncology Care: American Society of Clinical Oncology Clinical Practice Guideline Update. J Clin Oncol 2017;35(1):96–112. Available at: https://www.ncbi.nlm.nih.gov/pubmed/28034065.

32. Dans M, Smith T, Back A, et al. NCCN Guidelines Insights: Palliative Care, Version 2.2017. J Natl Compr Cancer Netw 2017;15(8):989–97.

33. Temel JS, Greer JA, Muzikansky A, et al. Early palliative care for patients with metastatic non-small-cell lung cancer. N Engl J Med 2010;363(8):733–42.

34. Bakitas M, Lyons KD, Hegel MT, et al. Effects of a palliative care intervention on clinical outcomes in patients with advanced cancer: the Project ENABLE II randomized controlled trial. JAMA 2009;302(7):741–9.

35. Bakitas MA, Tosteson TD, Li Z, et al. Early Versus Delayed Initiation of Concurrent Palliative Oncology Care: Patient Outcomes in the ENABLE III Randomized Controlled Trial. J Clin Oncol 2015;33(13):1438–45.

36. Temel JS, Greer JA, El-Jawahri A, et al. Effects of Early Integrated Palliative Care in Patients With Lung and GI Cancer: A Randomized Clinical Trial. J Clin Oncol 2017;35(8):834–41.

37. Zimmermann C, Swami N, Krzyzanowska M, et al. Early palliative care for patients with advanced cancer: a cluster-randomised controlled trial. Lancet 2014; 383(9930):1721–30.

38. Fadul N, Elsayem A, Palmer JL, et al. Supportive versus palliative care: what's in a name?: A survey of medical oncologists and midlevel providers at a comprehensive cancer center. Cancer 2009;115(9):2013–21.

39. Kavalieratos D, Corbelli J, Zhang D, et al. Association Between Palliative Care and Patient and Caregiver Outcomes: A Systematic Review and Meta-analysis. JAMA 2016;316(20):2104–14.

40. Grudzen CR, Richardson LD, Johnson PN, et al. Emergency Department-Initiated Palliative Care in Advanced Cancer: A Randomized Clinical Trial. JAMA Oncol 2016;2(5):591–8.

41. El-Jawahri A, LeBlanc T, VanDusen H, et al. Effect of Inpatient Palliative Care on Quality of Life 2 Weeks After Hematopoietic Stem Cell Transplantation: A Randomized Clinical Trial. JAMA 2016;316(20):2094–103.

42. Dionne-Odom JN, Azuero A, Lyons KD, et al. Benefits of Early Versus Delayed Palliative Care to Informal Family Caregivers of Patients With Advanced Cancer: Outcomes From the ENABLE III Randomized Controlled Trial. J Clin Oncol 2015; 33(13):1446–52.

43. Jordan K, Aapro M, Kaasa S, et al. European Society for Medical Oncology (ESMO) position paper on supportive and palliative care. Ann Oncol 2018; 29(1):36–43.

44. Basch E, Deal AM, Dueck AC, et al. Overall Survival Results of a Trial Assessing Patient-Reported Outcomes for Symptom Monitoring During Routine Cancer Treatment. JAMA 2017;318(2):197–8.

45. Nipp RD, El-Jawahri A, Ruddy M, et al. Pilot randomized trial of an electronic symptom monitoring intervention for hospitalized patients with cancer. Ann Oncol 2019;30(2):274–80.

46. Nipp RD, Horick NK, Deal AM, et al. Differential effects of an electronic symptom monitoring intervention based on the age of patients with advanced cancer. Ann Oncol 2020;31(1):123–30.

47. Grewal US, Terauchi S, Beg MS. Telehealth and Palliative Care for Patients With Cancer: Implications of the COVID-19 Pandemic. JMIR Cancer 2020;6(2): e20288.

48. Nipp RD, Gaufberg E, Vyas C, et al. Supportive oncology care at home intervention for patients with pancreatic cancer. J Clin Oncol 2021;39(15):6558.

49. Shapiro CL. Cancer Survivorship. N Engl J Med 2018;379(25):2438–50.

50. Blank TO, Bellizzi KM. A gerontologic perspective on cancer and aging. Cancer 2008;112(11 Suppl):2569–76.

51. Mohile SG, Velarde C, Hurria A, et al. Geriatric Assessment-Guided Care Processes for Older Adults: A Delphi Consensus of Geriatric Oncology Experts. J Natl Compr Cancer Netw 2015;13(9):1120–30. http://www.ncbi.nlm.nih.gov/pubmed/26358796.

52. Mohile SG, Dale W, Somerfield MR, et al. Practical Assessment and Management of Vulnerabilities in Older Patients Receiving Chemotherapy: ASCO Guideline for Geriatric Oncology. J Clin Oncol 2018. https://doi.org/10.1200/JCO.2018.78.8687. JCO2018788687.

53. Nipp RD, El-Jawahri A, Traeger L, et al. Differential effects of early palliative care based on the age and sex of patients with advanced cancer from a randomized controlled trial. Palliat Med 2018. https://doi.org/10.1177/0269216317751893. 269216317751893.

54. Nipp RD, Greer JA, El-Jawahri A, et al. Age and Gender Moderate the Impact of Early Palliative Care in Metastatic Non-Small Cell Lung Cancer. Oncologist 2016; 21(1):119–26.

55. Mohile S, Dale W, Magnuson A, et al. Research priorities in geriatric oncology for 2013 and beyond. Cancer forum 2013;37(3):216–21. Available at: http://www.ncbi.nlm.nih.gov/pubmed/25346565.

56. Mohile SG, Mohamed MR, Xu H, et al. Evaluation of geriatric assessment and management on the toxic effects of cancer treatment (GAP70+): a cluster-randomised study. Lancet 2021;398(10314):1894–904.

57. Mohile SG, Epstein RM, Hurria A, et al. Communication With Older Patients With Cancer Using Geriatric Assessment: A Cluster-Randomized Clinical Trial From the National Cancer Institute Community Oncology Research Program. JAMA Oncol 2019;1–9. https://doi.org/10.1001/jamaoncol.2019.4728.
58. Nipp RD, Temel B, Fuh CX, et al. Pilot Randomized Trial of a Transdisciplinary Geriatric and Palliative Care Intervention for Older Adults With Cancer. J Natl Compr Canc Netw 2020;18(5):591–8.
59. Kane R, Solomon D, Beck J, et al. The future need for geriatric manpower in the United States. N Engl J Med 1980;302(24):1327–32.
60. Williams GR, Weaver KE, Lesser GJ, et al. Capacity to Provide Geriatric Specialty Care for Older Adults in Community Oncology Practices. The oncologist 2020. https://doi.org/10.1634/theoncologist.2020-0189.
61. Vanbutsele G, Pardon K, Van Belle S, et al. Effect of early and systematic integration of palliative care in patients with advanced cancer: a randomised controlled trial. Lancet Oncol 2018;19(3):394–404.
62. Greer JA, Jacobs JM, El-Jawahri A, et al. Role of Patient Coping Strategies in Understanding the Effects of Early Palliative Care on Quality of Life and Mood. J Clin Oncol 2018;36(1):53–60.
63. Jang RW, Krzyzanowska MK, Zimmermann C, et al. Palliative care and the aggressiveness of end-of-life care in patients with advanced pancreatic cancer. J Natl Cancer Inst 2015;107(3). https://doi.org/10.1093/jnci/dju424.
64. Lees C, Weerasinghe S, Lamond N, et al. Palliative care consultation and aggressive care at end of life in unresectable pancreatic cancer. Curr Oncol 2019;26(1):28–36.
65. Bhulani N, Gupta A, Gao A, et al. Palliative care and end-of-life health care utilization in elderly patients with pancreatic cancer. J Gastrointest Oncol 2018;9(3):495–502.
66. Michael N, Beale G, O'Callaghan C, et al. Timing of palliative care referral and aggressive cancer care toward the end-of-life in pancreatic cancer: a retrospective, single-center observational study. BMC Palliat Care 2019;18(1):13.
67. Wang JP, Wu CY, Hwang IH, et al. How different is the care of terminal pancreatic cancer patients in inpatient palliative care units and acute hospital wards? A nationwide population-based study. BMC Palliat Care 2016;15:1.
68. Schenker Y, Bahary N, Claxton R, et al. A Pilot Trial of Early Specialty Palliative Care for Patients with Advanced Pancreatic Cancer: Challenges Encountered and Lessons Learned. J Palliat Med 2018;21(1):28–36.
69. Woo SM, Song MK, Lee M, et al. Effect of Early Management on Pain and Depression in Patients with Pancreatobiliary Cancer: A Randomized Clinical Trial. Cancers 2019;11(1).
70. Maltoni M, Scarpi E, Dall'Agata M, et al. Systematic versus on-demand early palliative care: A randomised clinical trial assessing quality of care and treatment aggressiveness near the end of life. Eur J Cancer 2016;69:110–8.
71. Maltoni M, Scarpi E, Dall'Agata M, et al. Systematic versus on-demand early palliative care: results from a multicentre, randomised clinical trial. Eur J Cancer 2016;65:61–8.

UNITED STATES POSTAL SERVICE ® Statement of Ownership, Management, and Circulation (All Periodicals Publications Except Requester Publications)

1. Publication Title	2. Publication Number	3. Filing Date
HEMATOLOGY/ONCOLOGY CLINICS OF NORTH AMERICA	002 – 473	9/18/2022

4. Issue Frequency	5. Number of Issues Published Annually	6. Annual Subscription Price
FEB, APR, JUN, AUG, OCT, DEC	6	$470.00

7. Complete Mailing Address of Known Office of Publication (Not printer) (Street, city, county, state, and ZIP+4®)

ELSEVIER INC.
230 Park Avenue, Suite 800
New York, NY 10169

Contact Person
Malathi Samayan

Telephone (Include area code)
91-44-4299-4507

8. Complete Mailing Address of Headquarters or General Business Office of Publisher (Not printer)

ELSEVIER INC.
230 Park Avenue, Suite 800
New York, NY 10169

9. Full Names and Complete Mailing Addresses of Publisher, Editor, and Managing Editor (Do not leave blank)

Publisher (Name and complete mailing address)

Dolores Meloni, ELSEVIER INC.
1600 JOHN F KENNEDY BLVD. SUITE 1800
PHILADELPHIA, PA 19103-2899

Editor (Name and complete mailing address)

STACY EASTMAN, ELSEVIER INC.
1600 JOHN F KENNEDY BLVD. SUITE 1800
PHILADELPHIA, PA 19103-2899

Managing Editor (Name and complete mailing address)

PATRICK MANLEY, ELSEVIER INC.
1600 JOHN F KENNEDY BLVD. SUITE 1800
PHILADELPHIA, PA 19103-2899

10. Owner (Do not leave blank. If the publication is owned by a corporation, give the name and address of the corporation immediately followed by the names and addresses of all stockholders owning or holding 1 percent or more of the total amount of stock. If not owned by a corporation, give the names and addresses of the individual owners. If owned by a partnership or other unincorporated firm, give its name and address as well as those of each individual owner. If the publication is published by a nonprofit organization, give its name and address.)

Full Name	Complete Mailing Address
WHOLLY OWNED SUBSIDIARY OF REED/ELSEVIER, US HOLDINGS	1600 JOHN F KENNEDY BLVD. SUITE 1800 PHILADELPHIA, PA 19103-2899

11. Known Bondholders, Mortgagees, and Other Security Holders Owning or Holding 1 Percent or More of Total Amount of Bonds, Mortgages, or Other Securities. If none, check box ▶ ☐ None

Full Name	Complete Mailing Address
N/A	

12. Tax Status (For completion by nonprofit organizations authorized to mail at nonprofit rates) (Check one)
The purpose, function, and nonprofit status of this organization and the exempt status for federal income tax purposes:
☒ Has Not Changed During Preceding 12 Months
☐ Has Changed During Preceding 12 Months (Publisher must submit explanation of change with this statement)

PS Form 3526, July 2014 (Page 1 of 4 (see instructions page 4))   PSN: 7530-01-000-9931   PRIVACY NOTICE: See our privacy policy on www.usps.com.

13. Publication Title	14. Issue Date for Circulation Data Below
HEMATOLOGY/ONCOLOGY CLINICS OF NORTH AMERICA	JUNE 2022

15. Extent and Nature of Circulation			Average No. Copies Each Issue During Preceding 12 Months	No. Copies of Single Issue Published Nearest to Filing Date
a. Total Number of Copies (Net press run)			157	137
b. Paid Circulation (By Mail and Outside the Mail)	(1)	Mailed Outside-County Paid Subscriptions Stated on PS Form 3541 (Include paid distribution above nominal rate, advertiser's proof copies, and exchange copies)	62	49
	(2)	Mailed In-County Paid Subscriptions Stated on PS Form 3541 (Include paid distribution above nominal rate, advertiser's proof copies, and exchange copies)	0	0
	(3)	Paid Distribution Outside the Mails Including Sales Through Dealers and Carriers, Street Vendors, Counter Sales, and Other Paid Distribution Outside USPS®	48	40
	(4)	Paid Distribution by Other Classes of Mail Through the USPS (e.g., First-Class Mail®)	0	0
c. Total Paid Distribution (Sum of 15b (1), (2), (3), and (4))			110	89
d. Free or Nominal Rate Distribution (By Mail and Outside the Mail)	(1)	Free or Nominal Rate Outside-County Copies included on PS Form 3541	31	29
	(2)	Free or Nominal Rate In-County Copies Included on PS Form 3541	0	0
	(3)	Free or Nominal Rate Copies Mailed at Other Classes Through the USPS (e.g., First-Class Mail)	0	0
	(4)	Free or Nominal Rate Distribution Outside the Mail (Carriers or other means)	0	0
e. Total Free or Nominal Rate Distribution (Sum of 15d (1), (2), (3) and (4))			31	29
f. Total Distribution (Sum of 15c and 15e)			141	118
g. Copies not Distributed (See Instructions to Publishers #4 (page #3))			16	19
h. Total (Sum of 15f and g)			157	137
i. Percent Paid (15c divided by 15f times 100)			78.01%	75.42%

* If you are claiming electronic copies, go to line 16 on page 3. If you are not claiming electronic copies, skip to line 17 on page 3.

16. Electronic Copy Circulation		Average No. Copies Each Issue During Preceding 12 Months	No. Copies of Single Issue Published Nearest to Filing Date
a. Paid Electronic Copies	▶		
b. Total Paid Print Copies (Line 15c) + Paid Electronic Copies (Line 16a)	▶		
c. Total Print Distribution (Line 15f) + Paid Electronic Copies (Line 16a)	▶		
d. Percent Paid (Both Print & Electronic Copies) (16b divided by 16c × 100)	▶		

☒ I certify that 50% of all my distributed copies (electronic and print) are paid above a nominal price.

17. Publication of Statement of Ownership

☒ If the publication is a general publication, publication of this statement is required. Will be printed in the OCTOBER 2022 issue of this publication.   ☐ Publication not required.

18. Signature and Title of Editor, Publisher, Business Manager, or Owner

Malathi Samayan - Distribution Controller

Malathi Samayan

Date 9/18/2022

I certify that all information furnished on this form is true and complete. I understand that anyone who furnishes false or misleading information on this form or who omits material or information requested on the form may be subject to criminal sanctions (including fines and imprisonment) and/or civil sanctions (including civil penalties).

PS Form 3526, July 2014 (Page 3 of 4)   PRIVACY NOTICE: See our privacy policy on www.usps.com.